CHANGE

EMBRACING YOUR TRUE POWER

BARBARA RATKOFF

ARNICA PRESS

The material contained in this book has been written for informational purposes
and is not intended as a substitute for medical advice,
nor is it intended to diagnose, treat, cure, or prevent disease.
If you have a medical issue or illness, consult a qualified physician.

Published by ARNICA PRESS
www.ArnicaPress.com

Written by Barbara Ratkoff
Illustration on page 410 by Georges Ratkoff
Cover and interior portrait photography by Ulrick Theaud

ISBN: 978-1-7336446-6-2

CHANGE

EMBRACING YOUR TRUE POWER

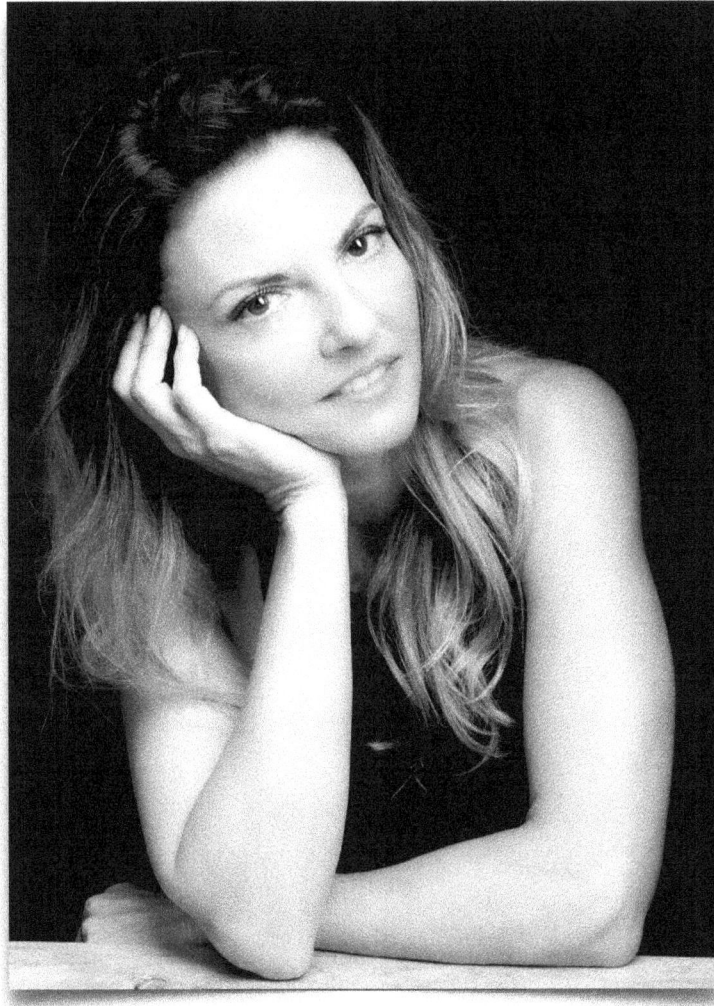

BARBARA RATKOFF

ARNICA PRESS

For YOU

CONTENTS

CHAPTER THREE
On the Path to Physical Transformation.....................199

CHAPTER FOUR
Change The Way You Work and Play.....................307

CHAPTER FIVE
Learning to Embrace Painful
and Unwanted Change

INTRODUCTION

When I think about it, the word CHANGE simply defines me. From a very early age, I constantly had to learn to adapt to new situations and environments. My mother was a historian, specializing in North American Indian First Nations. We were often on the go. When I turned 9, our life really took a decisive turn with her work taking us away from life in the big cities such as New York, Washington DC and Toronto, to smaller towns or Indigenous Canadian Reserves.

Canadian Ojibwe reserves to be more precise. Looking back today, it still amazes me and I can't help but wonder: what were the odds of this happening? The way I see it: 1 in 10 million, the same odds as choosing the winning lottery ticket. Now, don't get to thinking I was sleeping in tipis (or teepees) and horseback riding all day. It might come as a surprise to some of you but this has been a recurring question that people have asked me over the years. No, these were the 70s and 80s and we lived in homes and drove around in cars! But fortunately, although the "white man" had left its mark on the North American Indian First Nations, their sense of pride, pride of their heritage and of who they are, still subsided. History books tell you about the *defeated Indian* but as I bathed in their culture, their traditions, their legends, their arts and crafts and their philosophy of life, I was fortunate enough to grow up and see them with a different perspective.

At the time, I was homeschooled and spent most of my days reading books or being outdoors in nature. I read English and French literature but devoured and heard many Ojibwe tales as well. Many people have turned to Buddhism for its principles and to find inner peace and as I write these words I find myself thinking: why go so far when we have so much to learn from the enlightened and wise way of the North American First Nations? Indeed, I am profoundly convinced that the daily teachings I have received back then far outweigh anything I ever could have learnt on any school bench.

Reading played an important part in my childhood but so did my interaction with nature: both have taught me to treasure life, to observe and listen, to respect and see the beauty in people and all things. Thanks to them, I have come to the understanding of life's most important lesson: we are here to learn. Life is a path we take in order to grow and acquire wisdom, or so it should be…

The day I left the reserves, at age14, to go back to school in Washington D.C., I was forced, literally overnight, to face a new reality and view life through an entirely different lens. As I write these words, I am surprised to feel tears rolling down my cheeks. I realize how much I had cherished this part of my life and how much it had, in fact, affected me to leave it behind, and I can't help but wonder: what lies within these tears? Are they recalling the shock of the transition or is it that lost childhood that they miss? Probably a bit of both.

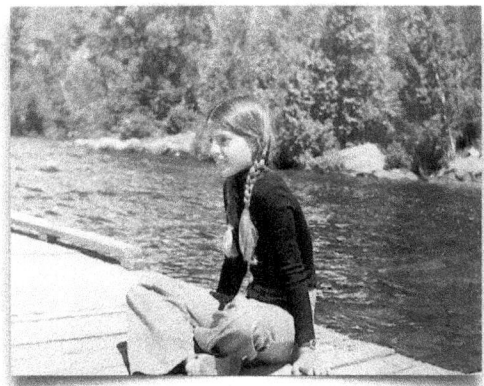

And so, in a moment of gratefulness, I sit back and feel the need to honor this past and choose to do so by taking a stroll down memory lane to relive a Pow Wow. For those of you who don't know, a pow wow (also powwow or pow-wow) is a social gathering held by many different North American First Nations; it's a big event where the indigenous people have the opportunity to meet and dance, sing, socialize, and honor their cultures and the traditions of their ancestors. The image of my friends dancing and twirling beautifully still remains vivid in my mind and I can also hear the pounding of the drum and the powerful cries of the men singing.

Occasionally, back in the day, I would join in. Although my heart felt totally at home, my light hair and fair skin, however, were a constant reminder that I was out of place here. I understood this. With everything these First Nations had endured because of the "white man", I learned to walk on eggs. Even though I lived on the reserves and had friends, I knew I had crossed a fine line and that I had to be very careful about what I did or said. I accepted this fact and took it as a true privilege to already be there.

This experience definitely was a life lesson and has taught me what it feels like to be the odd one out, the difficulties of integration and being accepted by a new community and thus the importance of respecting people's differences.

But it seems as though life had yet more changes in store for me. Indeed, with a historian, life is spent travelling and we seldom stayed put: frequently my mother would announce that we had to hit the road. These departures, I knew, meant leaving everything behind. In my head it was "goodbye home", "goodbye friends", "goodbye things I am used to", "goodbye places I used to visit"…and "hello" to starting everything all over again. I was going to have to adapt to a new place, meet new people, and do things differently.

Although deep down I am an adventurous person, it was hard at times. It hurts knowing you will never see your friends again and it's not easy to leave your "home" behind. When you settle down somewhere, you tend to create habits and slide into a certain comfort zone… and it's nice. Moving on means kicking in the butt everything you know. Each time we were about to leave, we always said: " I hope we'll come back soon", but deep down inside I knew we wouldn't. The moment I sat down in the backseat of the car and shut the door, it became clear to me that I was shutting out this life for good.

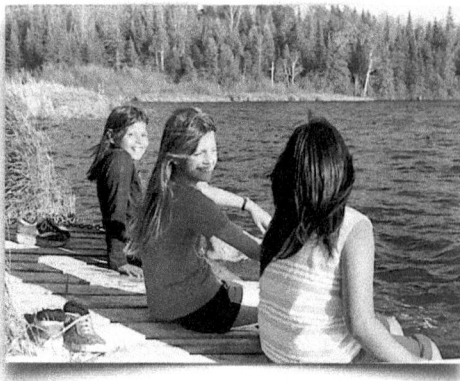

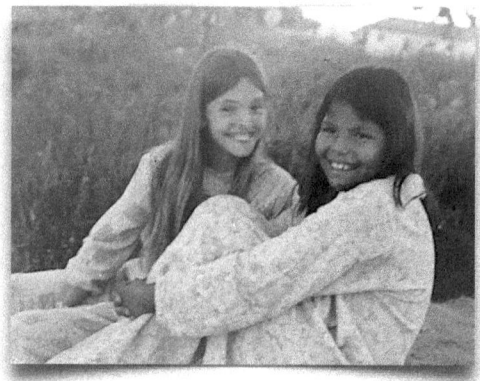

But when change occurs, one must remember that change isn't an ending. In fact, it's quite the opposite: it's a new beginning! As they say, when one chapter ends, the book isn't over, there are still many more chapters to write.

And so, each time we drove off and I could feel the tears starting to well, I would forbid myself from crying. I had to be brave and accept the situation: I was going to have to CHANGE.

Also, because of her unusual professional demands, my mother would sometimes drop me off into people's homes. The length of these stays ranged from a short sojourn to several years. Having to live with these different families, demanded once again to call upon my capacity of adapting to a new environment, as each and every one of them had their own specific way of doing things. I had no choice but to comply with their demands, their habits, their "laws"… in other words, I was constantly obliged to adapt and CHANGE.

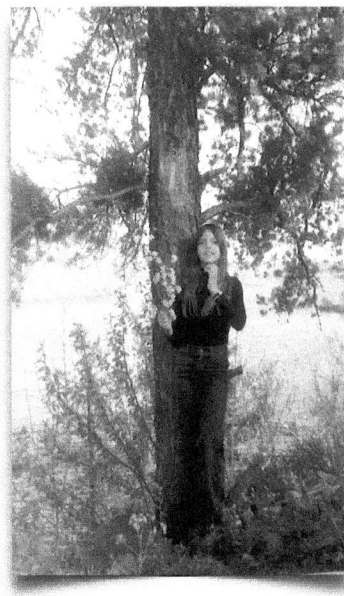

It may seem derisory, but every time I had to face the usual explanations: "We fold our towels this way, we put our dishes away that way." And, every time I had no choice but to conform to their wishes.

Here's just one example among many that I had to deal with: In one family, I was told to put the glasses away in the cupboard placing the bottom of the glass on the shelf. The lady whom I was staying with explained that over time the shelf gets dusty and we don't want to put the rims of the glasses down on the shelf, since we will be drinking from these rims later on. So "bottom of the glass" on the shelf it was.

Then I would move in with a new family. I remember the very first day I helped to clear the table and did the dishes. And as I was putting the glasses away, I automatically put them "bottom down" on the shelf. But to my surprise, I was told: "NO, No, no! You must always put the glasses away upside down or else dust will land inside the glasses and we would then have to wipe them every time before drinking. Hasn't anyone ever told you that?"

In both cases, the explanations were valid… there really is no right or wrong way of doing it. But it just goes to say that I had to put up with this for every little thing and Change became something natural and I learned to EMBRACE it.

In many instances we must endure changes, but sometimes it can be our very own personal wish: maybe losing a little weight, getting a new job or simply quitting a bad habit.

And so, we try, but most of the time we abandon the idea after a few months, sometimes a few weeks, or even a few days. In French, there is an expression that says: "If you try to chase away something that comes naturally, it will come back galloping."

But that is not always the case, and we have all seen it happen: someone we know has succeeded in losing all those extra pounds, they have been brave enough to start anew, or to totally quit a bad habit. How did they accomplish this? How come I can't? Why do I always fail?

For many of us, years seem to go by and yet we still remain at the same point in our lives, with the same unfulfilled goals:

"If I could just lose a few pounds, my life would be so much better",

"If only I could land a better job, I could take my family away on vacation",

"If only I could get fit, I wouldn't feel so tired all the time",

"If only I could save up some money, I could finally buy a house »

…. and so on and so forth.

One cannot fail to observe that most of us stagnate in our lives. Five, ten years may go by and aside from having a few more wrinkles here and there, nothing much else has changed. But you too want to change and you wonder: How can I achieve my goals?

Did you ever notice that Listen and Silent are spelled with the same letters? There just might be a reason for it!

As a child and adolescent, I was an avid observer. It wasn't always easy to live with a family that wasn't my own and it was often a wiser choice to just stay silent and not meddle into their various discussions. Many times, I was confronted with difficult family issues that I should not have normally been a part of, such as couple or parenting issues, arguments or financial difficulties. It was clear that my intervention would not have been appreciated. So what else could I do aside from listen, reflect upon the situation, make my own conclusions… of course all without ever saying a word or expressing anything. I believe these years of observation and reflection taught me more life wisdom than any school, or any education could have, and I am truly grateful for them.

SILENT
STENLI
TINLSE
NELTIS
ETNSLI
TLESNI
NISTLE
LISTEN

I was about fourteen and living with one of these families when I started goal setting. I remember one of the couples that had taken me in had frequent arguments. The woman was a little overweight and was often tired from having to juggle between her job, taking care of the house and raising her children. She was actually quite pretty, but made no effort whatsoever to improve her physical appearance. While I lived under their roof, the husband cheated on her and it created a big-time drama. It was sad to be there and see what they were going through… the crying, the arguments, the drinking to forget the drama and then the silence because communication between them, at one point, just simply stopped…. I am in no way condemning the woman because I know how hard and challenging it can be to juggle all those tasks the modern-day woman has to juggle with… but it was at that time that I understood that no matter what happens, it's important to take care of yourself.

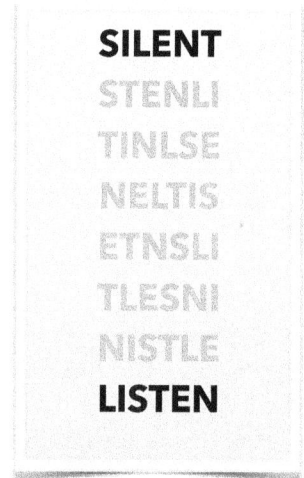

I always tell my children:
"You have two ears and one mouth.
As a rule of thumb, listen twice as much as you speak."

This woman totally lost herself to her work, her husband and children and never allowed some time for her own wellbeing. I believe it's important not to forget ourselves in our daily lives. It's not an easy task but everybody should have a little time just for one's self, each and every day. Anyway, it was then and there that something clicked in my head: I was determined that I would never forget myself… it was clear to me that this was a lesson and that I had to learn something from it. As the years went by, there has been like a post-it somewhere inside my head, and it stuck with me ever since. Even when times were tough, my goal remained undeterred.

Life is a gift
and the way I choose to handle it
is my way of saying thank you.

The way I see it, my life is like travelling on a boat moving forward. Now, I can choose to be a simple passenger and let someone else take the helm. In this case, I will just stay at the back of the vessel and chat with the other passengers, or stay inside my cabin. When danger or a storm arises, I will simply let someone else do the steering. Once in a while, I may fall down or go overboard. In either case, I will do what I can, I will struggle or ask for help.

There is however another option: I can decide that it's time to take the helm into my own hands, in which case I must position myself on the vessel in such a way that I have a clear view of what is coming. I must face forward. When problems occur, I can take control of the situation. I may make the wrong decision but it feels good to be the one that's pulling the sails out, giving the orders, and fighting the waves. Many times, I may have to navigate alone, but I will be the one doing it! If I am lucky enough, I might find someone who will be there beside me to help and sometimes I will be happy to hand over the helm or share it with him while standing by his side. So, who do you want to be on your boat? The deckhand, the leading seaman or the captain? And remember, you won't become a great sailor overnight: it's only by learning how to navigate that you will become a good one and eventually reach the position of the captain.

To conclude what I am trying to say: **You** must take control of your life. Face the fact that there is nothing you can do to change your past, but you most certainly can do something about your future. Stop making excuses and take action! At one point **you have to accept the responsibility of your own life**. Many times, people tend to find it more comfortable to blame their situation on someone else or an exterior factor, never shouldering the responsibility. I'm not saying that it is your fault that you were hurt, misunderstood, abused, or whatever hardship might have happened to you. However, it is your decision and within your control to decide whether or not you are going to react upon it. And come to think of it: what a victory over your past it would be if you did choose to take control of your life!

When I was in my early twenties, deep down inside I wasn't a happy person. So, a friend of mine recommended that I see a psychiatrist, maybe he could help me clear my mind. So, every week I had ONE appointment. The doctor was quite nice, but it was nerve-racking for me to have to face someone and talk about the things that had affected me in the past. Little by little the process eventually became increasingly more stressful. To summarize, this is roughly how it went: I knew I had an appointment on the following Wednesday and so by that day I absolutely had to find something of consequence to talk to him about. And so, in my head I went over each and every trauma I had endured thinking "Yes, I will talk to him about this" but almost immediately, I would conclude that it the chosen subject was either childish, not relevant or downright stupid…

And so, after only 3 weeks of this mind torture, I came to the conclusion that I didn't have any real problems that necessitated the help of a psychiatrist. I confronted him, told him how I felt, and that I wished to terminate the sessions. He was kind of amused by my explanation, but I can tell you one thing: I never felt the need to see a psychiatrist again! Believe it or not, as I walked out of my doctor's office, I left behind my issues and my excuses. It's as if I had come in with a set of luggage that burdened me, but now I chose to travel light. Evidently, this luggage, had been weighing me down. And now, without it all, I could finally stand tall and smile! I knew then and there that I had healed. That doesn't mean that I completely forgot my past. What it meant was that my past was no longer omnipotent, controlling me, or omnipresent, as in present at all times.

Before, the only way I would get some attention was by telling my story and have people feel sorry for me. After this realization, I could still tell my story, but with a decisively different approach: I was no longer looking for pity, I was proud to let people know that although I had my struggles, I no longer let them control me. "I " was controlling "Me". I had the will to CHANGE.

After this realization, my life totally turned around and I started to see that I could create the life that I wanted. But one key ingredient was still missing, and it came to me in the form of a quote:

> *"Ask and it will be given to you,*
> *seek and you will find,*
> *knock and the door*
> *will be opened to you."*
> *~ Mathew 7:7 ~*

I am not a religious person per se, however this sentence intrigued me and I really took the time to understand it and integrate it into my daily life.

ASKING

"Ask" means that you must ask for what it is that you really want.
To do so, you must have a clear image of what that is.

> *"A good goal should scare you a little*
> *and excite you a lot."*
> *~ Joe Vitale ~*

Avoid asking for something too difficult, too vague or general and try to be as specific as possible. This implies that you sit down quietly at your desk and grab a pen and write down your goal. Let's take an example:

You are currently working as a secretary for a company that you really enjoy. Your dream is to get promoted as a personal assistant. The job would be more gratifying and you would earn a higher salary.

Asking = Putting your goal down in writing

This leads us to the next step:

SEEKING

"Seek" means that you must find ways that will help you achieve your goal. If we stick to the same example: you could begin by finding a few books that are about becoming a personal assistant. You could also explore the web for videos on the attitude to adopt during a job interview. Since you will be requesting an appointment with human resources at one point, why not start getting ready for it now.

Here are two suggestions:

You can review your general presentation. How could you improve it?

Why not learn how to apply makeup, get a new haircut or try out a new hairstyle?

The options are limitless. And what about finding a few exercises that would improve your posture? Self-confidence is also an issue. You can use visualization techniques to boost it.

Find out what the requirements are for being a great personal assistant and work on them. Do you need to better your computer skills? Find a course, look online, read a book about it. Do you need to become more efficient or acquire excellent organizational skills? Research, research, research about it. The key here is to learn as much as possible. In your head you must already be that personal assistant. This seeking part implies that you take the time to break down your wish into as many different aspects as possible and that you work on them. Think of your goal as a puzzle with all its different pieces. Take the time to take it completely apart and find out what your goal is made of. Each puzzle piece is something that you can work on to get one step closer to achieving your goal. The more pieces you master, the closer you will get to realizing your objective and complete the entire puzzle.

Seeking = Dismantling your goal into different parts
and working on as many as possible

KNOCKING

"Knock" means that you have to be willing to get up and physically do things in order for them to happen. If your goal is to be a personal assistant, this would require you to physically get off the couch and apply for the job. You literally have to knock on doors and let people know your intention. If this is not possible in the company where you currently work, then maybe it is elsewhere. Look up for ads in the paper, send out your resumés and whenever possible, find the courage to hand them in personally instead of mailing them.

Knocking = Action

Every time I really wanted something, I made sure I went through all three of these steps. It's important to take the time to reflect upon what it is you really want, to find ways that will bring you closer to the realization of your goal and finally to get up and get it. As time passes, I can't help but notice how life always seemed to pull me in certain directions that were seldom taken by others. Life has always tended to be that way for me.

We don't always get to choose everything and things don't always go as we planned them. It's a rule of life and we must accept it. When I was pregnant with my second child, my son Enzo told me that he absolutely wanted a little brother and being only 3 ½ made it impossible for him to understand why it wasn't feasible to choose these things. One day, as we were at the fair playing one of those "capsule toy machines", where you place a coin in the machine and a random capsule roles out, I told my son: "You see, life is like a capsule machine, sometimes you get what you want and sometimes not." But still, I would often find my little Enzo all cooped up in a baby basket we bought for our second child, waiting for his little brother. At the time, Enzo loved Zorro and he never missed an episode. Now I don't know if you remember, but Zorro's civil name was Diego de la Vega and for some reason, my son Enzo decided that his little brother had to be called Diego as well. Maybe he would turn into some sort of superhero or have super powers! That name was not at all what my husband and I had in mind and so we tried again and again to explain to Enzo that it wasn't possible. But he was adamant and seeing that he was so looking forward to his brother's arrival, in the end we didn't have the heart to go against his wish. I often laugh thinking that if he had been watching Superman, Batman or Spiderman, our second son could have been called Clark, Bruce or Peter!

But let's get back to life choices….
After living over five years on Ojibwe Reservations, two years in Washington DC, I eventually moved to France to finish my final years of high school and attend university. I lived in Paris and then in Antibes and Nice in the South of France, and finally landed in Monaco.

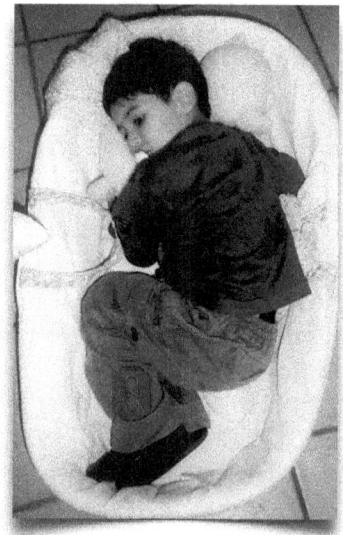

Enzo waiting in his little brother's basket:" When will Diego be here Mommy?"

In April of 2000, I got married in Monte-Carlo. For many of you that may seem glamorous, but in truth, my life was pretty normal. Monaco is a beautiful country and I love it. For those of you who don't know it is also a tiny one of 2.9 square Km, situated between the French and Italian border. It has a population of 38,000 people, of which ¼ - around 8,400 are actually Monegasque, which is the name given to the people who have a Monegasque - Monaco passport. 139 different nationalities live side by side and more than 100.000 people flow into Monaco every day to work or visit. They come mainly from France and Italy.

We actually struggled to pay our rent. Rentals in that part of the world are horrendously costly and what most Monegasque people do, is apply for an apartment that belongs to the state which offers special affordable rates. But once the application form is handed in, one is put on a waiting list and it can take years before you get a place. We wanted to have a child and since the cost for an extra bedroom was too high, we had no choice, but to find a place in France, where the rents are much cheaper. We would then commute back and forth every day in hope that we would soon get an apartment. But time went by, our first son was born and we were still waiting. With my husband working nights at the Casino and often finishing in the early mornings, it was difficult for him to sleep with a toddler waking up and running around at five a.m. every day. I guess it was time for me, once again, to embrace *Change*. As unusual as that may sound, we mutually decided that my husband would remain in our small apartment and I would move and live with my son on a boat in the port of Monaco. When I think about it today, the lyrics from that old 70s song by 10CC called "The things we do for love" starts playing in my mind… but back then, it seemed like the right thing to do. Although it was far from being a yacht, the boat was comfortable and big enough to live on, and with Monaco being so small, it was easy for me to get anywhere I wanted or needed to on foot.

We chose to call our boat "Lucky Charm" and many times as I would sit back at the stern of our ship and enjoy the view, I would get to thinking: what were the odds for me to find myself here at this very spot? I had been raised on Ojibwe reservations in Canada and today I was sitting on this boat overlooking the port of Monte-Carlo. I was aware that I was lucky; the toy capsules had been generous and kind to me.

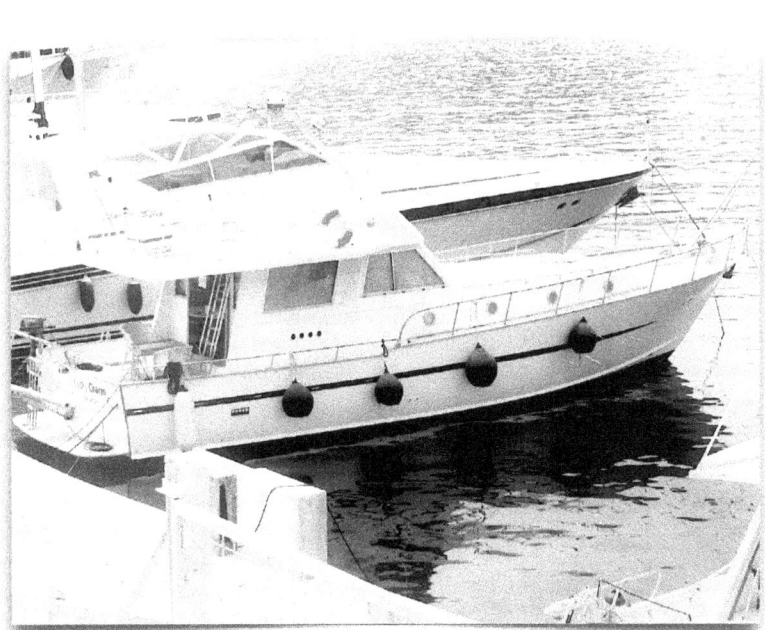

Living differently- on our boat "The Lucky Charm" in the Port Monaco

We did eventually get an apartment in June of 2005, just two days after the birth of our second child, Diego.

But life didn't seem to think that I should settle down just yet into a nice comfortable routine. In 2007, my husband started flirting with the idea that we should take the leap and homeschool our children. He had seen TV programs about parents who had done it, and it was something that really spoke to him as the right thing to do for our children. Having been homeschooled myself, I most definitely did not see eye to eye with him on this subject. But he was adamant about it and would go on and on, until I finally gave way and accepted to join him on this new journey.

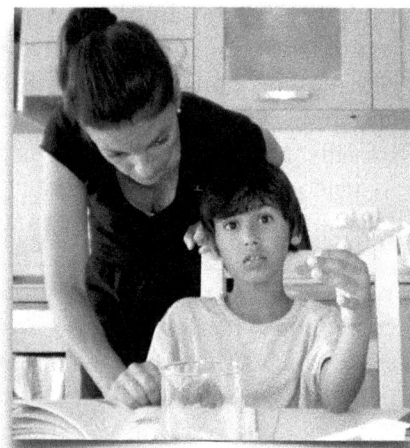

Homeschooling your children requires discipline, dedication, and patience.

Enzo had just finished 2nd grade and Diego had only done one year of kindergarten when we decided to grab them by the hand and take the leap towards new *Changes*. Now don't get to thinking it's an easy thing to do, because it really isn't. The resilience it took over the years to get the entire school programs done for two children of different ages, the mental strength it took to endure the judgments and endless critiques coming from other parents, the courage it took to face the questions I feared the most; such as whether I was capable and smart enough to educate them properly… it made me feel like I was running out into an endless ocean. I had accepted to leave the security of the shore and had no choice but to start swimming out into the waves not knowing what lay ahead. This was new territory, I was used to walking on solid ground and I now had to learn to adapt to sempiternal moving waters. Believe me, swimming while holding my two boys' hands was not an easy task. Once in a while the sea was calm and we embraced the joys of floating around on our backs. Sometimes the current would take us to an island and, in my mind, I felt serene and confident about my capacities and about the fact that we were doing the right thing. These were the times we travelled with our children and made them discover many beautiful and interesting places like Australia, Africa, the United States, France and endless other fascinating lands. But at times the ocean was also agitated, and I found myself amidst the waves of doubt, having to struggle against the storms that were going on in my mind. But all in all, I have to admit that I have this ability, maybe due to my childhood, whereby once I move forward, I don't waste too much time looking back or regretting my decision.

In 2011, we saw an advert about a cruise that was going around the world. The idea that we would be able to offer this opportunity to our children seemed totally out of reach. But it happened. We bought the tickets almost two years before the actual cruise and I must say that it was a great source of motivation to keep up the homeschooling and move forward. And on January 7th, 2013, we embarked the Costa Deliziosa for a 3 ½ month cruise, discovering almost 30 different countries while covering a total 34.764 miles, around 55 947 Km. We were still on the ocean, but I was no longer in the water swimming: I was cruisin'!

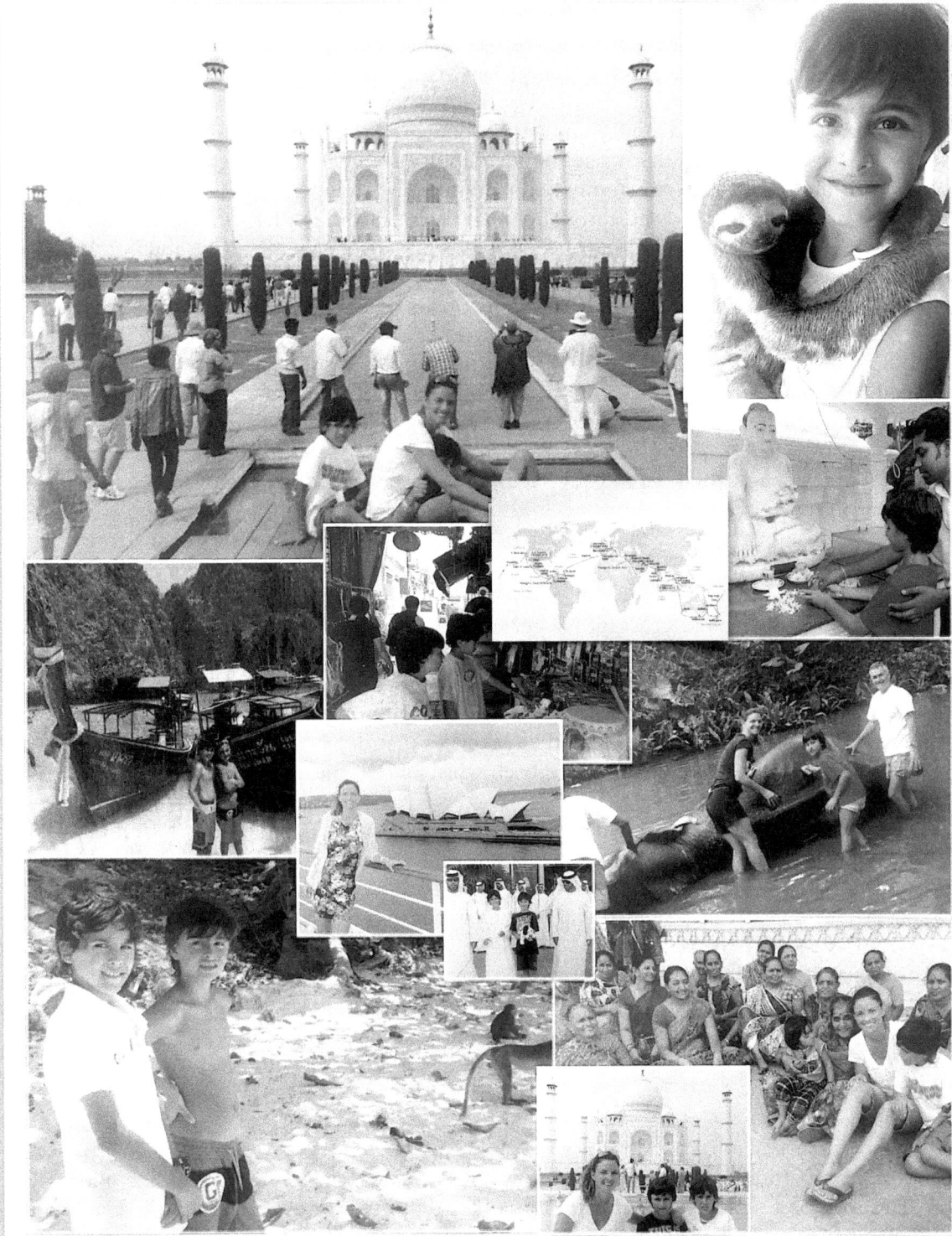

The itinerary we took during our Around the World Cruise. It was magical and remains one of the most beautiful and amazing experiences I have had the opportunity to embrace in my life.

Which brings me to another path life has put along my way: the writing path.

While I was cruising, I loved getting up very early every morning to watch the sunrise and write down all my experiences, everything I had visited and learned. I had a profound need to keep a written trace of it all. And as I sit here today and reflect upon it, it's funny how writing has always been an important part of me. Even when I was a little girl I loved writing stories. I once read that what you love doing as a child, or what you willingly do on your free time, is probably what you were meant to be doing as a job. I have to say, that writing has always followed me throughout the years in different forms, as diaries, blogs, stories and so on. However, I never once took it seriously or saw myself as a writer. When I was 28, out of the blue, the idea of a story came to me. I was totally thrilled by it and grabbed a piece of paper and wrote everything down. The words simply poured out of me, as if they were somehow given to me. In a way, it felt as though they didn't come from me at all, but from some exterior source. I talked about my idea with several of my friends, but it seemed as though no one was as thrilled about my story as I was. And so, I felt a little discouraged, and placed the manuscript on a shelf where it remains to this day.

The idea for the book you hold in your hands also came to me one day in April of 2016, as a gift, out of nowhere. I woke up one morning and the whole idea dawned on me: the outline, the chapters, along with hundreds of ideas to put in it. I sat down and wrote down enough material to fill out three whole pads. It was really strange: it was almost as if once again, the idea hadn't been mine at all, and had been somehow whispered to me. I guess this is what one calls "inspiration." Once I put everything down on paper, I wondered what I was going to do with it all. As the days went by, I pondered: "Could I do this? Could I actually write a book?" I let numerous questions commute back and forth in my mind until one day it hit me: "Who knows if I can write a book. But one thing is for sure, I can write a page and then another one and yet another." And so that day I grabbed my laptop, opened a blank page and typed in the title that had been whispered to me, in big letters: "CHANGE."

As I am writing these lines, the memory of that specific morning takes me back three years. Three years! Unbelievable! Very soon, my book will be available around the world! So many hours in front of the computer, researching, so many hours writing and organizing my ideas on paper… and I can't help but wonder what new changes still lie ahead?

But let's get back to the cruise and our world travels.

The cruise was convenient for homeschooling: no need to worry about travelling, finding places to sleep or fixing meals. Everything was taken care of. When out at sea we had lots of time to study, and when the boat would arrive at a certain destination, we would visit most beautiful sights.

After the cruise we embarked on many more trips, all of which were very enriching. But the children were getting older and the school programs increasingly more demanding. Basically, my days were as follows: I would wake up very early to work out and would sit down with one of my sons to start studying at 8 am. We would work from 8 to 10 and then I would sit down with my other son for two hours until noon. Lunch breaks meant fixing meals, cleaning up and maybe throwing in a few loads of laundry. Then, back to the studying for another 4 hours.

In the evenings I often had to prepare two dinners: since my husband had to be at work around 6:30 pm, he would often eat an hour earlier and with the kids that were often out doing afterschool activities at that time, we would usually eat later, around 7pm. I could sometimes relax in the evenings, but I frequently had more chores or lessons that needed preparing for the next day.

These were long days and although it had been my husband's idea to homeschool our boys, most of the work and stress lay solely upon my shoulders, and it took a real toll on our relationship. I started to increasingly feel that the situation was unfair: working for long hours, shouldering the entire responsibility of their education, with no pay at the end of the month, which meant I had no financial freedom whatsoever. I am not saying I was unhappy, but slowly, insidiously, I started feeling that the situation was out of balance, with my side of the scale tipping more and more with obligations and a sense that I was actually tied down and had completely lost all my freedom. Indeed, as the kids were getting older, the school programs got to be more challenging and required more work, research and preparation. Although I asked my husband for help numerous times, he was reluctant to lend me a hand, not because he was lazy - I honestly think he would have been happy to, but he wasn't confident about his own capacity to do it properly, and honestly believed that I was most likely much better at it.

The day I started talking about leaving him came as a complete shock to my husband. The way he saw it: I had the life of a princess and he had always made sure I had everything I needed, I had never been obliged to "work" in the past 17 years, and he had made it possible for us to travel around the world. Those were a few of his arguments and they were all valid and true. But isn't it strange to live side by side with someone under the same roof and yet live two completely different lives. He was totally oblivious to what I was going through, and my numerous explanations came to no avail. And as life has it, when one thing goes wrong, bad news tends to pile up and only a few weeks after telling him I was unhappy with our marriage, I was diagnosed with cancer. And from then on everything seemed to just spiral downwards. I was overwhelmed with putting the kids back to school, the numerous doctor appointments, followed by lawyer consultations to move forward with the divorce, but also going to job interviews. It wasn't an easy task to sell myself and be convincing with everything I was going through… and I won't even bother to describe the crushing feeling of guilt I felt all the while, because, after all, since I was the one to leave, it all ended up being entirely my fault.

But my decision was made, and never, even for a moment, did I waver, look back or regret it. Getting all of the blame annoyed me, and I couldn't understand that my husband and other people who were judging me so harshly couldn't simply recognize and accept that I couldn't put up with my life anymore as it was, and that things had to Change. And as I always say:

If you don't like where you are in life, move!
You are not a tree.

Why do we always have to blame someone when marriage fails, why not just accept the fact that life has its ways of changing us and we can either adapt or move on. I did my best to swallow these new capsules with acceptance and I kept my focus on what lay ahead.

One of the things I feared the most was not being able to have the time to move forward with my book, *Change*. But amidst all this chaos, the capsules of life put on my path a rather particular job. Once again, I wasn't going to do and live as everyone else: I landed a job as a night secretary. I would be working three nights a week, which would leave me lots of time during the day to write. I couldn't believe my luck and took it as a real sign that I had to move forward and continue with the writing of my book.

When going through difficult times, it's a struggle handling all that pain inside of you. I don't know whether you are aware of it, but **Pain is a FORCE!** Once you integrate this notion, you understand that you can channel this pain, you *must* channel it to bring something positive out of all you are going through. Take the pain, embrace it and use it to create something beautiful, whatever that may be for you. Perhaps it's writing poems or songs, singing with emotion, fixing up your car, training to rebuild your-body, taking pictures that have a meaning, creating a beautiful garden, or even writing a book. Find out what puts your heart at peace and pour all your pain into it. Keep faith, move forward with trust, without ever letting hatred settle down inside your heart. If you embrace the pain, I promise you, that at one point, when you lift your eyes to see what lies ahead, it will come as a surprise to see that you are no longer swimming, you will have reached the shore. You will look back at the ocean behind you in disbelief and smile, maybe even laugh when it hits you… that you managed to cross an entire ocean.

I watched my sons play this game numerous times and it got me thinking…

Be a Rock*: know what it is you want and walk with determination towards your goal.*

But also know when to **be a Paper***: that is to say when to be flexible and learn to accept things you cannot change. When something bad happens, try to see the lesson that lies within it.*

Finally, know when to **pull out your Scissors***: whenever possible "cut out" what is weighing you down. Sometimes it can be people but many times, I find, it's our very own negative thoughts about ourselves that harm us the most. So, cut it out! Focus more on doing things that you love like painting, exercising, gardening… whatever is your passion, and start seeing your real potential.*

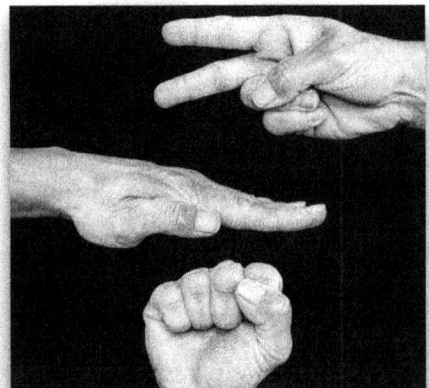

HOW TO READ THE BOOK "CHANGE"

According to the United Nation's latest "World Happiness Report" the United States is ranked 18th happiest country in the world. When asked why, many Americans said they felt less control over the choices in their lives.

Do we really have no choice? Wouldn't it be more correct to say that we have slowly, insidiously accepted to be somehow formatted into thinking that routine equals comfort and safety? Everything that deters us from our routinely lives is stressful, so shouldn't we do our utmost to keep things the way they are? Have you fallen into a routine rut? Are you leading the life of a robot, a life in which you just seem to be repeating the same day, over and over again?

Although many people dislike the way they live, when given options to escape their formatted lives, they always come up with a series of excuses. Just having to change one little thing in their daily routine, makes them feel very uncomfortable and actually really gets them upset. It's understandable: I mean let's face it, life is already hard as it is, right? Why on Earth would we want to complicate things by adding "CHANGES", to the picture?

When we think of it, it's true, every time something changes in our lives, we are forced to adapt, think things over, question ourselves and our abilities, reorganize, all of which puts us under a lot of pressure. If you were asked to take the time and look back at that specific moment in your past when change occurred, all you would recall are the negative emotions such as stress, feeling uncomfortable, agitated, while wasting time and energy. Everything that unfolds, after having experienced change, still bears a strong mark of negativity. Indeed, once we experience a negative emotion, it lingers on and it's not that easy to get rid of.

The key here is to prepare your mind, ahead of time, by reprograming it to start viewing CHANGE as a great amount of fun. Take a few minutes to step back, tear off those blinders, and start looking at the situation with a new set of eyes. It might not be easy to disassociate a state of fear or stress when a change occurs haphazardly, but what if you decided to be excited with the idea of incorporating changes voluntarily into your daily routine? What if you actually looked forward to provoking changes deliberately? How would you feel if you purposefully decided to change something, were totally prepared, and then did it with passion and excitement? What would your life be like if you looked forward to trying out new things, and started exploring unknown places? What if you stepped out of the box and challenged yourself to tasting surprising new flavors and textures and started doing things you never before thought were possible?

Yes, what would happen if you…. **embraced CHANGE?**
The idea is to start off by psychologically preparing yourself ahead of time. In order to be convinced that change is something positive, it's important that you stop making excuses, and dwelling on the past. Let's take this opportunity, here, to clear up one thing: It is absolutely essential that you understand that **your past experiences are the source of the inner wisdom you have within yourself today**. They were all lessons, in other words gifts that were given to enable your growth. They created the wonderful person you are today!

There is no need to look back anymore. Keep you focus on what lies ahead. The past is over and done with, but the future offers limitless possibilities. You can't create or recreate the past so why macerate in it? Why focus on the painful events of your life? Many people tend to climb into a slow cooker that's on very low heat, choosing to simmer in the past, in the midst of all those negative emotions.

Get up and wipe away the past which can easily be done by completely focusing on the clean slate you have ahead of you. That slate is all yours to create. It's like playing Minecraft: start creating a world in which your hands and imagination are doing the building. The way I see it: the life ahead is like a beautiful garden of opportunities. I see my future with joy in my eyes, anticipation in my heart and I move forward with open arms.

Being the creator of your world, by bringing changes into it, is not only exciting, it is also rewarding. Indeed, pretty soon you will be reaping the benefits. At one point, when you start being more open to Change, you will discover just how powerful it is and to what extent it can have a positive impact on your life.

So, spark up that inner flame. Yes, I know it's down there somewhere inside of you. Press the "Reboot" button and awaken the part of you that is dying to break lose, that is craving for more fun and excitement, and longing for a new life! Reignite your way of seeing life by infusing passion and love in everything you do… Come on, decide that once and for all, your life is going to CHANGE!

Let's enter your garden now and start imagining the big picture, in other words, the progress you could make over the period of one, two or three weeks, as you start seeing things differently. Understand that each day is another opportunity to improve yourself, every hour gives you the possibility to learn something new, and every minute offers you 60 seconds to improve who you are.

Some of you might argue that you tried to change in the past and have systematically fallen off track. Every time you attempted to bring something new into your life, such as eating a healthier diet or leading a more active lifestyle, you abandoned your goal, and felt as a quitter and a failure.

To this, I will say two things:

ONE ~ Be easy on yourself: relapses are totally normal

It is absolutely essential to understand that these *temporary relapses are totally natural*; they are in fact a part of the learning process. A surefire way of avoiding them, is to tackle very simple changes first: **Always make sure it is something very easy to do.** Many people dive into change with an "all or nothing state of mind". Be easy on yourself. Little changes can really go a long way.

Embrace change armed for success: expect these relapses, so that when they do occur, you can acknowledge and accept them, and then, quickly get back on track.

From now on, don't ever say that you quit or have failed: **you are in the process of learning**. On this path that you have chosen, there will be some ups and downs, where initial feelings of discouragement and loss of interest will be followed by moments of strength and confidence. Accept it. Be at peace with it.

When babies learn how to walk, they constantly get up and fall back down, over and over again, but they have the tenacity to keep on trying. Believe me, they don't waste any time thinking that it's impossible and that they will never succeed. Remember one thing: at one point you were that baby as well and you had that resilience to keep on trying.
So, what exactly happened? It seems as though, somewhere, along your way to adulthood, you have grown accustomed to the idea that making mistakes or having to try over again is synonymous with being a loser. But you are not. You are simply going through a learning phase and it's all perfectly normal.

TWO ~ Approach change with a positive mind and a passionate heart

To make this point clearer, let me start by asking you the following:

In the past, when you set your heart and mind on changing something, how did you tackle each change that you wanted to incorporate into your life?
First of all, what type of emotion did you feel in your heart when you engaged on this new journey? Was your heart filled with joy? Did you feel any passion? Were you excited by the forthcoming process?
You must embark on this ride with your heart filled with positive emotions. Don't do it out of anger or to seek revenge. Do it with faith and joy.
Every single day I got into the habit – and I encourage you to do the same - of taking the time to experience a series of positive emotions. I just shut my eyes and for a few minutes, I let "joy" in, allowing it to encompass and totally surround my entire mind and body.
After a few minutes, I choose another positive emotion, such as "faith", "gratitude", "power", "resilience", "passion" and I surrender myself to it completely and fully.
If you want to successfully bring change into your life, it's essential to fill your heart with as many positive emotions as possible.

Let's move on to your mindset:
What state of mind were you in when you approached change? How did you envision the whole process? Did you see it as something negative, as an obligation or a punishment?

Why is it that most people always have a tendency, after they decide to change something or reach a certain goal, to succumb to self-punishment or restriction?
I would like you to stop and think about this, and understand how resorting to this type of behavior is, in fact, counterproductive. You will only be setting yourself up for failure. I am sure you would agree that relying on frustration or resorting to force in order to reach a goal, will make it very difficult to maintain in the long run. You cannot embark on this road with a knife under your throat. You have to go lightheartedly. This is not a war or a battle that you must fight. Just let go of all of your negative emotions and surrender with joy. You have to engage on this path towards change with a peaceful and positive mind.

So, stop "negating" and start focusing on "adding" positive elements into your life. Change can only happen with a positive mindset.

In my twenties, I kept trying over and over again to become healthy. I would ban "bad food" from my closets, forcing myself to eat only the healthier choices. Most of my days were spent living either in frustration, because of all the food I wasn't allowed to eat or feeling guilty because I relapsed. Once I got into the habit of feeling proud of all my daily accomplishments and focused only on the positive factors I had undertaken for myself, a real shift occurred in my head. I felt like doing more and more good things for myself. I persisted with this thinking pattern over the years and today, in my fifties, I am proud to say that I am at peace with my "plate" and that I have a healthy mind in a healthy body.

Let's just say that you have decided to lose some weight, for example. As I said before, instead of following a restrictive diet or quitting all of your favorite foods, why not focus of bringing more positivity into your life. We don't want to "take away", "deprive" or "restrict" ourselves from doing something, quite the contrary: we want to "bring in something positive." All you have to do is select one healthy behavior and ADD it to your life, every day. To lose weight, you could choose to have a daily fruit, vegetable drink or soup. Look up Change n°14: *A Daily Dose of Goodness.*
Or you could make sure that one meal - either breakfast, lunch or dinner- is totally healthy. Look up Change n° 16: *One Special Meal.*
Or you could see to it that you simply start drinking water every day.

Now don't change anything else. Don't get all drastic and start spinning your whole life around. Go about your days as you usually do. You just want to make sure that you either drink that juice, eat that one healthy meal, or drink a sufficient amount of water!
You are probably thinking: "Well, that's not going to get me anywhere", or "I'm not going to lose any weight this way!"

But let's forget about losing weight. Let's focus on making sure that you get that one objective done. You have probably been wanting to lose weight for several years and haven't succeeded. So, let's just be a little more patient.
At the end of every day, you can reflect upon this and tell yourself:

> ### I am on the road to change and am proud of myself:
> ### today I did something that was good for me, I...
> *I had that fruit & veggie drink, had that healthy meal or drank enough water.*

The following week, you can add another positive element into your life. Let's say last week you choose to drink fresh juice, well, now you could ADD one healthy meal a day. Remember to keep that daily juice in the picture…it's slowly becoming a habit anyway.
The third week you could do some research about the benefits of drinking more water, find out what the best sources are, depending on where you live and what cost-effective solutions you have. Look up Change n° 13: *Hydrate.*

Do you see what I am getting at? After the very first week it looks as though nothing much has happened, but if you look at your progress over the period of three months, which is the time it would take you to complete an entire chapter, you could have integrated 10 to 12 positive new changes into your life and would now be well on your way to becoming a much healthier person!

And what if the 4th week you decided to discover or eat a different fruit or vegetable every day? Make it creative, original and fun! Cook it any way you want and discover new flavors! You will find more information about this in Change n° 17: *Try Something New.*

At the beginning of the 5th week, why not decide to find a few books about nutrition and healthy eating and commit to reading and learning about it every day. Look up Change n° 23 *Read! Read! Read!*

In the 6th week, you could decide to observe your eating habits. Check out Change n° 20: *Self-Observation*. Notice the amount and what kinds of foods you eat, your recurring eating patterns and finally, find out the reason why you have an unhealthy relationship with your plate.

By the time the 7th week arrives, you could choose to eat only when you are hungry and stop eating when you are satisfied. You'll find this in Change n° 19: *In Tune with Hunger – Ms. FULL-O-METER.*

Week 8: you could continue on the same path and make sure you learn to slow down while eating mindfully and really chew every bite. Look up Change n° 22: *Eating Mindfully.*

Week 9: you could read change n°21, *Rules Between Meals, and* decide to no longer eat in between meals and after 8 pm.

And why not incorporate visualization into week 10? Find 10 minutes every day to visualize yourself attaining your goal or simply feeling total confidence. If you tried the classic visualization technique and it didn't seem to work for you, why not try a new approach? Check out Change n° 18, *Visualize*, for more details.

By the time Week 11 arrives, you could be tackling "The Big 5 Challenge" and making sure that you are eating 5 fruit and vegetables every day. Explore Change n° 15.

And on your 12th week, you could decide to eat a variety of different foods and enter the "*11 Essential Vitamins and Minerals Challenge*". You'll find this in Change n° 24: *Add Variety.*

Do you realize how much closer to being healthy you could be over the course of a 3-month period and just how much you could change?

And if you keep at it, before you know it, six months will go by, but this time, these months were different: you managed to bring positive elements into your life and when looking back, you have something to be proud of.

You were active and were actually doing something for yourself. You got out of your comfort zone and accepted to CHANGE!

And pretty soon, you will see that, as you move forward, you will want to improve other aspects of your life.

What I find amazing about tackling life challenges this way, is that once you understand how it works and become accustomed to it, you can apply it to all areas of your life. When you truly integrate this notion, there will be no stopping you, and you will want to change many other different aspects and even start taking on some bigger challenges or setting higher goals.

This book contains 5 chapters. Each one proposes 12 Changes, which means that you have a total of **60 different Changes**:

Chapter One ~ Improve your Self-esteem
Chapter Two ~ Improve your Relationship with Food
Chapter Three ~ On the Path to Physical Transformation
Chapter Four ~ Change the Way you Work and Play
Chapter Five ~ Learning to Embrace Painful or Unwanted Change

Read on as I suggest and guide you through different ways to help you achieve these goals.

Understand that it's entirely up to you, you are totally free to focus on only one aspect of your life, such as improving your relationship with food - in which case you would essentially focus on Chapter 2 - or, if your goal is more general, and you wish to improve yourself overall to pick an element from one chapter the first week and then another, from a totally different chapter, the following week.

Here is a list of things you can do over a period of three months to generally improve yourself:

Week 1: Change n° 4: Try "The Confidence Walk "
Week 2: Change n° 14: Have "A daily dose of freshness"
Week 3: Change n° 27: Bring mindfulness in your workouts
Week 4: Change n° 2: Stand tall and Improve your posture
Week 5: Change n° 16: Have "One Special Meal"
Week 6: Change n° 53: Start Decluttering
Week 7: Change n° 8: Do "Your Daily Love"
Week 8: Change n° 36: Carry out an exercise challenge
Week 9: Change n° 49: Sleep more, or you can explore your romantic life in Change n°41.
Week 10: Change n° 51: Communicate with nature
Week 11: Change n° 13: Hydrate
Week 12: Change n° 12: Create your commercial

So, the next three months think about *YOU*! Commit to doing something for yourself! Bring a little bit of change and see how you can make your life more interesting, fun and colorful!

Once you have completed the initial 12-week Change transformation, you may continue to explore the changes you could bring into your life the following weeks:

Week 13: Change n° 22: Eating Mindfully

Week 14: Change n° 38: Take the leap and go back to school: take a course about nutrition, healthy eating or whatever you feel passionate about.

Week 15: Change n° 09: Challenge yourself to learning something new every day

Week 16: Change n° 07: Be Inspired by reading inspiring books, watching inspiring videos and meeting inspiring people!

Week 17: Change n° 56: Smile more

Week 18: Change n°… go on and on changing your beautiful self!

NOTE: Sometimes you will have goals that you can implement all year long (such as drinking enough water or walking 20 minutes) and at other times, you will have a goal that you will keep for only a week or so, such as an exercise challenge.

Start imagining today the person you are going to be in twelve weeks. Stop the quick fixes and start seeing all those weeks, months, years you have ahead of you as open possibilities to thrive. And remember, when you fumble along the way – because it will happen - stop saying that you have failed and just, simply, keep on trying. You will see, I assure you, that the length of time that you spend in a relapse, as well as the number of these relapses will decrease over time, until they become a rare exception.

I hope you understand that by adding positive elements to your life, you are adding a powerful dynamic to it. This plan of action will improve your self-confidence because you will be learning to set small goals and will actually reach them! It's important for you to see that it is absolutely possible to succeed. At the end of a year or at some point along the way, it will hit you that you actually have a secret power within you and that *YOU* CAN CREATE YOUR LIFE.

And here's a question for you:
What have you got to lose?
Why not just try?
You'll see, it's easy!
Don't you think you owe it to yourself?

How do *YOU* feel about CHANGE?

If you are reading this page, it's most probably because something about the word "CHANGE" resonated within you. As you reached for or clicked on this book, you were aware that your life needed to change.

Let's dig a little deeper to clear things up and enable you to know where you stand on this issue, how you truly feel about change.

When you hear the word CHANGE, what does it evoke for you?
What is the first thought that comes to mind?

Is CHANGE something POSITIVE or NEGATIVE? ~ *Circle your answer*

Does CHANGE ignite FEAR or EXCITEMENT? ~ *Circle your answer*

This book is here to help you EMBRACE Change, learn how to accept it whether it's "good" or "bad", whether it feels comfortable or not. Progressively, you will start opening new doors and tackling change with a totally different approach and quicker than you think, change will turn into something positive and exciting!

Think about it: in life everything is constantly transforming, transitioning, shifting, switching, developing, and adjusting. Of course, you will say, every second of the day, you are growing older and thus changing. Every minute of every day you are constantly adapting to new changes that come your way, nothing ever being exactly the same as the day before, even when it comes to routine. At times, changes are barely noticeable and at other times, change can feel like a major revolution, such as when you have to change jobs or move to a new place, when you are diagnosed with cancer, you are heartbroken or you lose a loved one.

Sometimes CHANGE comes unwanted, but then at other times it is your deepest desire for it to come into your life: you want to lose weight or quit a bad habit like smoking or biting your nails. Maybe you are dreaming of mastering a certain skill, such as language or a sport. Perhaps you have a beautiful voice and love singing or you are gifted at drawing and you would like to really develop this potential. These changes are like dreams you would like to see come true.

Opening up to bringing changes into your life on a regular basis when the good times are rolling, will help you remain stronger and more capable of embracing change when it's painful.

But first, let's focus on your dreams. What are your dreams? Tell me something YOU would like to accomplish, something you would really like to change and then fill out the next "HOW TO CHANGE" workpage.

I WOULD LOVE TO ACCOMPLISH THE FOLLOWING:

_____
_____
_____

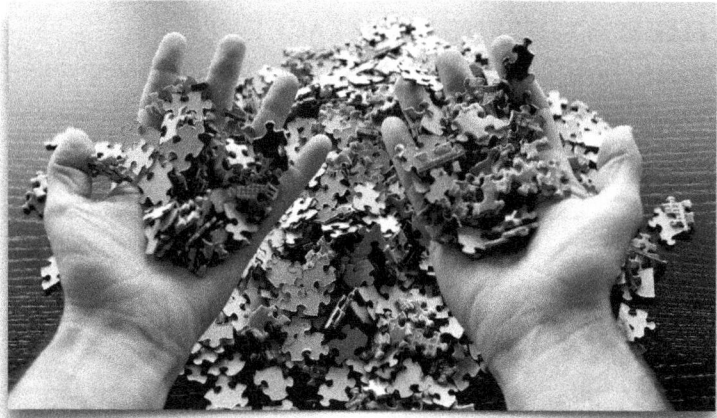

Get into the habit of dismantling your goal into different parts and then simply make sure you do at least 1 or 2, preferably 3 or 4 things every day, to get yourself one step closer to reaching this goal. Remember, little changes can go a long way.

Now, let's look at what you can do to accept change when it's difficult or challenging.

WHAT WAS THE BIGGEST CHANGE YOU HAVE EVER HAD TO OVERCOME IN YOUR LIFE?

_____
_____

WHAT MADE IT SO CHALLENGING FOR YOU?

Describe the emotion that overcomes you, when you think about it.

_____
_____

NOW WRITE DOWN 3 OTHER CHANGES THAT WERE DIFFICULT FOR YOU TO ACCEPT .

For example: It has been hard for me to accept to see my body changing, such as putting on weight, getting older etc. - It has been hard to accept my children leaving home. - It has been hard to see that the years have gone by and I haven't really achieved anything. - I am constantly struggling with my weight and it's hard on a day to day basis.

_____
_____
_____

When going through difficult times, remember: it's time to grow. Ask yourself, what can you do to turn this painful moment into something positive? Every day start by investing a few minutes into channeling your pain into something creative, whether it be gardening, singing, writing, composing, sewing, painting, giving some of your time, meditating, doing yoga or any type of exercise etc. pour your heart into it and progressively put in a little more time.

WHAT MADE THEM SO DIFFICULT TO ACCEPT?

Try to find two or three words sum up how you felt.

Example: When my children left home, I felt abandoned/useless

1. _____

_____

2. _____

_____

3. _____

WRITE DOWN WHAT YOU LOVE DOING OR WHAT YOU ARE GOOD AT

To help you, remember: "What you did willingly as a child, on your own free time, often tells you who you were meant to be or what you were meant to do."

1. _____

_____

2. _____

_____

3. _____

_____

CHOOSE ONE OF THEM. POUR YOUR HEART AND ENERGY INTO IT: DO IT MORE, BECOME BETTER AND WHY NOT EVEN EXCEL AT IT!

I CHOOSE TO IMPROVE:

_____

Now write down everything you can do to improve your personal skill

1. _____
2. _____
3. _____
4. _____
5. _____

And then get up and start seeing what can happen when *YOU* start embracing the *POWERS OF CHANGE!*

REFLECTING ABOUT CHANGE

Many of us waste an awful lot of time and energy trying to get rid of our bad habits. And then, when we quit trying, we spend our time feeling guilty, because we are incapable of changing. We will all be adamant in saying that our desire to stop smoking, over-eating or nail biting is very strong. So why is it that every single time we try, the only outcome seems to be failure?

Then, at other times, it's not that we would like to quit a bad habit. What we want is **to bring some changes into our lives, in a sense, create new healthy habits**, such as exercising regularly, having a healthier diet, and sleeping more. And we realize that creating a new habit isn't that easy and most of us end up quitting within a few months, weeks or even days from trying. Think about it. What changes do you wish to create in your life? To help you find out, I have listed a number of things that you might want to change:

- I want to be happy
- I want to feel loved
- I want to feel beautiful
- I want to have more money or be rich
- I want to speak up
- I want to change the way I eat
- I want to eat less
- I want to slow down: do less
- I want to have great abs
- I want to be more muscular
- I want to lose weight
- I want my posture to be perfect
- I want to sleep like a baby
- I want to be more confident
- I want to quit smoking
- I want to quit drinking
- I want to be more organized
- I want to stop biting my nails
- I want to exercise more regularly
- I want to have a great sex life
- I want to stop the munching
- I want to be more active
- I want to be better at my job
- I want to have the strength to say "No"
- I want to stop lying to others and to myself
- I want to stop criticizing/judging
- I want to stop bringing everything back to myself (being self-centered)
- I want to stop being jealous
- I want to stop being angry
- I want to stop being lazy
- I want to improve my relationship with my man/woman
- I want to take better care of myself

Which habits would you like to quit and which new ones would you like to make a part of your life?

I would like to change once and for all and quit the following habits:

_____

I would like to bring these changes into my life:

_____

If you take the time to really think about it, change has a lot to do with breaking old and creating new habits.

When I realized this, it got me thinking: so how does one create a new habit?

At first you do something. You might find pleasure or not in doing it. If it is pleasurable, you will then want to do it again. Later on, you remember this moment of pleasure and you wish to recreate it. This is how something as simple as drinking your morning coffee can turn into a necessity.
It has happened to all of us: We try something. We find it pleasurable. We associate pleasure with that specific experience. We then want to renew this experience over and over again, because it makes us happy and feels good.

Let's keep asking questions and look into this matter a little deeper. What can push you to change?

We can change immediately under strong emotions such as fear or anger. When you find yourself in a state of emergency, your entire being, mind and body reacts and you put all your uncertainties and fears aside. You change instantaneously. This can happen, for example, when we are diagnosed with a serious health problem and it's important to quit a bad habit at once, before our condition worsens or could become fatal. Some smokers, once diagnosed with emphysema, quit smoking overnight, and others, when diagnosed with type 2 diabetes linked to their obesity, take immediate action to lose the excess weight. A strong emotion *can* provoke change.

We are at a point in this sub-chapter where you need to stop and ask yourself the only essential question: do you really, truly want to change? Come on, you have to be true to yourself here: do you want this more than anything in the world? Is it something that you feel deep down in your gut?

If you really want to change something in your life, then just do it: CHANGE! Not tomorrow, not next week, not when you have the time or when your situation is better. This is your book to change right now. Quit the excuses. Stop coming up with a list of reasons why you can't do it now. If you want it, then the best time to start doing something about it, is NOW.

Are you still hesitating and coming up with some "good" excuses? Then maybe you don't really, truly want to bring this change into your life, maybe not as much as you thought you did, anyway.

Some of you will counter-argue that you are not in an urgent situation that requires immediate change and that it's difficult to create such a strong emotion. Deep down inside we know there is no emergency and life just has a way of tempting us out of our good resolutions.

Might I ask you then: "What's holding you back?" Could it be Fear? Often our desire to change is quickly choked up by some form of self-preservation. We start wondering what will happen if we actually do change. For example, you are in a bad relationship. You know that it has to end, but you just can't gather up the courage to break up. You tell yourself that if you leave them, you might not find anyone else. Or you remember the good old days and you start telling yourself that the situation could return to how it was before and…, in a way, leaving the relationship, isn't it kind of like giving up?

It's normal to ask yourself these questions. But what if you took the time to be really honest with yourself, to quit all the lying? Deep down inside we know what we have to do. Is there still some hope and a way of saving this relationship, or is it time to step out of our comfort zone and move on? Why is it that we tend to accept certain situations even when they are really bad?

I am going to ask you to stop right here and remember one fundamental truth: **you deserve the best**! So, if your situation is and has been painful for a while, then it's a clear sign that you have to move on: when deep down inside you are feeling unhappy and no longer in synch with yourself, it's time to start doing something about it.

In order to thrive, one needs to feel good on the inside. If you don't, then life is sending you a message that things have got to change. Why this ingrown fear of the unknown? The fear of what lies ahead most definitely is what's keeping many of us from changing.
Are you unhappy with your present situation? Look ahead: a clean slate lies before you. Put your fears aside and start seeing your future as a huge garden full of opportunities. Be brave! Get up! Don't look back! Now is the time to focus on your new future! I am not saying it's going to be easy. I am saying that you can no longer accept this situation you are in and it's time to move on.

Some of you will contest that you are not unhappy and then ask: Why bother changing when it's so much easier to stay within my comfort zone? And I hear you. Indeed, change requires you to get back to square one again, with all that it implies: questioning yourself, having to learn again, feeling awkward and uncomfortable and so on. Sometimes it's just so much easier to leave things the way they are. There is a certain form of comfort in staying lazy.

I am going to repeat myself here… and ask you again: do you really want to bring this change into your life, Yes or No? If your answer is a big fat "YES" then decide to change NOW.

One day, Jesus faced a crippled man and gave him an order: "Get up and walk!" You, right now, are like that crippled man. Your excuses cripple you from achieving the things you really want to do. It's time to get up and act now. Start walking and see how all your excuses crumble to the ground. Don't let anything or anyone stop you anymore. Keep that one change in mind and tackle it with all your might!

Still haven't run off to change something in your life?

Ok. Then come with me: I would like you to consider looking into the following five aspects:

~ The importance of knowledge ~
You have to know and understand what you are undertaking.

~ The importance of passion ~
What room have you left for passion in your life?

~ The importance of slowing down ~
Is there a possibility that you might be under too much pressure
to handle any more change?

~ The importance of faith ~
You have to move forward with confidence and believe that life has your back.

~ The importance of placing a smile on your heart ~
When facing change undertake it with a happy heart!

~ The importance of Knowledge

When you wish to bring some form of change into your life, it's a bit like trying to master something new. And what better way to do so than to try and become more knowledgeable in this area of expertise. Many people, when they decide to tackle a new goal, dive into it blindly without taking the time to research or plan things out.

Why don't you start by asking yourself a few questions: What are the benefits? Why do you want this change? What could you do to improve your overall knowledge about it? Do you know of anyone that could help you and is knowledgeable in this domain?

Let's take an example: You would like to improve the way you eat, become a healthy eater. Everyone knows that fruit and vegetables are good for you. But do you know why? Do you actually know the benefits of each and every one of them? And then turn the question the other way around and put the focus on the junk you eat. Why not try to have a closer look at these foods and find out why they are bad for you. Start reading labels, watch short videos, read books, ask your doctor or a fitness expert.

When you start watching videos to see how chicken nuggets and other processed foods are made, when you start researching to know why you should go organic, and you begin reading labels to understand what ingredients to avoid, you are actually opening your conscience up to the reasons why you shouldn't be eating certain foods. It's not an overnight process, but the more you are aware of what you are actually putting into your mouth, the harder it becomes to continue eating this way.

So, from now on, when you wish to bring some form of change into your life, remember to do your research. Keep in mind that becoming more knowledgeable is an important part of the whole process.

~ The importance of Passion

Ask yourself the following question: Why did you sink into that bad habit in the first place? Why do you overeat, indulge in sweets, drink too much, or criticize others?
Let's take a closer look at your life. What's it like? How are things going for you at work? How is your love relationship? Are there moments throughout the day when you partake in an activity with great passion? Are you passionate about anything at all? Do you jump out of bed excited about the new day? Do you live your life with enthusiasm? Or, on the contrary, could it be that are you are bored and your life has become somewhat of a routine, where you simply repeat the same day over and over again?

Think about it: how many times a day do you feel enthusiastic about what you are doing?
For me, every single day is a bit like Christmas Eve: Who knows what today and tomorrow will bring? The prospect is exciting, almost exhilarating.
How about you, do you live your life this way?
If you live passionately, put your heart into what you do, find joy in the big and little things, love your job or enjoy listening to what people have to say, if you see life as a garden of opportunities... then your mind and heart are too busy being happy and curious to waste any time creating or indulging in new "bad habits."

Because let's face it, if you are overeating, heading to the bar after work, finishing your evenings as a couch potato in front of the TV with a bag of chips, it's only because you are trying to fill a void: that emptiness you feel inside.

So, if you can't quit your bad habits cold turkey, why don't you begin by finding ways to bring back that inner spark into your heart? Why not create inner passion? Find that inner light that is craving to come alive? Your heart's passion can help free you from your worst habits. If your attention is fully centered on what you are doing and you feel pleasure or passion while doing it, you will no longer resort to all those bad habits of yours.

Just simply remember the last time you were in love, how your focus was almost completely channeled towards that one special person. Nothing else really mattered, right? When falling in love, very often people have a tendency to lose weight. Have you ever noticed this? Why? Because their attention is focused on that special someone and no longer on food.

And this got me thinking - I always tend to find messages everywhere – that maybe the act of falling in love actually came with a coded message attached to it. Maybe the whole purpose of falling in love is there to teach us what it feels like to live with passion. And so, I ask you: why not recreate this passionate feeling and pour it into your daily activities? Reconnect with your work and find ways of making it more interesting again, learn new things to improve yourself, be professional at all times, start by asking more questions and why not even try to get a promotion? Bring more passion into your home: learn to listen to your spouse again, to your kids, make your meals with love and then share them with your family in a pleasurable atmosphere. Try to bring back that flame between you and your special someone. And then, why not find something that you feel passionate about and then do everything to excel at it.

Quit the routine lifestyle and start living your life at its fullest. Embrace every instant.
          "If you only had one more hour to live, what would you do?"

Think about it. Is it possible to live that way? Making the most of every single second, hour and day. If you wake up thrilled and live each moment with passion, there will no longer be room or desire to partake in activities that bring you down.

Do things passionately. Bring passion into all aspects of your life and start seeing it change. What makes life worthwhile? LOVE. You are not a robot so don't live like one. Start putting more love into what you do.

Find time to do the things you really want to do. My days are quickly filled up with training, writing my books, reading, enjoying the company of my boyfriend or a friend, sharing a special moment with my kids, eating, meditating… there are so many things that I want to do every day, it just seems as though there aren't enough hours to get them all done. The way I see it:

Life is a gift.
What I choose to do with it
is my way of saying "thank you".

~ The importance of Slowing Down

We often hear people say that they have no willpower; it's a flaw they have. Just like some tend to be unkind or lack generosity, others, according to them, come without any willpower.

Do you share this belief as well?

Let's stop here a minute or two and think about this: What if I told you that you have just as much willpower as anyone else? Then why, might you ask, is it that certain people are capable of setting a goal and successfully managing to follow it through while you can't?

Maybe you are looking at this from the wrong angle. Step back and reflect on your days: are most of them spent running from one activity to another, juggling between work, kids, chores, friends? Are most of your activities done under a lot of stress? Haven't you noticed how we spend our days always rushing? How can we be efficient at work when we are constantly interrupted by phone calls, emails, colleagues and so on? No wonder we have stomach ache and heartburn: we seldom eat peacefully, often doing something else during our meals like texting, watching TV, or working. For some of us, eating has become a necessary burden and for others a comfort from all the stress we have to handle.

So, tell me something: how on Earth do you think you can successfully add one more thing to this stressful context? Your body and mind are craving for a moment to relax and here you are talking about setting a new goal?

Have you ever taken this into consideration?
What if you slowed down? What if you did less? What if next time you started saying "no" instead of taking on even more? What if you simplified your life… what would happen?

Try it. Start by making the important moments in your life, such as eating, or spending time with your spouse or children, really count. Try putting certain chores off to later and use this time to relax. Forget about cleaning up the whole kitchen, leave a little earlier for work and go have yourself a nice cup of coffee in a special café before tackling your day. As much as possible do your best to stop stressing yourself with the list of things you have to do. Learn to slow down. Make "happiness, love and peace" your top priority and start focusing on feeling good and making more of your moments *happy*.

Notice, after a while, how you no longer need willpower, how things you have been longing for start happening naturally. By doing less you will have far more energy and desire to do the things you decided to accomplish and do them appropriately. You will start wanting to exercise more often and you will be less likely to eat for the wrong reasons. Slowing down and doing less, will also have you even-tempered and you will no longer be wasting as much time looking for things, getting upset for no reason, or feeling completely exhausted at the end of the day.

So, slow down, do less and see how, in fact, you get more done. To much surprise, you will notice that many things that once seemed important, aren't so anymore. Relax and feel more confident that things will unfold in your favor and then see how they fall into place and your life will become so much easier.

How can you, in your right mind, expect to change anything if you keep on living under so much stress, on a day to day basis? Because let's face it, your life is hectic!

And, in what way can forcing yourself to change be beneficial? Indeed, "to force yourself" already implies, somewhere along the line, that you are reluctant to doing it.
What if, instead of forcing yourself to change, you did your best to create the ideal situation to bring about some changes into your life? Why not do your utmost to reduce the amount of stress you live in and replace it with passion, as many moments as possible? I am sure that this way, you will succeed in positively changing many little things that previously seemed totally impossible.

One thing is for sure, it's far easier to focus on doing less while engaging in more things that make you happy, than to force yourself to change.
So, slow down. I mean really slam the breaks and do your utmost to clear out stress. Make time for more passion in all areas of our life by really paying attention to what counts, such as listening to others and becoming more knowledgeable in different areas that could have a real impact your life.

I'll tell you one thing: It can't hurt to try: why not start *right now*?

~ The importance of Faith

Faith is absolutely essential. You have to move forward, every single second, every single minute of the day with confidence, with the inner conviction that you are here to learn, that the "downs" in your life are only lessons and that this life you were given is your most beautiful gift.

Every self-help book I have opened talks about manifesting your desire, seeing what you want as already there. But your faith, I mean truly believing deep down inside that you are here for a reason and that you have an actual hand on "your" story, that is the true key.

I mean, what's the point of imagining your ideal future, even if you add the emotions to make it feel real, if throughout the rest of the day you believe that you are lousy, that you are a loser, that you will most probably never achieve that desired weight, meet that special someone, or land that dream job you have always wanted? Most books say: your mind can't see the difference between your imagination and reality, you can fool it with creative visualization and positive emotions. But what about your heart? Can your heart be fooled?

The answer is clearly "no!" Many of my friends visualize on a regular basis, create vision boards, repeat affirmations, but to no avail.
It's important to understand that if you want to obtain something, you have to nurture that faith in your heart. You can't just sit down and visualize the ideal situation and then go about living your life feeling miserable and full of doubt.

If you want your wishes to manifest themselves, you need faith.

Without faith, you are simply imagining things, daydreaming. It's as though you were building something but didn't bother to set up a proper foundation. It's like writing a whole book and then letting all the pages scatter randomly in the wind.

At one point in my life, when I was going through very difficult times, I would spend my days, whenever possible, meditating to reconnect with myself. I would go for long walks with a determined mindset, stand very tall, smile at every opportunity that was given to me, swim in the ocean to be in touch with nature, and do as many things that I loved as possible… Although I often cried along the way, deep down within, I *knew*, that I was going to be ok. It was only a question of time. I had faith!

Many of my friends encouraged me to consult a psychiatrist or go on medication for depression, but I refused to go down that path. I chose action and faith to help me move forward: I accepted the fact that all I was going through was a lesson, a necessary process. Although it was very painful, it was clear to me that I was on this path towards change for a reason. So, I kept my focus on what lay ahead of me, knowing that pretty soon I would be embracing a new life, a life in which I would be so much stronger and happier.

But then, you might ask, what if you don't have this faith? How can you awaken it?
Faith can be built. One of the best ways to work on that faith is by getting up and smiling, by doing things that make you feel good, enrich you, make you vibrate and love life, and make you want to get up tomorrow and do it again. This is the way you build your faith. Bring joy in your heart, take care of yourself inside and out, have dreams, do things that really matter… and make your life worthwhile.

The day you step out your front door embracing your day with faith in your heart, and belief that you are worthy of receiving, then you are one step closer to manifesting your dreams. It's at this point, I believe, that you can start considering visualization. For this reason, I feel like saying: stop dreaming your life and focus on making your present moment as happy as possible. Do the things that really matter, that bring joy to your heart and one magical day, you will see, you will set your foot down in the morning with a smile on your face, knowing with certainty that faith has finally come.

~ The importance of putting a Smile on your Heart

When tackling something new, instead of stressing, letting yourself be submerged by fear or focusing on what others might say about you, why don't you decide to change your mindset: learn to stop in your footsteps, press the pause button and place a smile on your heart. Commit, no matter what it is you have to do, to do your best to have more fun in the process.

Our job environment can be very stressful. Indeed, it is not always easy to be, at the same time, professional, quick and efficient and then maintain that high level throughout the entire day, five or more days a week. When I first started my actual job, I know I would go through my entire day stressed and scared that I would make yet another mistake. At the end of the day, I would leave either relieved to have made it through the whole day without making an error or like a total failure because I had been a disappointment.

Why is it that we always have a feeling that we are the only ones to make mistakes or that it is such a bad thing to make one? Once I got past the fear of losing my job - understanding that it would not be the end of the world if I did - I was able to tackle my days differently and intentionally shifted my mindset: I went to work with a big fat smile on my heart! Instead of wasting my time worrying and stressing about my flaws and mistakes, I directed my energy toward doing the best I can, helping others as much as possible and constantly trying to learn and improve myself.

It became crystal clear to me that if I wanted to be good at my job, I had to find ways to make my job more interesting and have more fun in the process.

And so, I worked on strengthening my concentration and organizational skills, took a weeklong course to master WORD, EXCEL and POWER POINT, started reading as many incoming and outcoming letters as possible to get a better understanding of the business in general, opened closets and files to become more knowledgeable and respond quicker…and all the while, I did it with a happy heart. Now don't get me wrong, as I write these words today, I am fully aware that I have yet to improve on a lot of things and I do still falter along the way, but I don't feel like a failure anymore as I immediately pull myself together and get back to work. Believe me, it doesn't take long before my heart starts smiling again.

What I am trying to say is this: when you have to face change or a challenge, stop in your tracks and ask yourself: "Can I tackle the situation in a more lighthearted way? Can I change how I see the whole picture and find a way to make the whole moment more fun and enjoyable? In short, how can I dedramatize the entire process?"
A quick shift in your mindset is often all you need to make the path toward change more pleasurable.

So next time you have to tackle something new or you want to bring some form of change in your life, start is by placing a smile on your heart and then do whatever it is you have to do with a happy heart.

To conclude, I encourage you to let all of these thoughts linger on inside your mind. Plant these seeds and let them grow. I hope they lead you to an "AHA!" moment as they did me!

One final thought: why not decide to go one step further and decide to no longer set any goals at all: why not, from now on, let yourself go and be totally confident in what lies ahead. Slow down, put love and peace in your heart, and from now on make sure your focus is on being happy and feeling good. Chances are all those things you have been struggling with, or wishing for, will come to you in the most natural and easy way.

Wishing you all the best of luck on your journey to Change!

CHAPTER ONE

~

IMPROVE YOUR SELF~ESTEEM

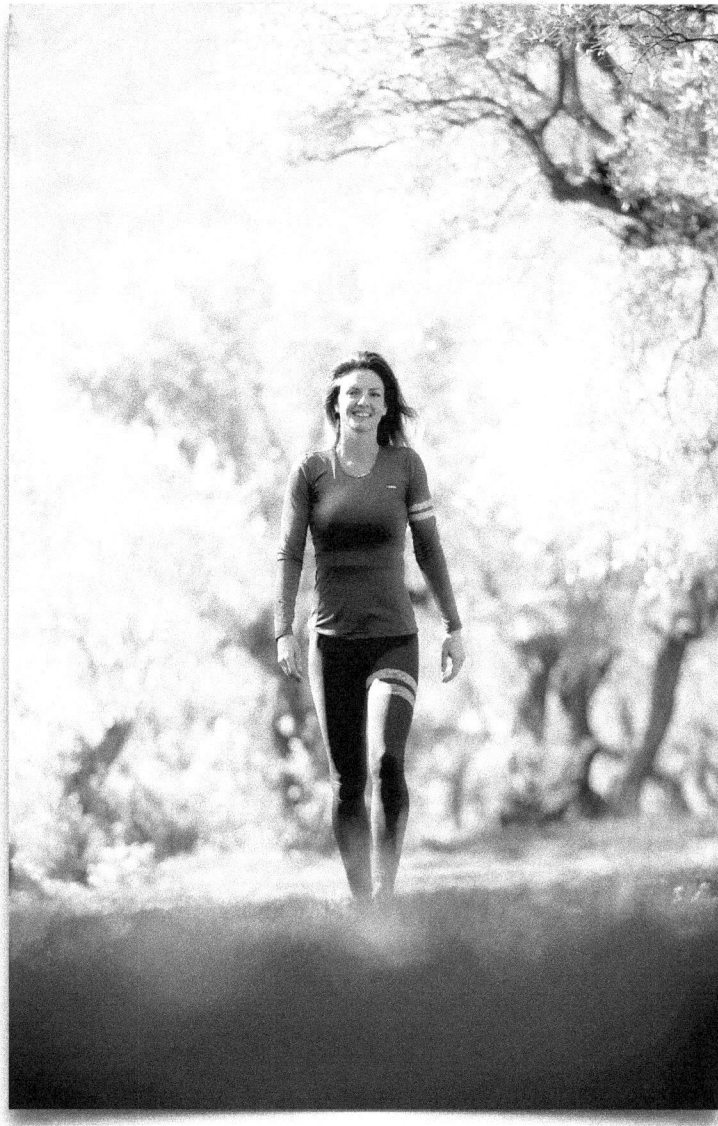

They were just thoughts
that danced through my little head…
about Aging.

When I was a child, my mother's job as an historian brought me to live on several Ojibwe reservations. Since she was often busy for long hours at a time, my favorite way to escape was to read…. I remember that I particularly enjoyed legends and tales of North American Indian First Nations: they were all about lessons to be learned, of having to surpass yourself. They also took me away on adventures and made me laugh.

One day, as I was reading these legends, it occurred to me, to what extent our society had changed. Indeed, the Elders in these stories were respected and looked up to. Frequently the younger generations would consult them to seek for advice. The moment they would step out of their tent, the children would gather around them and beg for stories or a joke. The elderly were always wise and calm; no words or action was ever wasted.

Today, aging is something our society rejects…. We don't want to get old and we no longer respect the elderly. For many, as they reach their old age there is this feeling of having lost their sense of purpose, and it makes me sigh…

But when as a child, I read these stories, I remember thinking how wonderful it must be to grow old and wise. It was inspiring and kind of like a dream you wish could come true. Shouldn't our whole life be a process in order to acquire this wisdom?

This thought never left me and I decided I wanted my life to be that way: I imagined that as I would get older I would become wiser, more open minded, more tolerant, I would have learned how to slow down, how to listen to others and stop the judging. And of course, in the end I would have attained a certain inner peace.

Think of it, living life this way would make growing old an amazing process; it would be a goal we would all like to reach and a person we would like to become.

So, these were the thoughts that danced through my little head…

These thoughts still dance today, and I know they will never leave me.

Change n°01
YOUR "DAILY POSITIVE CHECKLIST"

Change n°02
STAND TALL

Change n°03
YOUR SELF IMAGE

Change n°04
"THE CONFIDENCE WALK"

Change n°05
BELIEVE IN YOURSELF - CREATE YOUR VERY OWN P.E.T.

Change n°06
YOUR EMPOWERING BOARD

Change n°07
BE INSPIRED

Change n°08
YOUR DAILY LOVE

Change n°09
7 RINGS TO LEARN 7 DIFFERENT THINGS

Change n°10
RESPECT YOURSELF

Change n°11
LOVE MORE

Change n°12
YOUR COMMERCIAL

*There are many things that you can do to improve the way you feel about yourself
and here you will find a list of possibilities.
You will notice that I do not mention "exercise" as one of the options.
My entire Chapter Two is dedicated to this purpose.*

Change n°01
YOUR
"DAILY POSITIVE CHECKLIST"

1.

A. Creating and Using Your Journal

a. My Journaling Experience

As a child, I created my very own journal: Being homeschooled and having a lot of free time on my hands, I just loved to write down all the lyrics of my favorite songs, do some drawings, write my thoughts, but also paste in postcards and pictures from magazines and so on. My journal was my companion.

I spent hours flipping through all the pages and spending time with it. As the years went by, I kept up with this habit but its usage somehow changed along the way. I've created and wrote:

• Fitness journals
• Diaries
• Blogs
• Pregnancy journals
• Motivational journals
• Short stories
• My book

Each journal has been a great source of motivation for me: it takes only about 10 to 15 minutes a day, but those few minutes are the time that I spend self-motivating, reflecting, logging my achievements and thinking about how I can achieve my future goals. I strongly encourage you to begin creating one now: write down your goals, make a note of your accomplishments and remember to add photos. Take some alone time and you will move one step closer to achieving your goals and getting to know yourself!

b. What You Need:

• A notebook
• Colorful markers
• Scissors, scotch tape, glue
• Magazines
• A camera or phone camera
• My "Daily Positive checklist"

The first thing to do is go out and buy yourself a notebook. No need to get a fancy or an expensive one, any one will do. The key here is to make this notebook your very own and super special by writing in it – either one or two full pages - every day.

c. How to Use It

Every day have fun filling out your pages. Since the purpose of this chapter is to boost your self-esteem, you'll want to write down all the positive things you have experienced each day, and also what you have done for yourself and others!

Examples:

• I had a healthy snack and ate an apple for my 10 o'clock break!

• I went to bed early and slept 8 hours last night and I felt fantastic today!

• This nice guy held the door for me with a huge smile: That made my day! Or: I held the door for someone today and they gave me a huge smile in return, and it made my day!

• We went for a walk with the kids after homework: it was really nice to share this moment with them!

• I had a light dinner and went to bed feeling good about myself!

• I am doing Change No 17 this week. I have decided to try one new fruit or vegetable every day and today I ate fresh lychees! I had never eaten them fresh before! It was so cool! And my husband and kids are really finding this goal a lot of fun as well. We are already planning on going to the market next weekend to choose new ones together!

• At the restaurant today, I only ate half of my meal and boxed up the rest to finish it up later tonight. I was so proud, and I felt really good all afternoon! Plus, that's two meals for the price of one!

Focus on the positive:

Stop feeling guilty because you didn't go to the gym or you had a hamburger. Start focusing more on all the healthy food choices you made such as eating five fruits and vegetables, the different rounds of exercises you completed, (you walked to work and went twice up those five flights of stairs). Be also aware of the happy moments you've had throughout your day, like taking a singing lesson or finding the time to play with the kids or your pet.

Remember to be grateful:

And why not also add a line or two about what you are grateful for today. It puts things back into perspective when we take the time to see how lucky we really are. Appreciate the big things like your job or your home but also the little ones such as "I was in a hurry and a man noticed how stressed out I was while queuing and he let me go ahead of him. It was so unexpected! I'll make sure I do the same thing next time I see someone in my situation."

Pray or close your eyes and meditate:

Whether you're religious or not, take the time to pray or simply close your eyes and clearly define what it is you really want in life.

To move forward, remember that it's best to travel light: in other words, it's time to forgive those who have hurt you, as well as ask forgiveness for your mistakes. You can be totally honest and sincere: you are all alone. No one is here to judge you, so pour your heart into it. Then, begin observing and noticing how, all of a sudden, things seem to go your way: doors start to open, things become easier and you begin to get "lucky". Try it and write down all the positive effects of prayer and meditation. Keep track of all the wonderful little things that have happened to you. See just how lucky you really are and how you are transforming yourself into a much more positive person.

Taking the time to write a journal on a regular basis, is empowering.
Flip through your notebook every once in a while: look at the colors, read your notes, check out your accomplishments, smile at your silly photos!

d. A Few Tips On How To Create Your Own Journal

- Make it colorful by using colored markers or pens.

- Add in lots of positive stickers. You can find great ones online.

- Cut out quotes from various magazines. I type a whole page of them in different fonts, color or sizes and print them out.

- Flip through magazines and cut out a batch of motivational pictures for later use. For example: photos of beautiful fruit, healthy meals, fit or confident looking people, a recipe that you would like to try out, and also places you would like to visit, and store them in an envelope for future use.

- Give your notebook a name: My special Journal, My "Me Time", My Happy Book, My Success Book, My Goals, Dear Diary, My Sunshine Book, My book to success, Dear_____ (put your name) or whatever you want to call it.

- Paste some good photos of you. I am sure you can find a few where you are exercising, smiling or laughing out loud, eating healthy food, a group exercise photo at the end of a biking class or when sharing a moment with the kids… If you need to create a few "happy" photos have fun with a friend and ask them to take some nice shots. Paste in some silly photos of yourself, maybe sticking out your tongue or making faces with the kids. Why not include some "dirty" photos of you covered in mud after a mud race, or all sweaty after a long jog or walk?

- If you really don't want to put up a photo of you, you could take pictures of your shopping cart filled with good food, or your hands as you are picking vegetables at your local farmer's market. You could take a photo of your local gym, your gym equipment or your feet with your running shoes on. I personally like to tape in photos of the meals I have prepared. The list is endless, but I believe it's important to make it personal and select pictures of items or occasions that you can relate to, and that are a part of your world. They are things that you have done and that you can be proud of.

- Take a picture of your accomplishments, big or small or a shot of when you have successfully reached your goal and immortalize it! Today you ate a healthy lunch, why not take a photo of the actual meal? Did you go to the gym and have a killer workout? Take a picture of you before, after, or during your gym session!

- Print out the "How to Reach my Goal" document in the introduction chapter entitled "How to Read the Book "CHANGE.""

Take a look at the puzzle and imagine it as your ultimate goal. You will notice that there are many different pieces.

Now, write down *your* goal at the top of the page and do the exact same thing, in other words, take it apart. Try to find as many different ways as possible to reach your goal and write them down. Now that you know what actions will allow you to move one step closer to your goal, all you have to do is make sure that you do at least one of them every single day.

B. The Power of Writing

a. A simple note

Often, when I am confronted with a problem or feel that I have a message that needs to be clearly expressed, I will take the time to sit down, think about it, grab a pen and paper and lay down my thoughts. I believe problems need to be addressed and internal messages need to be expressed.

The other day, I had a problem with a colleague of mine at work and it was really troubling me, because *she* was the one I was looking forward to seeing every time I was at the office. For some unknown reason, she was upset about something and although I tried to break the ice, things didn't seem to get any better.

One night, as I sat on my bed and thought about her, I grabbed a piece of paper and wrote: "Help me solve the problem with Francine." I spent a few moments staring at the words and really wishing that things would get better.

The very next day, for no special reason, she came up to me, and said she was sorry. I was so happy to have my friend back.

Another time, I had gone through a difficult period after enduring a heartbreak. Weeks and months had gone by and although I tried my best to move on, I could feel that it still wasn't possible for me to meet someone. Not just yet.

But slowly, slowly, I started smiling again, and no longer felt as though I had something weighing me down. I observed as couples walked by hand in hand and I missed the feeling of closeness. One night, as I sat on my bed ready to go to sleep, I felt a sudden urge: I grabbed a pen and paper and wrote these three words down: "I AM READY", meaning that I was ready to move on, I was ready to meet someone. I looked at the words and felt serene. I really was ready.

Three days later, a friend of mine wrote to me that she just happened to be in the company of a longtime friend of hers, who was a coach about my age, currently writing a book just like me, and she was wondering if it was ok for her to give him my number. I said "yes". And a few days later, when we met, we both hit it off immediately.

Don't underestimate the power of words. Taking the time to write them down is like breathing life into them. Remember however, you need to be totally honest. It's no use lying to yourself, and there's no lying to the Universe either. Believe me, although you might be able to fall for your very own lies, the Universe will never be fooled. Only by being truthful and honest will you receive the keys that can unlatch closed doors.

b. Try a writing ritual
One day, my best friend offered me a wish box. I never even heard of such a thing and was intrigued. As I opened the box, I saw that it contained a little ceramic bowl, a box of matches and a small leaflet with blank sheets of paper that could easily be torn off. It was a sort of ritual box and I instantly loved the whole idea of it.

That very night I sat down and tore out one of the pages from the leaflet. On a tiny sheet of paper, I wrote down what meant the most to me, and placed it into the ceramic bowl. Then I struck a match and took my time watching it burn while I imagined that the smoke rising from the paper contained all my words and that they were all spreading out into the Universe.

The way I see it, smoke is to the sky, what seeds are to the ground. I had just planted my wish into the sky. No need to buy a ritual box, for you can very well create your own. Remember, however: words can be just words, but they can also be very powerful if you speak the truth, say them with intent, express your thoughts with all your heart whether out loud or in writing and finally, if you take the time to let the words resonate within you.

C. Your "Daily Positive Checklist"

a. A Powerful Tool! One day, I decided to write a list of all the little easy things that I could do for myself each day, that would be positive and could help me lead a healthier lifestyle while feeling better about myself. That's how I came up with the idea of a "Positive Checklist". It was incredible how powerful this checklist turned out to be for me. Every day, I would take some time to fill it out and put check marks in the tick boxes. The first few days I realized that I wasn't ticking that many, but somehow, it all became fun. Soon, I found myself consulting the list several times throughout the day, to see how many points I had acquired and kept organizing myself to get more of them done. Quickly it became a game and I loved it and felt better, because of all these positive things I was doing for myself.

Below is a sample of *"My Daily Positive Checklist"*. You are free to copy it and use it, or better yet, let it inspire you to create your very own, tailored to your specific needs. The one I propose is composed of 40 positive things that can be done every day. At the beginning, you might tick only a few boxes each day, but as you get used it, you will eventually start ticking more and more. Your goal? To tick as many boxes as you possibly can each day, keeping 20 as your ultimate goal. Start today: it's easy, rewarding and fun!

My Daily Positive Checklist

Here are 40 different things you can do right now to feel better and improve yourself.
Set a goal to tick at least 5 boxes every day. Your ultimate goal: to tick at least 20!

- I stood tall and worked on my posture (ex: Stretched to improve my posture 5mn)

- I worked on my self-image by_____

- I stood tall and worked on my posture (Stretched to improve my posture 5mn)

- I drank 1 2 3 4 5 6 7 8 9 10 glasses of water

- I went to the bathroom 1 2 3 times

- I practiced walking tall and I maintained great posture the entire walk

- I exercised_____

- I meditated

- I listened to my P.E.T. (Positive Empowering Tape)

- I did a commercial about myself or watched it

- I read an inspiring book

- I did something kind for someone_____

- I took the time to do or go over my Accomplishment Board

- I took the time to improve myself on the inside

- I took the time to improve myself on the outside

- I slept more: 1 2 3 4 extra hours or at least 7 hours

- I did something I love today _____

- I learned something new today

- I consulted a specialist to help me improve_____

- I had a junk-food free day

·℘· I ate a healthy meal: Breakfast - snack - lunch - snack - dinner

·℘· I brought some change in my sex or love life

·℘· I reached my goal of walking at least_____ steps

·℘· I watched a video to improve my self-esteem

·℘· I wrote in my special notebook

·℘· I prayed with intention

·℘· I pampered myself (hair, nails, face, body…)

·℘· I got a massage or I massaged myself (legs, feet, arms, face…)

·℘· I hugged someone

·℘· I took some time off to embrace "nothingness"

·℘· I had a "party night" and I ate and did exactly what I felt like without feeling guilty

·℘· I communicated with nature

·℘· I spoke up and / or said "no"

·℘· I tried a new activity, tried something different

·℘· I ate fruit 1 2 3 4 5 6 7 8 9 10 11 12

·℘· I ate vegetables 1 2 3 4 5 6 7 8 9 10 11 12

·℘· I juiced

·℘· I took a cold shower

·℘· I finally succeeded in doing_____

·℘· I took my time to enjoy my meal and ate slowly

·℘· Other_____

Remember that this is a gradual process. At first you will only tick in a few boxes, but quickly you will see how fun it becomes and you will be trying to tick as many as possible. Remember that your goal is not to force or punish yourself to change. Focus on bringing positive elements into your life, such as doing things you love or that make you happy and proud. Renew with your inner child and rediscover the joys of learning…. because to Embrace Change means enjoying the ride!

b. The Question

It's essential and quite helpful to frequently ask yourself throughout the day the following question:

What can I do, right now, to feel better and improve myself?

At first you will have to browse down the list to see if there is something that you can do. But quickly, it will become second nature and you will get an immediate response, such as:

- I could drink a glass of water
- I could eat an apple or another piece of fruit
- I could go twice up and down the stairs of my building
- I could take a cold shower
- I could stretch 5 minutes to improve my posture
- I could listen to my P.E.T. - Positive Empowering Tape, check out Change n° 05: *"Believe in Yourself - Create your very own P.E.T."* and tailor it to your needs!
- I could do something kind for someone, like give them a call, send a text, get a coffee for a colleague
- I could read something inspirational or watch an inspiring video

Pretty soon after starting this experiment, I was ticking 20 boxes every single day! It was easy but also involved some challenge and it turned out to be a lot of fun! I felt increasingly prouder of myself and all my daily accomplishments!

Sometimes, I would reach the end of the day having ticked only 10 boxes and would tell myself: I have another two hours before heading to bed… I could look at my vision board, meditate, stretch and go to bed earlier… that would be another 4 checks. And so, I would set out to do four more positive things for myself!

After only two months, I noticed that I no longer needed to fill out my page: my mind automatically remembered to do these things and, systematically, throughout the day, I would catch myself asking: "What can I do, right now, to feel better and improve myself?" and I would set out to do it!

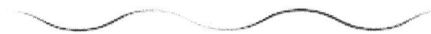

Change n°02
STAND TALL

2.

Take a few minutes to view yourself in the mirror:
- First, look at yourself standing naturally
- Now pull your tummy in, lift your chest up, pull your shoulders back and if your head is slightly protruding bring it back into spinal alignment
- Now look at yourself again
- Finally, add one more thing to this picture: your confident, determined and beautiful smile!

This simple exercise takes only one minute, but it enables you recognize what other people see when they meet you. Which one of the two positions exudes self-doubt and which one makes you appear self-confident and happy?

You have to keep in mind that posture tells others who you are and how you feel about yourself. If you stand in a slouched position you convey a negative message: one of an unhappy person, who is somewhat uncomfortable in their own shoes; perhaps even somewhat depressed.

According to the American Posture Institute (A.P.I.), "Self-esteem is measured as an overall positive or negative attitude toward oneself. Global self-esteem consists of two aspects, the first is a sense of social worth or 'self-liking' and the second is a sense of personal efficacy or self-competence." One must keep in mind that self-esteem doesn't only have to do with how one feels about himself, indeed, what others think about you is also important, especially when socializing or at work. Also, according to the A.P.I. "A tall posture is directly correlated to a higher level of self-esteem and an uplifted mood."

Why don't you decide this very moment to become a "Posture Specialist" and find out everything there is to know about having a correct posture and how it can improve your self-awareness. At this point, we are going to see what the benefits are of having a good posture, what solutions you can bring in order to improve yours and in how your posture can improve your self-esteem.

A. What are the Benefits of Having a Good Posture?

a. Back Problems
Did you know that back problems are one of the biggest health problems in the US? People tend to sit for long hours at the office, slowly creating back discomfort or various aches and pains. In fact, you may not know this, but sitting is actually worse than standing as it forces your muscles to work more. In her excellent book *Posture, get it Straight*, Janice Novak tells us that when you are in a seated position there is 40% more pressure on your lower back discs than when standing. Maintaining good posture will eliminate pressure on discs as well as the pain associated with it.

b. Numerous Other Benefits

There are many other benefits to standing tall. Have a look at the list below to see what else you will gain by focusing on changing your posture:

- Straightening up makes you instantly look taller but also slimmer. Take two minutes to look at yourself in the mirror, observe your tummy and see what happens when you straighten up. Your waistline actually loses a few inches
- You will reduce pain in your lower back, neck and shoulders and may actually help eliminate your headaches. Remember, by letting poor posture settle in, your condition can only worsen
- Directly linked to the preceding point, improving your posture can reduce your chances of getting an injury
- When naked, you will look more attractive
- You will have more allure and look better in clothes
- You will look more graceful
- You will feel and look more powerful
- Your lungs will actually have more room to breathe and your other organs will have more space as well
- You will look younger. A hunched over posture is associated with being old whereas a tall, strong posture is associated with youth
- It can help you in making important decisions by giving you added control
- Lifting your chest up gives the impression that it is bigger
- If you are feeling down, depressed or unconfident, chances are that by simply modifying your posture, you will change how you feel

B. What Solutions Will Improve Your Posture?

a. Here are Just a Few Ideas You Can Look Into:

- Get a good mattress and a good pillow, you don't want them to be either too soft or too firm
- Take breaks when you are at work. The A.P.I. (American Posture Institute) suggests taking 30 second breaks every 20 minutes
- When sleeping, try to alleviate the load on the spine: it is recommended to sleep on the side, fetus style, because your back stays aligned. You can place a pillow under your neck and one between your legs to keep your whole body in alignment
- Get some new shoes with good arch support. See a podiatrist to learn exactly what you need
- Avoid wearing heels and if you do, the lower the better
- Refrain from wearing shoes that are too narrow. Your shoe has to feel roomy and comfortable
- How do you carry your handbag or your backpack? Over one shoulder? This creates imbalance and you can actually end up with one shoulder lower than the other. Try to even out the weight by properly carrying backpacks on both shoulders or by occasionally switching your handbag from one side to the other. There are lots of nice and professional looking handbags that can be carried as a backpack

- When you want to lift or carry something heavy, do it the proper way. Everybody knows the technique but no one does it: bend your knees, lower yourself down with your back straight, grab the heavy object and then straighten your legs out again
- See a posture specialist and learn what he can do for you to help correct your posture. You will get an assessment and he will suggest a few strengthening and stretching exercises
- Buy a book about posture and evaluate for yourself what are your weak points? Practice the exercises that are recommended for your problem
- Watch Posture DVD's
- Take bar or dance lessons. All the exercises promote good posture
- Try Pilates, excellent to get your whole body elongated in proper form

C. Trying Out Different Postural Techniques:

a. Open Up and Stand Tall and Why Not Imagine You are Somebody Important

There is no need to be boastful, make the word "happy" your motto and go conquer the world. Just simply remember "Open Wide and Stand Tall": Pull your shoulders back, open your chest, suck your tummy in, bring your head up, look forward. You have to feel as though a string is pulling you up. Now smile and go for a walk. See how people look at you. Others feel your confidence. Try practicing regularly! Check out change n° 04: *The confidence Walk*. The feeling is so empowering you will love how you feel and will want to do it more and more. If you are a little shy at first, bring your P.E.T. (Positive Empowering tapes) with you and listen to them for an added boost while walking. Check out Change n° 5 to learn how to create your own.

b. Soak Up the World's Energy!

Stand tall and open up your arms as wide as you can to the side as if you were embracing life completely. Breathe deeply and soak up all of the world's energy that is readily available and just waiting for you.

c. Fist Clenching Technique

Stand tall and place yourself in front of a mirror. Your arms are hanging loosely by your sides. Bring your chest up, pull your shoulders back, contract your arms and shoulders and then tightly clench your fists.

Next, let your arms come up in front of you until they reach your ears (superman style), then bring them down still contracted and then raise your arms to your sides, bringing them up to your ears once again. Look up to the sky and bring your arms back down.

Repeat the whole process at least five times. Feel how all the stress disappears in your upper back and shoulders and how you feel so much stronger. If you are feeling stressed, breathe deeply and then try yelling or saying some Power words out loud such as "I can do this" "let's go" "do it" "yes". Remember to always finish with a Smile!

If you are feeling stressed, breathe deeply and then try yelling or saying some Power words out loud such as "I can do this" "let's go" "do it" "yes". Remember to always finish with a Smile!

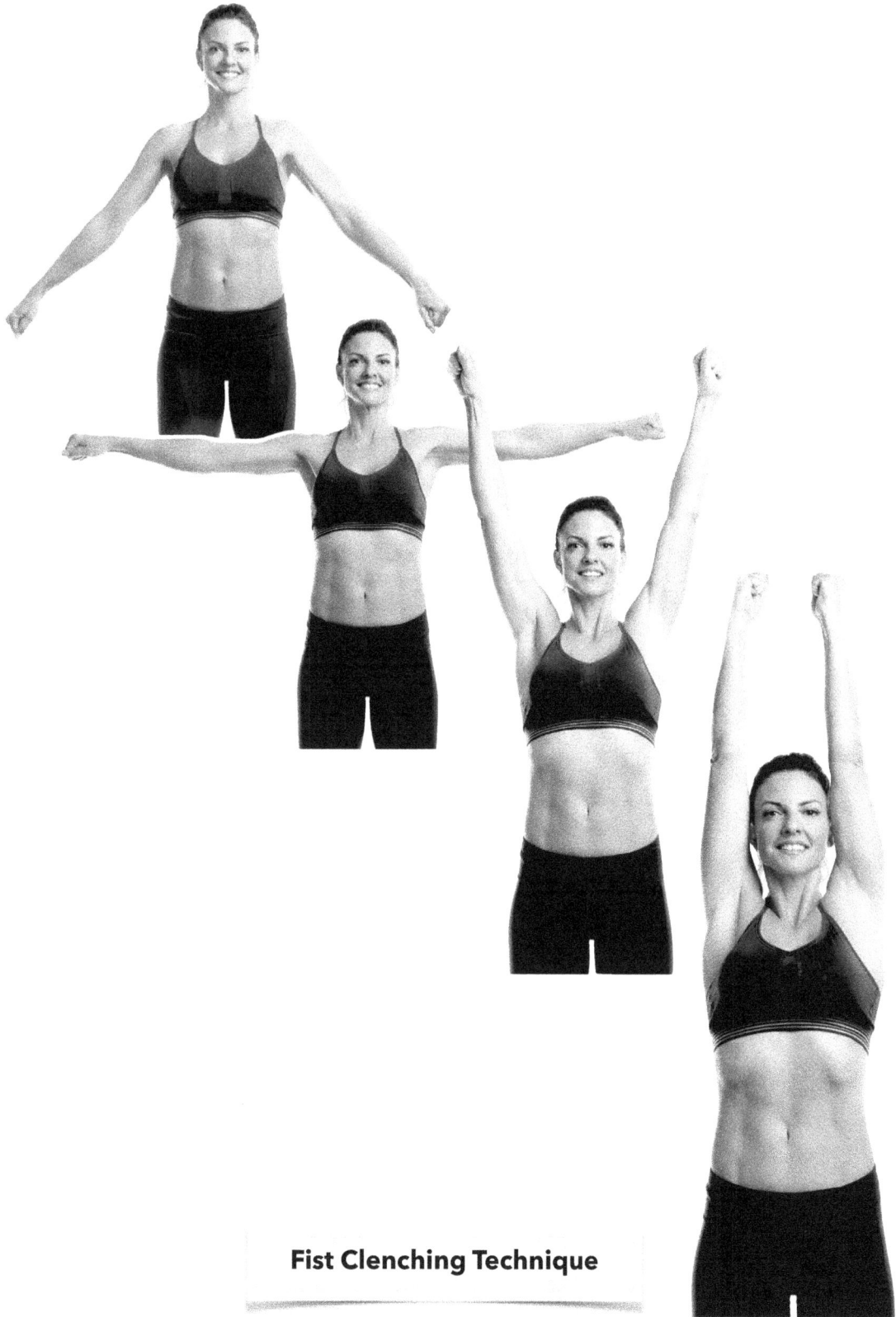

Fist Clenching Technique

D. **Your Posture Affects Your Energy Field, Your Aura**

Everything is energy. Each and every one of us is comprised of energy and whether we acknowledge it or not, this energy emanates from us, creating an "energy field" that is constantly changing according to our mood, our thoughts, and our interactions with others. Many times, throughout the day, I like to step back and be aware of how I feel and what type of energy I am conveying. I often ask myself: If I had to choose a color, which one would represent how I am feeling right now? Would it be a greenish or more of a bluish one, would it be red, or more like a dark black? This really helps me become more aware of my emotions and quite often, I realize that I have to "stop", close my eyes, calm down and breathe for a minute or two. If I feel that my energy field is "expressing" negativity - such as anger, resentment, or even if I am simply dwelling on things - I will imagine that my aura is pink or surrounded by some other soft, warm colors. Very quickly I feel a sense of relief and am then able to put things back into perspective.

If we take a closer look at poor posture and the reason why we carry ourselves the way we do, it is obvious that it is due to bad postural habits but it is also linked to emotional factors: do you live in fear, feel depressed, suffer from low self-confidence or lack of love? Often these negative emotions are stored up in the heart or solar plexus region. Indeed, lack of self-love, being heart broken or rejected or any other emotion related to the heart and love agglomerate within the heart and emotions that turn around fear and anger concentrate themselves within the solar plexus. Slouching over becomes a way to protect ourselves, to shelter both these parts of the body in which we often bottle up most of our pains.

If you take the time to observe someone that is walking with rounded shoulders, you will often notice that the head will be tilting downwards and the eyes looking down as well, which sends out a negative image of this person.

Isn't it time for you to start looking up again and being proud of who you are? When you stand up nice and tall, your blood flows easily and arrives abundantly to your heart. When you stand up nice and tall, your lungs expand, receiving more oxygen. When you stand up nice and tall, you are more open to receive what life has in store for you, and you become more receptive.

It's not always easy remembering to straighten up. Here is a technique that might help you that I call the "Posture Checkup":
• Stand with your back up against a wall
• Pull your shoulders back until they actually touch the wall
• Maintain the natural curvature of your lower back and keep the abs contracted
• Then leave the wall but make sure to maintain this posture for as long as possible. Repeat this exercise throughout the day, whenever you can

Posture has its importance indeed, but so does the energy you convey. You can't just pull your shoulders back and think that's all there is to it: you also have to be authentic because if you aren't, your energy field will reveal it.

Let me share with you a story, to help explain my point:

I was in my early twenties and I had just finished work. As I returned home and reached the front door of my building and pushed the key into the keyhole, all of a sudden, my entire body, froze, literally from head to toe. I managed to turn my head and right behind me stood a handsome young man, dressed in a suit and tie, smiling back at me. As I stood there looking at him somewhat perplexed, I felt fear but at the same time I was impressed by this man's presence, smile and good looks. The man walked past me and stepped inside the building. Hesitantly, I followed behind him as well. A few seconds later, to my bewilderment, he attacked me and threw me up against a wall.

Luckily, in that very instant someone came through the door and my attacker was obliged to stop and take off. But it served me as a good lesson, that I absolutely have to listen to my instincts: this man's aura, his negative energy field clearly warned me of his intentions, but his allure, his great posture and good looks had conveyed confidence and managed to fool me. Even without being aware of his presence something inside of me instinctively sensed that I was in danger. My eyes had betrayed me, I had accepted to be fooled by conventions.

The point here is for you to understand that just standing tall won't do: your vibrations have to be in it as well. Although most of you don't have bad intentions, your inner malaise transpires into negative vibes. You might then ask me: how can you convey positive vibrations when your inner state is full of sadness, anger and resentment?

The answer: press the "pause" button. Slow down. STOP! Take the time to breathe and meditate. Give yourself undivided attention. Open yourself up to love and peace. Let "LOVE" flow through you: Learn to embrace and then release it, allowing it to spread all over. It won't happen overnight but if you ask for it – I mean truly desire it - you will receive it. Remember: Love is energy and it should not be contained, so let it flow freely.

Having an upright posture and emitting positive energy vibes is empowering and it conveys a high level of self-confidence. If you make sure, throughout the day, to regularly check your posture, practice specific strengthening and stretching exercises, slow down and meditate in order to project positivity, you will quickly start noticing big changes in the way you feel about yourself, and how others perceive you as well.

Change n°03
YOUR SELF~IMAGE

3.

When you start looking into self-image I feel it's important to take two things into account:
• What you think about yourself
• What image you project
I truly felt a difference in how I felt about myself when I acknowledged both these aspects.

A. Changing within

a. Ask yourself the right question and find out why your self-esteem is low

At one point in my life, when I first started to consider changing my self-image and improving my self-esteem, I realized that I was going to have to look on the inside to see what I actually thought about myself. I reflected upon this and realized that although I would often downsize my capacities, deep down inside I really believed that I was a good person. What that meant was that my foundation was good but the problem laid within my thoughts: indeed, my negativity stemmed from my mind. This realization was like a revelation.

I then questioned myself what exactly happened to make my mind start having negative thoughts about myself. Why do I depreciate myself? Answers started to pop up in my mind: "because at many different occasions I was told that I was no good", "because I was always average at school", "because I had attempted to do things and had failed", "because I had never received compliments or encouragements when I most needed them. I had always had to rely solely on myself."

Then I wondered about my failures and just how many failures were necessary to be really good at something. I couldn't help asking myself: "Won't there always be someone better than I am but in a different way?" "Won't there always be someone who has had more experience than I or more opportunities?" We are all unique. Although there might be some similarities, no one else has ever lived my life, no one else will ever experience the exact same things that I have or feel precisely the same way I do now. We really are all unique. I knew all of this of course but I somehow "integrated it" at that very instant:

> **"Failure or trial and error
> are a necessary part of any process towards success,
> but they don't define who I am....
> but if I stopped trying, however, they would."**

Viewing things this way made it all seem so logical and took a huge burden off my shoulders: no use comparing myself to others anymore, I only had to focus on doing the best I could. Failing became acceptable if I got back up and kept on trying.

"I have not failed. I've just found 10000 ways that won't work."
~ Thomas Edison ~

Now it's your turn to ask yourself how and why you see yourself the way you do at this very moment. What was your spontaneous answer? Was it positive? For example: "I am proud of myself. I have this goal and I am doing my utmost to achieve it!" Or was it negative? "I hate my body. I keep telling myself to do something about it, but I have no willpower at all. I am a lost cause, no use trying. I will most certainly fail again."

It's pretty obvious that if you fall more into the second category, the conditions are not optimal for you to have a positive self-image.

b. Opening your doors and windows

I like to compare a person who has a negative self-image to a person that is trapped within himself. It's as if he is trapped within his own home, literally locked inside. He keeps busy by routinely going from one room to the other, the windows and doors are shut with no fresh air circulating, meaning that the same negative thoughts are lingering on inside of him. But what if this person opens a window to let in some new ideas or even goes a step further and opens the front door to step outside and seek new opportunities?

The very first thing to do is stop your negative mindset from controlling you and who you are. Observe how you let all these negative ideas creep in and control you. Open your eyes/windows and your ears/doors and let new ideas come in: then start seeing life as it really is.

c. A few tips to help you change from within

- You have to examine what can be done to improve yourself. Focus solely on this and accept that there are certain things that cannot be changed. Stop blaming others for your problems and start taking action. Start seeing everything life has to offer and believe me it will turn into something beautiful… a land of opportunities.

- To help you see life this way, it's important to find what you love in life, then do it, and really give it your all. Who do you want to be? What are you passionate about? What are you good at? How can you contribute to the world: in what way can you help? For example, even though I was going through a difficult year in 2017, I was passionate about writing my book. Deep down inside, I really felt, that by sharing my experiences and knowledge, I could help other people believe in themselves too.

- It is essential to boost your self-confidence: I can't stress enough the importance of reading. Find self-help books or a few articles that will help you develop a higher self-esteem. Watch online videos done by today's mentors: Anthony Robbins, Eckhart Tolle, Joe Dispenza, Vishen Lakhiani or whoever you admire and that have had an impact on the way you feel about yourself. They will all contribute to empowering and inspiring you to succeed. Write yourself an empowering message in which you believe in yourself. Tape it and listen to it every time you have the opportunity. Check out Change n° 5 for more details about creating your very own Personal Empowering Tape. This technique has turned out to be really helpful for me. When recording, make sure your tone of voice is loud and firm but also full of kindness and empathy.

- Be assertive. Put intonation while reading your text. Stop, breathe and take pauses while you read. You have to believe what you are saying and should sound as convincing as possible. When you are out walking, stand up tall, smile and play your tape and...go conquer the world!

- As much as possible, avoid being around people who depreciate you and surround yourself with people who have a positive attitude and mindset: observe them and soak in their positivity. Don't think it's natural or innate for them. It all started somewhere in their mind which means that you can reprogram yours as well.

B. Changing on the outside

a. Relooking

Changing your self-image also means changing your outside image. Some people say that it is best to change how you feel *within* first, before changing your exterior appearance. However, the way it happened for me, was the other way around. A friend of mine was setting up her business as a Relooking Coach and she asked me if I would be willing to be her guinea pig. I was thrilled with the idea. She took the time to explain what colors best suited me, taught me how to apply make-up, booked an appointment for my hair and spent a whole day going in and out of shops to make me try on different types of styles and outfits. The whole process boosted my self-confidence. I felt fantastic, strong and empowered. I started walking with more self-assurance and my eyes began to shine with a renewed sense of confidence. It just goes to say that without losing any weight or doing anything drastic, in as little as a few hours, you too could feel like a totally new person.

b. The mirror exercise

If you are tempted by the relooking, which I highly recommend, try the mirror exercise before and after you do it: look at your image in the mirror, see how you feel about yourself and then ask yourself why you feel that way. Note what it is that you like and dislike and write it down on a piece of paper. Chances are, that after the relooking you will find more things to like about yourself than before.

At first, you might have a say about many different parts of your face and body. Keep looking however. Try to imagine you are your very own dear friend. What would this friend tell you? How would they talk to you and what would they say about those parts of you that you dislike? Our true friends accept us the way we are and are far less critical than we are towards ourselves. Try, as much as possible to be your own best friend and don't be so hard on yourself.

c. Start taking action NOW

After having taken the time to look at yourself and expressed a bit of kindness towards yourself, look again and see what improvements you could bring. There are little things that you could do immediately (such as hair, nails, makeup or the way you dress) and there are others that will take more time but can be accomplished with a little perseverance such as losing or gaining some weight, improving your posture and having more charisma. Write everything down on a piece of paper so you don't forget and begin today, by focusing on those improvements immediately and addressing them, NOW.

Why not treat yourself to your very own home spa, or, if you can afford it, visit a real one. Book an appointment, NOW! Start focusing on everything you can do to improve your self-image. If money is an issue, there are loads of things that you can do to improve your self-image, that don't cost too much or virtually won't cost you a cent:

- Take a bubble bath: soak up all the benefits of this relaxing moment. Start visualizing everything you are going to do to improve your self-image.
- Wash your hair, have a mask, do your nails. While doing this, play some of your favorite music, songs that will get you going, fill you with energy and make you happy.
- Call a friend you love and tell her about your project and ask for assistance, or even better, why not program a self-care day together and have some fun experimenting with makeup, doing each-others hair, window shopping and even trying on different outfits. Why not take turns taking photos?
- Accessorize: sometimes a new accessory is all you need to revamp your look. This cuts down the costs and adds a special touch to a look that may sometimes seem bland. Women, can try a colorful handbag or shoes, a new necklace, scarf, a new shade of lipstick or smoky eye shadow. Men can accessorize as well: with a nice back pack, a tie or cool shoes. They can wear jewelry: a fashionable watch, necklace or bracelet. And what about glasses and hats? Sunglasses are a great accessory whether they are simple or glamorous. Some of you might not be daring enough to put on a hat, I know I am that way! But I have to admit that many times I have seen someone walking by wearing one and it can really liven up the whole look.
- You could accessorize with hair or eyelash extensions. I don't do it all the time but I have done it on certain occasions: it can be a real plus and a head turner.
- Teeth : now that you are on your way to transformation, have you thought about getting your teeth whitened? You can either have it done by your dentist or there are specialists around that do it as well. There are also quite a few over the counter products that you can buy that serve the same purpose. Before buying anything, have a look online to see what other people are saying about that particular product and compare with other ones proposed on the market.
- Have you ever considered waxing? Many women (and men!) hesitate fearing the pain! Waxing was one of the things I tried during my makeover and now it's a must every three weeks: I am bikini perfect! Some of you men might be considering getting rid of torso or back hair. That's entirely up to you and whether this hair is a problem for you. I personally think men come in a variety of ways: some are hairy and some aren't, and both are beautiful. Honestly, I personally find that the focus should be more on hair or beard: what hairstyle or beard style really suits you: remember what makes one person look fabulous doesn't suit everybody else. That's why I hate trends: people tend to follow them because it's the *new* thing but omit to look and see whether it really suits them or not. This, for me, is so annoying: a star comes up with a new haircut and then every single guy around has got the same one!!! Well, so much for individuality! Welcome to globalization! Urgh!! Fashion trends can become a real turn-off for me. If a guy came up to me with "the look of the moment", I swear, all I would be thinking of is: "why don't you, first, go and get yourself a personality and then we'll talk!"

• Try something new: Why not be a little daring? I am not talking about going over the top but simply trying one thing in the way you dress, that you have never done before.

As an example, I never wore heels. I was always a sporty kind of person and believed in living comfortably with cushiony shoes. As I was in the midst of my relooking experience, I started to question this point. Heels obviously embellish one's figure, so why shouldn't I give it try. It felt awkward, at first, but I kept at it and ended up enjoying having them on. I started with small heels and gradually added a little more height. The added height and the fact that it made me look better and gave me added presence was a definite positive factor for my self-esteem. So, if your motto is "Flat is better" put on some heels once in a while and see what it does for you.

I mention heels, but if you're the type of person that always wears pants, why not try skirts or a dress for a change? Chances are you might just like it… and others may as well!

I am obviously addressing women here, but men can also change things: how about wearing a different type of shoe or make a little effort to look a little smarter. If you're the type that always wears running shoes, why not buy a classy pair? Whether you realize it or not, your appearance is important, so make the extra effort and try to look nice. Do it for you, you owe it to yourself!

> **CHANGING THE WAY YOU WALK AND TALK MIGHT BE JUST THE THING YOU NEED TO BOOST YOUR SELF CONFIDENCE.**

Initially, this was only one change, but there is just so much to say about improving the way you walk and talk, that it quickly became necessary to split this point into two different parts. You will find "Talk and Listen" in Chapter Four under change n° 39.

There are many different things you can do in order to improve how you feel about yourself. Taking the time to learn to love who you really are or at least to be more accepting is already taking a step in the right direction and the funny thing is, when you start liking yourself, well others start liking you too. Your positivity radiates. Your aura literally glows and attracts people like a magnet.

Take care of yourself, believe in yourself: you deserve it… and see how your life changes for the better, how opportunities arise, how you have new encounters, and how you start attracting more and more positive things into your life.

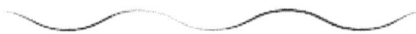

Change n°4
THE CONFIDENCE WALK

When I was 20, the simple act of walking in the street or eating in public was a challenge. I was totally self-conscious, scared of what others might think and it was impossible for me to relax and be myself. Anything could set me off into an inner panic: a run in my stocking, someone wanting to start up a conversation, being clumsy, you name it.

It's at that time, that I met someone who was my total opposite: he was totally laid back and couldn't care less about what other people thought of him. He did a world of good to me and gradually I learnt to laugh about my clumsiness or about being a little uptight and closed off. If I found a run in my stocking, well it was O.K. and I accepted it. He loved being out in nature, enjoyed simplicity and being around his friends who were just like him. In the end, it didn't work out with him, but he helped me put things into a healthy perspective.

Sometimes a person you meet doesn't end up being the love of your life, but will teach you a lesson and help you grow. Have you ever thought about that? It might be interesting to sit down and try to see what each relationship, the good *and* bad ones, have brought you. What did you learn from them? Turn these past relationships into something constructive and positive. Even though stories end, try to be grateful for what each person brought you, and this goes for friendship as well. Give it a try and see how some of your answers might just come as a surprise. One thing is sure, it will most certainly help you make peace with your past.

A. Why Change The Way You walk?

According to Olivia Fox Cabane, author of the must read, Charisma Myth, the first few seconds you meet someone are key: indeed, within that very short lapse of time, you are judged, categorized, classified and filed away in a person's brain according to that split second analysis. Just a simple glance, enables us to determine each other's social and economic level, our level of education and even someone's level of success. Within that short time frame, we also decide whether we like and trust this person or not. These first impressions are very hard to erase and are often indelible. So, don't minimize the importance of leaving a good first impression.

People are quick to judge you and for this reason, the way you walk and talk is of utmost importance. Many of us believe that we cannot change the way we are and that if we do, we will appear unnatural. This however is untrue: you may feel a little awkward at first, when standing tall and walking with confidence, but others won't notice it. They honestly don't care. What's important here is to avoid putting a superior look on your face. You can very well stand tall with your shoulders back while smiling sweetly or having a kind expression on your face. This week, observe how one simple thing, such as your walk, can change the way you feel about yourself for the better.

B. Tips and Ideas on How to Change the Way You Walk

There are a number of things that you can do to improve the way you walk, so if you want to stand out and be seen as a confident person, follow these simple tips:

• Comfy shoes

The very first consideration, obviously, is to have comfortable shoes. Make sure you have the right size and that you are at ease with the height of your heels. If your feet are nice and snug, your walk will come across as being effortless and natural.

• Your stride

Your stride must be comfortable: avoid making giant or tiny steps.

• Your pace

Your pace must be comfortable. Confident people are not running late. They are in control of their life and take their time. Walking fast or fidgeting will make you come off as being nervous or insecure. Relax into the rhythm of your walk, and slowly it will turn into something totally natural. Try to walk, act and talk slowly as though you have all the time in the world. To give you an idea, why not compare James Bond and Mr Bean. Observe how one walks, pauses before acting and always seems in control of the situation while the other is constantly fidgeting, not knowing what to do with his hands and arms and self-conscious, constantly looking around to see if someone has noticed him.

• Walking in heels

If you are walking in heels or flat shoes, remember to put your foot down "heel first" and then toes. Avoid putting your foot down flat, as if you had hooves. Some, actually, call this the "horse step". Remember that if you are walking in heels you want to look tall, strong, confident and beautiful! Many times, I have seen women walking with very high heels and my immediate thought was that a little shorter hill would have made them look at ease and natural.

If you feel that your heels make your head jut out, try to lean back slightly to keep your head in line with your spine.

It might take a little time getting used to, but keep practicing, practicing, practicing; very soon you will feel confident about your strut. I recommend finding an open space with a big mirror. Bring some friends along, put on some good music and have fun practicing and encouraging one another.

• Look up, look ahead

At first, it may seem challenging or pretentious to you as you may have always walked looking down. Remember that you are not trying to feel superior but confident, so make sure you adjust your attitude accordingly. The last thing you want is to come off as being arrogant. An issue I had when I first started looking up (yes, I used to walk looking down at my feet as well!) was, that I felt uncertain about what to do with my eyes. I didn't feel comfortable looking at all the people coming my way. Just do your best to relax, be yourself, show kindness, smile, or at least have a neutral gaze.

Another suggestion here would be to look as if you are looking at something that lies straight ahead of you. This technique will allow you to avoid all eye contact. And if that doesn't work, you can still resort to wearing sunglasses! So, from now on, look up, be more determined with every step and keep your focus on what lies ahead.

• How to Breathe
I think it's important, at least at the beginning, to focus on your breathing: breathe in deeply and keep it slow. It will help you to relax. Keep one thing in mind: you think everyone is looking at you and you may feel silly at first, but you will quickly get used to it and come to realize that you have a right to be where you are at that very moment, just like everybody else.

• What to do with your hands and arms
Fidgeting with your hands and arms or walking with your hands in your pocket are a big "no-no". It's really important to loosen up, look ahead and keep your hands to your sides in a slow, very slight swinging motion. If you really don't know what to do with them, hold onto something: a folder, a little bag or a clutch can offer a simple solution.

• What to do with your shoulders
Bring your chest up and push your shoulders back and down. When trying to find the perfect posture, I like to inhale and expand my chest, immediately creating an upward movement of the torso. Only then do I pull my shoulders back and down. Try to keep this position and to constantly remind yourself throughout the day to repeat this little procedure. Not really sure how far back your shoulders should go? Try the following exercise: Stand up against a wall, pulling your shoulders back until they are both in contact with the wall. Now focus on your upper spine: is it touching the wall as well? If not, just relax slightly until it does. You now have your reference point.

• Your Abs
Suck your abs in, contract them, make them participate in your walk.

• Your Style
How you dress and the image you convey are of utmost importance. No need to dress up: just make sure you are clean and that you are properly dressed. This is not the right time to try out a new style of clothes: you are focusing on your allure and it's enough work already as it is, so no need to waste time and energy on feeling self-conscious about how you are dressed.

• Learn to walk with confidence
See your mood improve. It will make you look powerful, as though you have things under control. You will look taller. You will make a strong first impression. So, keep your head up and look ahead. Bring your chest up and then pull shoulders back and down. Try to maintain a firm core. Let your arms move freely. Walk with determination at a normal pace. If necessary, wear sunglasses. As much as possible, wear a smile!

• Highlight your best feature

If your legs are your best feature, then highlight them as much as possible, enhance them by wearing clothes that flatter you and exercise regularly! But what if your legs are the last thing you want to showcase? In that case, put your best feature in the forefront: it could be, for example, your hair or your eyes. Make sure they are always flawless. Is fashion your thing? Do you love accessorizing? Take the time to prepare your look, ahead of time, so you will insure a positive first impression. Just make sure you feel absolutely comfortable when you walk past your front door.

• Take lessons

Take walking, poise or posture lessons. Look online to find any lessons nearby. I will also be programming workshops for hands on training. Check out my website for dates.

• Visualize yourself going on stage

Take the time to see yourself up on stage, walking the catwalk or the red carpet. See yourself walking with ease and charisma. Hear people complimenting on your allure. Feel the pride as you walk towards the stage, climb up the stairs and step up on the platform. Why not add a huge round of applause from the audience as you turn to face them!

• Observe others and learn

Observe others on the street, in movies or in online videos. You can learn a lot by simply looking. See how certain people walk with their shoulders rounded, slouching forward or are not comfortable in their shoes. Then notice how to the contrary, others are breezy and walk with ease.

• Practice walking on a straight line

Find a straight line and practice walking on it: this means your feet have to cross each other slightly, with your toes pointing straight ahead. It actually gives you a nice and sexy allure from a distance as your hips sway. Have someone film your walk and afterwards view the videos to learn from your mistakes. Keep imagining you are walking on an imaginary line until it becomes second nature…and remember, keep that lovely head of yours up and looking ahead!

• Take Catwalk Lessons

You could greatly benefit from learning how to walk this way: it would definitely bring you added self-confidence. You would never want to walk on the streets the same way as a model on stage however. You would look odd and come out as downright silly.

Let me share with you a personal experience. It might help you understand the benefits of cat walking. A few years back, I signed up for a weekend fitness boot camp. Part of the package was to learn how to walk on stage. Although, I had no intention of competing, I participated in this activity and boy not only was this hard, it was downright terrifying! There were at least 30 other women there, I had never seen in my life. I had to walk in front of all of them like I was "hot stuff". I have to admit that I probably didn't look "hot" at all but I did do it! And in the process, I learned two things: not just how hard it is to walk like a model or a fitness competitor, but also just how affected I was by what other people might think about me. It was a great life experience and I totally recommend it!

• Walk with a Book On Your Head

Remember how back in the day, women were taught to walk with a book on their head? So, I looked into it and most articles state that you have to be stiff in the shoulders in order to walk this way. I nevertheless decided to give it a try and found that it really helped me to keep up straight. So, I decided to take up the challenge of practicing my walk every day, with and without heels and with a book on my head. I really found this method to be very beneficial. As with everything, it's all a question of trial and error. Give it a try and always remember that what works for one person might not work for you.

• Create and listen to your P.E.T. (Positive Empowering Tapes)

Create an empowering tape! For more details, check out Change n° 5: *Believe in Yourself - Create your Very Own P.E.T.*. This may seem silly, but I have used this technique time and time again to boost my inner confidence when going through a challenging moment. Write down your empowering text which encourages and boosts you to walk nice and tall. Make sure you add in lots of compliments and phrases that show that you believe in yourself, and then go out into the world, play the tape and walk with confidence. You may also want to check out Change n° 27: *Mindful Workout.*

You cannot walk with confidence if your mind is constantly processing negativity. Banish all thoughts of doubt and fear and replace them with their opposite. Talk to yourself, listen to one of your P.E.T.s, repeat affirmations (for example, simply saying the word "relax" or "I am totally relaxed" will help you slow down and feel more comfortable). An idea might be to see yourself as "higher status", (not superior to others), but simply as someone truly worthwhile!

So now just get out and go conquer the world with your fabulous walk and then, why not check out Change n° 39: *Talk and Listen* and start thinking about changing the way you talk.

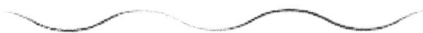

Change n°5
CREATE YOUR VERY OWN
Positive Empowering Tape ~ P.E.T.

5.

There is no doubt that a person who has a positive mindset is a happier and more successful person. But how is it that certain people tend to always see the positive in life whereas others, even when things are going smoothly simply have to find something to complain about? Why is it that these negative thoughts tend to come up automatically and incessantly, leaving us with the feeling that we have no control whatsoever over them? Can we reprogram our minds to think in a more positive way? Many people tend to believe that they are the way they are, and they cannot change. But that idea is erroneous: we can take action by observing ourselves from the outside, doing some introspection and becoming increasingly aware of this internal destructive pattern we created. Furthermore, by taking the time to be grateful for all the things we have, reprogramming our minds with empowering tapes and finally by really building up a desire to change this negative pattern, we *can* change our perception of things and become a truly positive person.

You can't get rid of all your negative thoughts, and in a way, you wouldn't want to. Indeed, negativity is not *all* bad. It's an instinct we have that is essential to help us preserve and protect ourselves from any upcoming danger. To sum things up, some of these negative thoughts need to be addressed immediately, whereas others are simply fear and imagination acting up in our minds. It's these later emotions that need to be worked on.

A. Why Are We Self-Destructive?

Our lives make us who we are, and we react the way we do today because of what we have endured in the past. A good place to start is to try and define yourself: what kind of thinker are you? Are you more of a positive or negative thinker? If you have chosen to work on this point, chances are you find you have too many negative thoughts.

This month, why don't you decide, once and for all, to program your mind into becoming more positive. Many times, in my life I have been confronted by situations where my thoughts were real nightmares and a living hell. Over time, I tried out different techniques that have enabled me to regain control.

The way I see it, we come into this world with certain tools: a body, heart, brain, our character and temperament. It's up to you to decide whether you are going to let these "tools" control you, or *you* are going to control them. Every single second, YOU can decide.
Who decides what comes into your mouth? You decide!
Who decides how you will react to any given situation? You decide!
Who decides to have a fantastic life? You, you, you.

a. What kind of thinker are you anyway?

Krishnamurti and on how to handle thoughts:
In his numerous books Krishnamurti explains that we are slaves to our habits whether it is smoking, over-eating or fostering negative thoughts in our minds. When we realize how enslaved we are, we try to get rid of this bad habit by fighting and struggling against it. But the habit seems to resist relentlessly. The more we fight it, the stronger it seems to get. The key is to step back, observe and be fully aware of our habit as well as our attitude towards it. Self-observation is essential throughout the entire process:

- **Example n° 01**: Stop the questioning! Quit the excuses! Smoking: Observe yourself smoking your cigarette, opening the pack, taking the cigarette into your hand, taking the lighter, placing the cigarette to your mouth, lighting it up, puffing up the first puff and so on. What you want to do from now on, is *every time* you smoke a cigarette, carefully observe yourself through the whole process of smoking that one cigarette. Don't condemn yourself, just be fully self-aware. Now read on and reflect upon the following: When you feel like doing something, let's say you want to play soccer, you simply get ready and go play soccer. You don't ask yourself: "How do I play soccer?", you just do it. So, why is it that when you want to stop a bad habit, you always begin by asking yourself: "How do I stop?" Asking questions is just a waste of time, it's in fact an excuse and a way to delay action. But if you see your bad habit for what it is (just a bad habit), if you really observe yourself and understand how this habit is controlling you, if you analyze your attitude towards this bad habit and give it your all, you *will* find a way to free yourself from this bad habit forever. Think of it: when you don't know how to do something that you really want to get done... you always find a way. The same thing holds true for a bad habit: you have to really want to stop, no questions asked, no excuses!

- **Example n° 02**: Eating: Observe your behavior and how you feel when you are eating: the hunger, the salivation, the sensation in the mouth, how you feel after the meal. Take the time to eat, enjoy the process, pay attention to your taste buds, breathe, feel your stomach and its sensations, look at your food, smile, and so on. If you really relax and pay attention, you will progressively slow down the entire eating process and will most certainly start to eat a lot less. Self-observation is the first step towards bringing more peace to your plate and learning to make it a lot lighter!

- **Example n° 03**: Negative thoughts: Observe what really happens when you let your mind wander off into negativity: how you in fact accept it, live it, play with it, add on to it. I know that sometimes I would let my mind wander off so far that it felt as if I was actually going through the situation I feared the most. And I would find myself crying the same way I would cry, had the situation really occurred. With time I have learned to say "NO." The second a negative thought pops up in my mind I immediately forbid myself, even though I feel tempted at times - and yes, *you too* will be tempted - to continue down that path. I know better now: I will only hurt myself and there is really no point in wasting my time in doing so.

Krishnamurti, who has been for me an "eye opener", in his book *THINK ON THESE THINGS* writes not to condemn yourself and see what you are doing as something "bad" or "wrong": He advises us to simply observe how the habit takes place. At one point, the moment suspends itself in time and you have an instant of self-realization. In order to move forward, you need to experience such a moment. It might take a little while but keep at it. To come back to my example n°03, I came to a profound realization when I asked myself: Why *do* I nourish these negative thoughts, am I really trying to protect myself, to prepare myself for things that might come or am I just deepening my self-inflicted pain?

b. Self-observation

Begin by observing yourself throughout the day and notice how negative thoughts keep recurring again and again. It might be a good idea to have a little pad and quickly jot them down. No need to write a paragraph, just between 3 to 5 words to define your thoughts. For example: I imagined Peter leaving me again, I saw myself arguing with a friend, the old memory of the crash returned to haunt me, I criticized myself and so on. You will slowly notice your recurring thinking pattern. Try to find a word to define what type of thinker you are:

- The thinker that can't help criticizing others, events
- The thinker that is constantly fearing and imagining a bad outcome of their future
- The thinker that is constantly criticizing himself, telling himself he will fail or be a disappointment
- The thinker that plays the same movie over and over again. This is when you obsess about an idea and keep pressing the "replay" button in your mind
- The thinker that has angry thoughts. Events have occurred leaving you with hatred and anger in your heart and you keep harping on the past
- The thinker that lives in regret of their past. Not necessarily angry but harping on old grievances
- There are numerous other types of thinkers that I haven't listed. Feel free to define what type of thinker you are

c. Learn To Change Your Thinking Pattern

Why don't you decide to change your thinking pattern to become:

- A positive thinker who sees others and situations in a positive manner, without systematically criticizing
- A grateful thinker, who appreciates all the good things that happen every day
- A bold thinker, one that overcomes fear and does it despite them, because deep down inside you tell yourself: "what have I got to lose? I am going to give this my best shot!"
- A "go with the flow" thinker that lives in the moment, absent of constantly fearing the past or the future. One that recognizes negative thoughts and places them in the adequate drawer in their mind and moves on

Now that you have determined what type of thinker you are, try to see in what way you can handle the negative aspects of your thoughts. Paying attention to your thinking patterns is the very first step towards taking positive action and eliminating your mind of all negativity.

Here are a few examples:

<u>Example 1:</u>
Your previous negative thought: Every time I see someone, I can't help criticizing the way they dress, look, or behave.
Taking action: every time this happens, take a moment to find out what is nice about the person/situation you are criticizing. You may not like the way a person is dressed but they may have beautiful eyes or hair. From now on, try as much as possible, to focus on people's positives rather than on their negatives. Then as you get better, take it a step further and compliment people when the opportunity arises. Most of the time, people respond positively to compliments and this will only make you feel better, make you appreciate them even more and want to continue on this positive path.

<u>Example 2:</u>
Your previous negative thought: you have a problem and you can't help obsessing over it. For example, things are not going well with your spouse/lover and you can't help imagining the breakup/separation.
Take action: find a positive affirmation and every time you catch yourself thinking in a negative way, quickly repeat your positive affirmation or simply say the word "STOP!" At the beginning you will be repeating the affirmation many times during the day. Try to do it each and every time this negative thought pops up. Then slowly as time goes by, you will be able to predict the recurring pattern and will automatically replace your negative thought with the affirmation the moment you feel it coming. I love the book by Susan Jeffers, *Feel the Fear, and do it Anyway*. In it, the author tells you to acknowledge your fear, in this case the fear of being dumped, and say: "No matter what happens, I will handle it." Because let's face it, at this very instant, things are still ok, so why stress about it? Why waste my time living in fear of an event that might not even happen? Repeat to yourself that you will handle the situation, no matter what it is, when and if the time comes. But right now, you two are still together.

B. Positive Empowering Tapes

a. How To Handle Your P.E.T.
I like to make myself a Positive Empowering Tape in which I define the problem I am going through and then wipe it out with positivity.
• To begin this process, it's a good idea to write things down. Ask yourself what the real problem is and what is the recurring negative thought that always seems to pop up in your mind. Then, next to every single negative thought, fight back with a positive outlook
• Write a short empowering text in which you annihilate all those bad thoughts that you have, and literally eliminate them with positive, encouraging, motivating words
• Once the text is done, take your phone and record it. Try as much as possible to play with your voice: make it determined, assured, positive. Yell, laugh, encourage, cry: put in lots of emotion. Make it an experience! Give yourself orders. Tell yourself what your problem is and then say "STOP, that's enough! It's over!!!" about whatever is troubling you. Finally compliment yourself, enumerating your values, and your qualities. Tell yourself you are ready to take action and list all the positive, empowering things you are going to do.

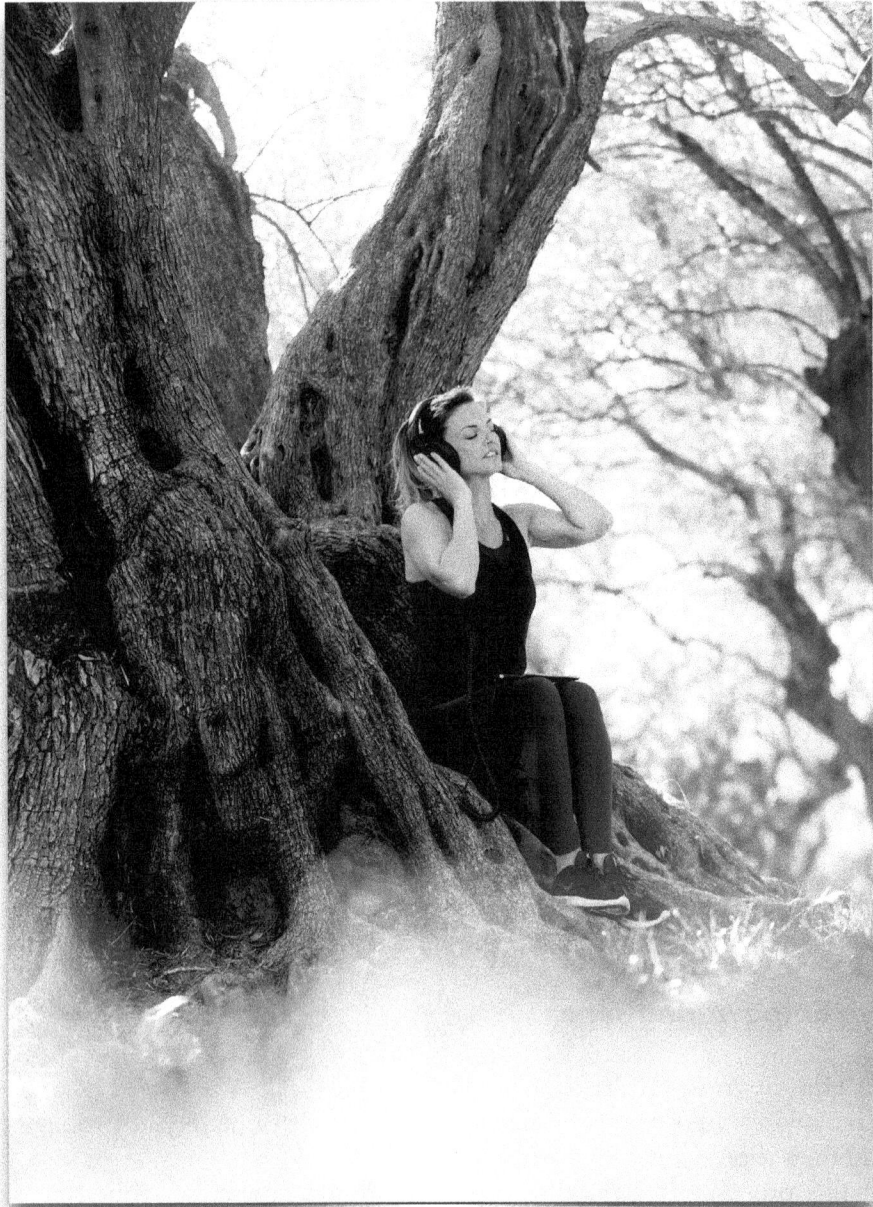

**I am open to change.
I accept to receive the very best
of what life has to offer.**

- Remember to make it personal. You can also find ideas from various inspiring books that you have read
- Now, listen to it. Is your tone of voice loud, strong and affirmative? If it is, then your Positive Empowering Tape is ready for use!
- All you have to do now is go out for a walk and listen to it. Stand tall, open up your chest and embrace every word

I have created many different empowering tapes depending on the problem I was facing, and I have always found that this technique has really helped me when I felt things were getting tough. These tapes vary between one, three, or four minutes. I often play them several times in a row and each time, I feel more empowered, in control and positive about the outcome of my situation.

b. A Personal Example

At one point in my life, I created a self-empowering tape to help me feel proud of myself. I never enjoyed being the center of attention and always felt comfortable being in a position of inferiority when compared to others. I did not want to stand out or be better than anyone else. It was sort of a contradiction, because for example, on one hand I trained a lot to be fit, but then I didn't dare stand straight, fearing that people would notice me. I was aware of this, but I simply felt uncomfortable standing tall and looking confident.

So, one day I decided to create a tape that would empower me, help me feel confident and encourage me to finally stand nice and tall. I would go out for a walk and listen to the tape several times in a row. It was gradual, but I started to stand tall, put my shoulders back and look straight ahead and I could feel the confidence coming. With time, I didn't need the tape anymore. The minute I would hit the sidewalk, my shoulders would be back, I would be standing tall and my confidence was there. It became second nature.

C. Create your very own P.E.T. (Positive Empowerment Tape)

As I mentioned before we are far more demanding with ourselves than we would be with anyone else. One thing I found that really helped boost my self-esteem was to create my very own P.E.T.s (Positivel Empowering Tapes): the idea is to create an inspiring recording via your phone's Dictaphone that states your goal or problem and that empowers you to achieve it or helps you to push past certain difficulties or challenges. This technique allows you to listen to it any time throughout the day, whether you are on your way to work, going for a walk or enjoying a bit of time on your own.

First start off by establishing your problem or goal and write it down on paper.
Then write down all the emotions that are associated to this goal/problem: fear, self-doubt, pain, anger and so on.
Finally, write kind and encouraging words next to each emotion. You know, the type of things a best friend would tell you.

There are many different ways of creating a P.E.T. One of them, as you will see in the example below, is to have a conversation with yourself: express what you feel and then let your "inner friend" respond back to you with a firm and yet supportive, understanding, and positive tone of voice. I usually write my dialogue down on a piece of paper and then I will read it out loud while taping it.

A little piece of advice: *On some of my tapes, I like to repeat the positive sentences so that they resonate in my mind when I listen to them: I find that it gives the whole process far more impact. Try it for an added boost!*

Below, you will find a sample of a conversation you could use, let's say, if you are struggling with self-doubt. You want to lose weight, for example, but you have a hard time imagining that you could achieve such a incredible goal. You have already lost some weight and some members of your family are not supportive of your efforts and others, you feel, are jealous of what you have achieved. You want to succeed but you don't want to be left out or rejected. This is just an example. Of course, yours would be different and it should address issues that concern *you* specifically and be tailored to your needs.

I named this P.E.T.: **"I am allowed"** and created one very similar to it at a time I was scared that others would reject me for succeeding. Remember to date it, this way you will know when you started using this technique.

I AM ALOWED

Am I allowed to succeed?..Of course!
Do I deserve to succeed?...YES!
Am I allowed to feel confident? ....Absolutely!
Can I succeed in the challenges I have set myself?...Yes!
Do I deserve to be successful?..Of course, I do.
Am I allowed to stand tall?...Yes!
Can I be proud of myself?...Of course!
Can I succeed? ....Absolutely.
Can I be a role model?...Yes, I am a role model!
Do I deserve to be an inspiration? ....Yes, I am an inspiration!
Do I deserve to reach my goals?..............Of course, I do! I deserve to reach my goals! YES, YES, YES. I am reaching my goals
Can I excel in what I love? ....Of course. I excel in what I love.
Is it ok to succeed when others don't?...Of course it is.
Is it ok if others don't accept it?..Yes, it's ok.

I have the right to show my best and most powerful self. Once I have achieved my goal, I could help them in turn to succeed. But first I have to let my true powers show. I must stand tall and be proud of myself! Yes! From now on, I stand tall and I am proud of everything I am achieving. I am allowed to be proud of who I am, to be successful and strong. I am allowed to succeed and feel good about myself. I am allowed to succeed even where others have failed. It's ok. And it's ok if people don't love me. It's time now to stand up tall, to lift my chin up and move forward. Yes! I am doing this.

Another piece of advice: You could actually listen to this tape while looking at yourself in the mirror. Stand tall, shoulders back, feet firmly planted into the ground and open a little wider than shoulder width apart (military stance) and face the mirror. While staring at yourself, play the tape, repeat a few of the affirmations out loud and look determined

If you are not much of a writer, you could look for an inspiring passage in a book, tape it and play that passage when you are feeling in need of a boost. Try to put enthusiasm into your voice and don't hesitate to repeat the words or phrases that have a strong impact on you. Here is another one:

"This is the beginning of my new life!
And this new life is going to be *amazing!*
Come on! I stand tall. I am strong.
I lift my head up, open my chest and pull my shoulders back.

This is it! *I* am *moving forward* with my life.
I am strong, my *mind* is strong, my *heart* is strong, my *body* is strong!
From now on I focus on my goals and I seize every opportunity I get to move *one step* forward. I want to achieve my goals and I *will* achieve them *all.*
No one can stop me.

And I will be fearsome. I *am* fearsome.
For this reason, I have decided to say "YES" to life
"YES" to my future, "YES" to opportunities, I Say "YES"
Yes! I am now *open* to change. I decide to be the creator of my life.
Doors around me start opening and opportunities start coming my way.
Hey! I *believe* in the powers of change!
I am strong, come on, shoulders back, Yes, my chest is open, and I stand nice and tall.
From now on *I* am focusing on my goals,

Yes! I am allowed to succeed and be proud of who I am
Yes I am successful in reaching my goals
Yes good things are coming my way.
My eyes are wide open and I seize every opportunity that arises!
It's time to move on with my life.
I cannot, I will not let myself be affected by what people have to say or think.
I deserve to be happy!
I look and feel fantastic and I feel that the entire Universe is working in my favor.
I walk taller than I ever have before and I feel strong and confident

Never let go. Never waiver. Those days are over now. Ok? *They are over!*
I can do this! I know I can! I know I freaking can!
So, I lift my head up high, I pull my shoulders back, my abs are tight.
I Add a smile to my face. I am a winner!
From now on, I Act like the role model I want to be.
I am that role model".

C. Becoming A More Positive Person

Aside from observing yourself and your thoughts, repeating positive affirmations and listening to an empowering tape, there are a number of other things that you can do to help your mind see things in a more positive way:

a. Read! Read! Read! Learn! Learn! Learn!

I keep insisting on this point because reading inspiring books about inspiring people or self-help books that nourish your spirit and mind with positive thoughts, can have an amazing impact on how you feel about yourself and life in general. If you hate reading, check out the hundreds of videos and podcasts online that are there to inspire and push you to achieve your best.

To become more positive, you have to live positive and this means you have to read positive, breathe positive, act positive; you have to make room for 100% happiness in your life.

b. Be around positive people

I can't insist enough on this one. If you are constantly surrounded by people that are putting you down, it's time to have a chat with them or find new friends. If these people really care, tell them how you feel about their comments about you. They will either leave or make the extra effort to be supportive. Sometimes, people tend to repeat the same unkind remark that hurts over and over again: addressing it will make them stop, changing your life for the better. It could be a remark about your looks, your weight or a bad habit that you have. You don't need to be constantly reminded of it. Let your friends know how you feel. If they keep at it, then it might be time to question their friendship.

I remember years ago, I had a friend who would systematically compare herself to me and tell me how she was so much better than I was: her hair was thicker and longer than mine, she was taller, her breasts were bigger… I don't know why, but she just simply had to put me down. It was a problem for me because although I didn't mind her being "better" than I was, I felt uncomfortable that she was constantly making comparisons as if we were in competition. After a while, I told her how I felt. She completely denied it and kept going. At one point, I simply decided to stop calling her. Although I felt a little guilty… I never really missed her.

c. Meditate!

By taking the time to meditate, you allow yourself to slow down, have some time alone and feel more centered, which in turn helps you clarify your thoughts, such as: what you want, what you don't want, what you need, and so on. Knowing what you want is already one step towards reaching your goal(s). So, stop making excuses, stop searching for tips and techniques. Free yourself from everything you have read or learned: just simply walk, sit or lie down, close your eyes (or, if you prefer, keep them open), breathe and observe.

Your thoughts will come and go and you will get the fantastic opportunity to discover who you really are. Thereafter, it's all a question of being honest with yourself. Understand that your thoughts will sometimes be selfish, or they might even be lies you are trying to convince yourself of, fibs of your imagination, or, to the contrary, they might be revealing unresolved fear, pain or sorrow.

d. Stay active!

It is proven that exercise has a positive effect on your mood and how you feel. You may not enjoy doing it (yet!) but the state of wellbeing you'll experience once you have done it, is simply priceless. You don't have to visit the gym, you don't have to train for one hour. Just go out and have fun: roller skate, play basketball with your kids, go for a walk, do a nature trail, or put on your favorite music and dance in your living room!

e. Be there for others

It may not be the first thing that pops up in mind when trying to bring more positivity into your life, however, helping other people that are in need, being there for a friend or offering random help to someone can actually make you feel so much better. There is so much joy in giving and making others happy. Try it!

f. Do more of what makes you happy!

This point is key and is fully developed in Change n°8: *Your Daily Love*. Make a list of all the things that make you happy: beginning with little, all the way up to the big things. It could be talking to mom over the phone, going to the farmers market, cuddling with the cat, taking a nice hot bath or going to the movies, buying clothes and helping others. The more you do things that you love, the happier you will feel. Even a little event can make your whole day worthwhile. A good idea is to stop and ask yourself, every once in a while, in what way are these moments positive and what makes them so special?

EXAMPLES

Example 1: What Makes My Morning Coffee So Special?

Think about the coffee you had this morning in a nearby coffee shop. In what way did it make you happy?

Your answer:

The coffee there is so good. I love the atmosphere of that little café. I like the people working there. I like how, even though it's crowded, I can just sit down and concentrate on my work. I love how I feel there: I can really relax. Sometimes it's sunny and in the winter it's so nice to soak up a little bit of sun and at other times, when it's a hot summer day, there is a breeze there that simply feels amazing. When I am there, I am happy.

Example 2: What Makes Going to the Movies So Special?

Why do I enjoy going to the movies?

Your answer:

I love the fact that I can watch something without being interrupted, which never seems to be possible at home. I love the atmosphere and the fact that it is a secluded area: I can give it my undivided attention. I love the emotions I feel while watching it. I love letting go of my emotions like (crying, laughing, freaking out). I love the smell and taste of popcorn and the reclining seats that some cinemas offer. I love sharing this moment with my family and how, when the movie is over, I am still in the experience.

Example 3: Ask Yourself what makes you happy and why

What makes you happy, why and what do you love about it?
You will see that you need to be aware of your emotions.

Your answer:

If I do more things that bring about positive, strong emotions, are mentally engaging in a positive way, help evoke peace of mind, are fun, make me laugh and vibrate with joy, keep me interested and focused, then I am well on my way to a more positive mindset.

g. Writting a gratitude journal

Taking the time to write down everything that you are grateful for can actually help you put things into perspective. You may be going through tough times right now, but perhaps it's not all that bad? Try to focus on the little details. You can't always expect amazing things to happen to you.

Was someone nice to you today?

Did something unexpected happen to you that made you happy?

Did you have the opportunity to laugh or share a special moment with someone?

Write it down. And if you find that nothing positive is happening then create it: watch a funny movie with the whole family or alone, call a friend and go share a coffee or a walk together, meditate on gratitude and take the time to see everything you have and thank the Universe for being so blessed.

These are simply a few propositions. At this very moment, we are all going through different things and it's important to adjust ourselves according to our own thinking patterns.

Our thoughts define who we are, they affect how we are reacting right now and the decisions we are going to make. Do you realize how much control they hold over you? Learn to see the importance of positive thinking and give less value to all of those negative thoughts that keep popping up in your mind. O.k. We know their mission is to warn you of a possible hazard in the future or remind you of who you are and what you have endured in the past. Thank these thoughts for being there to help you. You will not forget them, they are part of who you are today... But you must also tell them that now is the time to move forward, now is the time to acknowledge your fears and grab your positive thoughts by the hand. And, just as Judy Garland did in the Wizard of Oz, as she walked down the yellow brick road arm in arm with her friends "courage, heart and brain" you must tell yourself that you are hitting your sunshine road as well; the one that leads you to the land of pOZitive self-esteem!

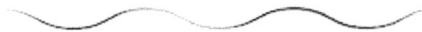

Change n°6
YOUR EMPOWERING BOARD *6.*

Many of you have already heard about Vision Boards. The idea behind this one, however, is not only to paste all of those things you would like to accomplish in the future, but also to put all of your past accomplishments as well. Being able to visualize your past successes on a daily basis and also pasting beside them what you wish to accomplish in your future, can really help boost your self-esteem.

A. How to Create an Empowering Accomplishment Board (E.A.B.)

We are going to divide this Accomplishment Board into different parts:

a. List Your Past Accomplishments

In this first part, you are going to take the time to post all of your past accomplishments. Dig into all of your old photos and take the ones that show your past accomplishments. It doesn't matter whether the accomplishments are big or small: riding your bike without training wheels, receiving a medal, creating something beautiful, winning a prize, passing an exam, your best drawing, you name it!

If there are too many, you could group them together and take a single shot of them. This way you will have several accomplishments in a single photo.

If you don't have that many which was my case as well, focus on eventful moments when you were particularly proud or happy, such as getting married or having a child, when you went on stage, negotiated an important contract at work, and so on. If you don't have any photos, find some on the internet that remind you of this event. You could even include a few difficult moments that you were able to overcome.

Try to remember your emotions linked to these events.

What did you feel: Happiness? Pride? Were you on top of the world?

What other words come to mind: Success? Achievement? Willpower? Determination?

You can either write them with a colored marker, type them or find the words in magazines, cut them out and paste them on your Accomplishment Board.

Next, find some quotes that have to do with what you have accomplished. If you choose willpower, for example, you could choose the following one:

> **Willpower is like a muscle,**
> **the more you train it, the stronger it gets.**

Words have power, so choose ones that inspire you, have a special meaning, motivate you and feel just right.

b. Pasting Your Future Goals

In this second part, stick on your board the things you wish to accomplish. You could either do this on the reverse side of your board, if it's a small one, or you could split your board in two, with half of it devoted to the past and the other half, to the future. Again, you will have to find images that correspond to what you want. The idea is to paste the photos of your future accomplishments that you wish to achieve (you can find them in magazines or on the internet) and replace them with yours every time you achieve a goal. You can either stick your achievements on top of the initial picture or simply replace them.

Now that your Empowering Accomplishment Board is complete, you can either put it away in a drawer and let things unravel, or, if you prefer you can keep it close at hand. I, personally, like to hold on to it, look at it with intent, read it with conviction, smile at it, as I imagine these images soon coming my way or because I am grateful for all the good things that have happened to me throughout my life. It can be a powerful reminder of all the positive things that have come to you in the past.

There are two ideal moments during the day to take the time and look at your E.A.B.:
• First thing in the morning, as it will help you start on a positive note, and
• Right before you go to sleep, knowing that these last thoughts will remain in your subconscious mind throughout the night. The way I see it, the more these images stay with you, the better!

B. Understanding Why E.A.B.s are powerful

a. An E.A.B. is a Powerful Tool

I believe that the real power of an Empowering Accomplish Board resides in the fact that you sit down and take the time to know what you really want in life. By doing this, you are creating a clear idea of how you envision yourself in the future, you are being proactive and doing something that is getting you one step closer to reaching your goals.

Note that in order to achieve something, it's important to:
• **Have a clear idea of what you want: KNOW!** By asking yourself what it is you really want and searching for photos and quotes, you will know what it is you want in life.
• **Really desire this idea to come true: WANT!** This is the part where you take the time to hold your E.A.B. and visualize yourself achieving your goal to strengthen your "Want."
• **Move towards reaching your goals: ACT!** There is always something that you can do to get one step closer to reaching your goal. So, get moving and make things happen!
• **Have total faith that the fulfillment of your desire is coming your way: BELIEVE!** It's essential to believe that this goal is possible and within your reach. Relax your body, put faith in your heart and belief in your mind and see how things start happening to you.

Start Cooking!

Once you have finished your E.A.B., ask yourself what other action you could do in order to get another step closer to making this dream come true. Make a list of all the little and big things that you could do and start crossing them out, one at a time. When I am hungry for food, I don't just sit down and wait for it to come. I am no longer a child. I get up off the couch and I prepare it, myself. It's the same with your goals. Do you want to reach them? Well then get up and get your list of ingredients ready. List the things you can do to reach your goals and then, start cooking!

Change n°7
BE INSPIRED

7.

To start things off, let's define the word "inspiration." What does it mean to be a source of inspiration or inspirational? Biographyonline offers one of the best definitions:

To be "Inspirational is to offer something valuable, uplifting which motivates others to bring out the best in themselves."

"To be inspirational is to lead by example and encourage others to feel there is something worthwhile to become and do."

Being inspired can go a long way. How many times have you heard stories in which a person, an event, a book or a movie inspired people to change their way of life?

When you feel inspired it's like adding wings to your soul and there is no stopping what you can do.

So, this week, why not decide to cultivate your inspiration? The way I see it, books, people, conferences and movies are a type of fertilizer that can make things grow exponentially inside of you, put faith in your soul and bring a sense of meaning into your life.

A. Benefits of reading

If you ever go to the Library of Thèbes in Greece, as you walk in, this is the inscription you will read:

> ***Books are medicine for the Soul.***

My home is full of books and ever since I can remember they have been an important part of my life. Books are powerful and can greatly impact how you feel and make you question all your beliefs: some of the books I've read have been a revelation and even life transforming.

a. Benefits of reading books in general

Let's begin by listing the main benefits of reading in general.

• First of all, did you know that **most important people read a lot**? This, in itself, might be a motive to get you to read more. For me, life wouldn't be the same without my books and I never leave home without at least one in my handbag. You just never know when you might have a few minutes to read a few pages. When I am waiting in line at the bank or riding on the bus, I am also accompanying an adventurer through some wild tracks, sharing someone's first passionate kiss or am perhaps hanging breathless in the middle of nowhere wondering what is coming up next…

But reading will also:
- increase your vocabulary
- improve your language
- improve your writing style
- improve your reading skills
- increase your general knowledge
- improve your spelling

b. Benefits of reading autobiographies, biographies and true stories
To make things clear, let's define the words "biography" and "autobiography" and see in what way they differ.
"Bio" originates from the Greek word that means "life"
"Graphy" comes from the Greek word "graphos" which means to "write".
In other words, a biography is the account of the series of events making up a real person's life, not the author's, and an autobiography is when someone writes their own life story.

The way I see it, books are pure magic: they have this incredible power over you and can actually influence how you feel. Opening a book is like opening a door to the unknown: When you flip open the cover page and start reading "Chapter 1" you don't know yet what type of emotion you are going to experience: will it be fear, grief, suspense or admiration, joy and compassion or perhaps anger or disgust. That is why one must be careful when opening that door, because when you set that book down, the words you read still linger in your mind and can affect you for hours, days and sometimes for a lifetime.

Let's face it, when the book is good and you are totally captivated by the story, you are literally transported into another world. For this reason, if you want to bring more positivity and change into your life it is essential to select your reading material carefully. I have found that reading self-help books can really help give you some tools on how to bring about certain changes. But what I find most inspiring is to read biographies or autobiographies. There is something in the fact that these stories are not only inspiring, but they are also true. Every once in a while, as you are reading along, you can simply stop in amazement while realizing that all of it actually happened in real life. You might read about someone's incredible path to success, but you will also discover what they had to endure to get there. Read *Anne Frank*, *I am Malala, the girl who stood* up for education and was shot by the Taliban, or *Unbroken* by Laura Hillenbrand, *Midnight Express* by Billy Hayes, *I Forgot to Die* by Khalil Rafati, *Wild: From lost to found on the Pacific Crest trail* by Cheryl Strayed, *Into the Wild* by John Krakauer, *Walden* by Thoreau…and get inspired!
Let the author's words linger in your mind and ask yourself: "Could I do the same thing?" I am sure you are expecting me to give you the typical answer: "Yes, of course, if you set your heart to it". But I feel like saying: "Who wants to live the exact same life as somebody else? You are a different person with a totally different life path. For this reason, you have to be the author of your very own book, you must write your own story, turn your very own pages, struggle through the ups and downs of *your* own chapters.

Reading real life stories can truly be inspirational. When we read about certain peoples' lives, it's simply amazing to see what they have been through but also what they have accomplished. It seems that some have literally lived several lives in one.

What theme inspires you? Successful Men and Women? Politics? Success in business? Charisma? Sports? Actors/actresses? Read about the lives of people whom you admire. If you are into a certain type of sport, then read the biographies of famous athletes, if you are into science, then choose books about famous scientists… you get the idea.

If you are not much into reading but still feel that you could benefit from biographies, why don't you check out children books. When my kids were homeschooled, I loved buying biographies for them and ended up reading them myself. They are quick easy reads yet still inspirational. Check out by name the "Who is" "Who was" series of books and explore reading all that interest you.

Reading these types of stories makes you realize that man is capable of great things. These inspirational people are human beings just like you and I. If they can do something great, so can you; if they can fulfill their dreams, well then you can too. Find out what you are passionate about, give it your all and why not become *yourself* a source of inspiration.

Depending on the biography, autobiography or true story that you read, you will enjoy an array of benefits, some of which are listed below:

- You will **increase your knowledge** of history, various cultures and religions.

- Bios and Autobiographies are often **fascinating**. Let's face it, some of these people, like Napoleon Bonaparte and Richard Branson have accomplished in one life things that most of us couldn't even dream of accomplishing in nine lives. Others, such as Gandhi, have the capacity of bringing people together. He single-handedly managed to bring a nation together by questioning the rights of the authority in place.

- The people you are reading about can be viewed as **mentors**; they are people that you can look up to. How is it that certain people manage to accomplish the unimaginable and change the world's destiny?

- What really matters is not so much the fortune that certain men or women have amassed, but **the values** they have instilled: faith in what they were doing, resilience to keep on going, loyalty towards others, being true to themselves, faithfulness in love, and so on. Take the time to ask yourself what values make this man or woman incredible. Why don't we all try to live according to these same values? Or better yet, why don't you set out to find out what YOUR core values are and set your foot down next time someone questions them. These values are a part of who you are. Chances are that if you live accordingly your kids will look up to you, maybe not while in their teens, but later when they realize that your values have probably kept your family afloat.

- These men and women can be **a source of motivation** and push you to accomplish things for yourself. "Hey if this guy can do this, well then why couldn't I do….. ?" I will let you fill out the blank for that one. If their dream came true, why couldn't yours?

- You will **learn from other people's mistakes** and question what could work on your life path. When I was young and living on Ojibwe reservations in Canada, I loved to read their legends. They always told a story but the main purpose of each and every one was the teachings you learned from the main character's trials and errors. All great men and women made mistakes along their path, but that doesn't make them less credible. While reading about their experiences you come to realize that they are just normal human beings like us and that it's okay to falter along the way.

- **You will develop your sense of empathy** and become more understanding about how people live their lives and why they've made certain choices. You will get a different perspective and the opportunity to understand and respect situations you might not have in the past, thus learning to be more accepting, becoming less intransigent. Often when you are reading, it is an opportunity to put yourself in someone else's shoes and express empathy.

- You will be **more appreciative of what you have,** express more gratitude in your life and towards the people you live with. When you read what Anne Frank or Nelson Mandela went through, you can only feel grateful for what you have and for all the simple things in life, such as running outdoors and knowing that you are free to go wherever you wish.

- You get the **opportunity to "visit" a famous person's mind**. When you think of it, how cool is that! How did this person think and what are their general views? How did they react in certain situations? How did the main character get through the ups and downs of life? What was their love life like and how did they behave with common people? Were they respectful or arrogant?

Final thought:
Researching about biographies and autobiographies got me thinking about "authors" in general and I wanted to encourage you, next time, before reading any book, whether it be fiction, a thriller, a love story or what not, to take a few extra minutes and get to know the author by browsing through their bio. You might get a little insight on certain events that occur during the story and what instilled the author to write about them.

c. Reading self-help books to find inspiration

Reading inspiring and motivational books puts you in the mood for success because let's face it, taking control of your life can be scary. That's when reading these types of books can make a difference: in a sense they will permeate your mind with positivity, make you understand that change is possible and pretty soon you will be totally boosted into taking action!

Read below to learn in what way reading more self-help books can be a great source of inspiration:

First of all, most people who have already read a personal development book, will tell you that, when they set the book down, they **felt more positive, happier with a real sense of relief**. Indeed, reading, seeking and reflecting brings peace to your heart and mind.

These types of books will help you make the difference between what is essential and what is not: **they help you put things into perspective**.

We all tend to act like know-it-alls. **Personal development books make you question your beliefs**: "The way I see things… could it be that I am wrong?"

If the self-help book is good, **it will give you the needed push to get moving**, it will turn you into a go-getter. Self-help books can really help you understand that the solution to your problem lies within you and certainly not by trying to change other people or hoping they will change.

You might be a firm believer that you do not need to read personal development books, or you might contest the validity and necessity of reading these kind of books. For many of you, I am sure that you already know, intuitively, what most of these books have to say. But, I know that I **feel appeased** when reading them: the same way I feel after praying.

Some things are beyond our control, such as other people's reactions and their beliefs. Many of us spend an awful lot of time feeling frustrated and complaining about others. As we read these books, we start to understand that **the only person we have any control over, is ourselves** and that if something needs to change, it's up to us to do something about it.

Depending on the amount of time you have available, decide ahead of time how much you will read: One chapter a day, one book per week, one book per month? You decide. However, make sure you read every single day! If this is your goal this week, I suggest you read an entire book this week or dedicate enough time to reading at least one whole chapter every day.

When starting something, get into the habit of doing it 200%. Engage your mind 100% by giving it your full attention but be active as well. When you are reading self-help books, make sure you apply the principles and do the exercises. Take notes, underline the passages that really speak to you or copy them down onto a piece of paper, glue them inside a special notebook or stick them on your wall.

d. Watch Inspiring Videos and Films

If you aren't much of a reader, why not check out movies and online videos as a source of inspiration. Many of these videos are extremely powerful and motivational. Why not decide, over the course of this week, to take a few minutes to watch one of these videos every day.

e. Meeting Inspiring People

Has anyone ever inspired you? Maybe a teacher, a family member, your coach or have you ever heard someone deliver an inspirational speech? Take two minutes and ask yourself what makes that person inspirational? Below I have listed some of the qualities of an inspirational person:

• Great communication skills
• They know how to listen
• They have principles
• A challenge doesn't scare them
• They are passionate
• They radiate positivity and faith
• They make you believe that all things are possible
• They have a sense of purpose
• They have a clear vision of what they want
• They are there for others and are not scared to roll up their sleeves
• They have an aura, a special something about them
• They are humble
• They are authentic. They are for real.
• They find joy in the process, not only in succeeding

So why not decide to get out there and start meeting new people? We tend to stick around the same crowd of friends. But I feel like asking: why should we? Why not change our connections? Think about your goals and then start setting out to meet people who are in-line with them. Do your research in book stores and online. Observe, listen, read and then let the words thrive within you; watch as your goal starts to come alive.

Why not push things a little further by becoming a source of inspiration for others? You could start taking better care of your appearance: look your best, stand tall, be clean and fresh and remember to get enough sleep and exercise.

Be happy and start seeing things in a positive light. Bring more passion into your life by doing more things that you love. Be yourself and be proud of who you are: try to be spontaneous by letting others see the real you. Take the time to find out what your true values are and fight to live accordingly. Last but not least, remember to be there for others. Do I have to add "with sincerity" and make a point of being a good listener.

f. Go to Conferences, conventions, talk shows, debates

In my days as a personal trainer, I was constantly saving up some money to go to personal training conventions. It was so inspiring and motivating. I always came back completely boosted and couldn't wait to apply all the things I had learned.

Just recently I was asked to go to a book presentation for a book is called *Mind over Matter* by Philippe Lamache, the French title being *La Pensée au Coeur du Corps*. It was so inspiring to hear the author explain the importance of engaging one's mind while exercising, training with total focus, being fully aware of our body and the movements as we perform each and every one of them. I came out of this presentation totally energized. Although concentration has always been an integral part of every single one of my training sessions, the author's words and demonstrations managed to really stimulate my convictions.

What is your dream? What subjects interest you?
There are conferences out there on just about anything: sports, cooking, nutrition, history, medical topics and so on.
Check out churches, museums, theaters, art expositions, but also search the local weekly newspaper to see what is going on in your region. Look on internet, if the city where you live in doesn't have much to offer.

There are also debates, book presentations, concerts, you name it, it exists. And if you are into music why not check out different concerts. Many places offer free concerts. Listening to a variety of different kinds of music can be interesting, uplifting and inspiring.

B. Over 100 different sources from which you will find inspiration:
It might be a good idea to ask yourself what *your* goal is and to find inspiration in this area of expertise, whether it be through books, articles, videos, conferences, podcasts, you name it. Make sure you choose to read, watch and listen to things that inspire *YOU*!

Find inspiring biographies, autobiographies and true stories:
• *Becoming* by Michelle Obama
• *What I Know for Sure* by Oprah Winfrey
• *Into the Wild* by Jon Krakauer, an inspiring story about a young man who tries to survive on his own in the wild
• *Steve Jobs* by Walter Isaacson
• *Loosing my Virginity* by Richard Bronson
• *One Click Jeff Besos* and the rise of Amazon.com by Richard Brandt
• *Shoe Dog* by Phil Knight, the inspiring story of the rise of Nike
• *Wild* by Cheryl Strayed: about a young woman who decides to hike the west coast of the United States alone. Follow her on this therapeutic walk during which she unravels her life and discover how step by step she slowly heals her life wounds and finds her life purpose
• *The Autobiography of Benjamin Franklin*
• Booker T. Washington's *Up from Slavery* tells about his struggle for equal rights in America
• *Unbroken* by Laura Hillenbrand. It's not a biography but a true story
• *Mother Teresa of Calcutta*
• *Mutant message down under* a novel of Aboriginal Wisdom by Marlo Morgan
• *Mutant Message from Forever*: also by Marlo Morgan
• *Audrey Hepburn by Barry Paris*. I have always loved Audrey Hepburn and I found her life truly inspiring.

- *Enchantment: The Life of Audrey Hepburn* by Donald Spoto
- *De Niro : A life* by Shawn Levy
- Bob Dylan: *Chronicles*
- *Elvis: last train to Memphis* Peter Guralnisk
- Michael Jackson
- *Born to Run* by Bruce Springsteen
- *Mozart: A life* by Paul Johnson
- *Unfinished Journey: Twenty Years Later* by Yehudi Menhuhin
- *Tiger Woods* by Jeff Benedicts
- *Breaking Night: A Memoir of Forgiveness, Survival, and My Journey from Homeless to Harvard* by Liz Murray
- *The Virgin Way* by Richard Branson
- *Little House in the big woods* by Laura Ingles Wilder
- *Krishnamurti's journal* by Jiddu Krishnamurti
- *Into the magic shop* by Dr James R Doty, A neurosurgeon's true story of the life-changing magic of compassion and mindfulness

These are all famous people, but why not search for inspiring men and women who have accomplished amazing things and who are not necessarily famous. For example, I have read, *Around Africa on my Bicycle* by Riaan Manser. This guy crossed 34 different countries while riding a bicycle around Africa; that's 36 500 km! He was alone for two years, two months and fifteen days. I was not only amazed by his courage and determination, I also loved his writing and his view on things. A must read!

Find inspiration for your career, work and Business:
- *Little Bets, How breakthrough ideas emerge from small discoveries* by Peter Sims
- Adam Grant's two books: *Originals* and *Give and Take*: about how to become more creative at work and why giving is an essential component of success
- Richard Branson: *Like a Virgin: Secrets they won't teach you at business school*
- The biography of Steve Jobs
- *The accidents of Billionaires: the founding of Facebook: A tale of sex, money, genius and betrayal* by Ben Mezrich
- *Oprah*: A biography by Kitty Kelley
- *One Click* by Jeff Bezos and the rise of Amazon company
- Mary Kay Ash: *Miracles Happen*
- *The Widow Cliquot*: The story of a Champagne Empire and the woman who ruled it. By Tilar Mazzeo
- The *"E myth"*
- *The slight Edge, Turning simple disciplines into massive success and happiness* by Jeff Olson and John David Mann
- *The Magic of thinking big* by David J . Schwartz
- *Pulling your own strings – How to take control of your life* by Dr Wayne W. Dyer
- *Crucial conversation – Tools for talking when the stakes are high* by Patterson, Grenny, McMillan and Switzler

- *The 7 Habits of Highly Effective People* by Stephen R. Covey
- *The War of Art* by Steven Pressfield: how to finish what you have started. Many of us are dabblers and not completers and tend to start something and never following through their project to the end. This book gives you the tools to get things done!
- *Life in Motion* by Mindy Copeland (if you are into dancing)
- *Raising the Bar* by Lauren Kessler (if you are into dancing)

Find inspiration reading peoples' Adventures:
- *Around Africa on my bicycle* by Riaan Manser
- *Mind of a survivor: What the wild has taught me about survival and success* by Megan Hine
- *Annapurna the first conquest of an 8000 meter peak* by Maurice Herzog
- Ray Mears' Extreme Survival series

Peoples' values as source of inspiration:
- Gandhi: *The story of my experiments with truth*
- *Freedom in Exile* the autobiography of the Dalaï Lama
- *Walden* by Thoreau

I also recommend reading Krishnamurti's books: they often relate encounters he has had with people like you and I and many are presented in a question and answer format. These dialogs will question many of your beliefs, habits and principles.
- *Think on these things* by Krishnamurti
- *This light in oneself* by Krishnamurti
- *On mind and thought* by Krishnamurti
- *On education* by Krishnamurti
- *Facing a world in crisis* by Krishnamurti
- *The Network of thought* by Krishnamurti
- *On love and loneliness* by Krishnamurti
- *Freedom from the Known* by Krishnamurti
- *The first and last freedom* by Krishnamurti
- *The only revolution* by Krishnamurti
- *The book of life* by Krishnamurti
- *On truth* by Krishnamurti
- *The flight of the eagle* by Krishnamurti

Find inspiration to change your life:
- *Who moved my cheese? An amazing way to deal with change in your work and in your life* by Spencer Johnson
- *Choose to live Peacefully* by Susan Smith Jones
- *Choose Radiant Health and Happiness* by Susan Smith Jones
- *Choose to live each day fully* by Susan Smith Jones
- *The Artist's Way* by Julia Cameron – A spiritual path to higher creativity (A course in discovering and recovering your creative self)
- *The simple Living Guide* by Janet Luhrs – a sourcebook for less stressful, more joyful living. Discover simple living approaches to time, money, inner simplicity, work, simple pleasures and romance, virtues, families, holidays, cooking and nutrition, health and exercise, housing, clutter, gardening, travel

- *The last lecture* by Randy Pausch
- *Choosing simplicity* by Linda Breen Pierce – Real people finding peace and fulfillment in a complex world
- *Girl, wash you face: stop believing the lies about who you are so you can become who you were meant to be* by Rachel Hollis
- *Girls, stop apologizing* by Rachel Hollis – A shame free plan for embracing and achieving your goals
- *The Power of now*, A Guide to spiritual Enlightenment by Eckhart Tolle
- *As a Man thinketh* by James Allen – Purity of mind leads to purity of life
- *The Secret* by Rhonda Byrne
- *The Power* by Rhonda Byrne
- *Conversations with God* by Neale Donald Walsch
- *How to stop worrying and start living* by Dale Carnegie
- *How to win friends and influence people* by Dale Carnegie
- *The four agreements* by Don Miguel Ruiz
- *Ultimate Confidence* by Marisa Peer
- *Creative Visualization* by Shakti Gawain
- *The Charisma myth* by Olivia Fox Cabane
- *Be Healthy Stay Balanced* by Susan Smith Jones. If you can, read all of her books!
- *Thinking Fast and Slow* by Daniel Kahneman, a whole new look at the way our minds work, and how we make decisions
- *Solitude : In pursuit of a Singular Life in a Crowded World* by Michael Harris
- *Unapologetically YOU, Reflections on life and the Human Experience* by Dr. Steve Maraboli
- *Life : the Truth and Being Free* by Steve Maraboli
- *The Charge by* Brendon Burchard
- *Make time : how to focus on what matters every da*y by Jake Knapp and John Knapp and John Zeratsky
- *Tiny Buddha's 365 Tiny Love Challenges* by Lori Deschene
- *Women who run with the wolves* by Clarissa Pinkola Estès
- *Ask and it is Given learning to manifest your desires* by Esther and Jerry Hicks
- *You are awesome* by Matthew Syed
- *Non violent Communications* by Marshall B. Rosenberg
- *Presence is power* by Gudni Gunnarsson
- *Becoming Supernatural* by Joe Dispenza
- *You are the Placebo* by Joe Dispenza

Find inspiration to quit an addiction… or never succumb to one:
- *I, Christian F, 13 years old, on drugs and a prostitute*
- *I forgot to die* by Khalil Rafati
- *Recovery 2.0, Move beyond addiction and upgrade your life* by Tommy Rosen
- *Video workshop: the 5 things that stop us from overcoming addiction* (and what to do about it)

Strengthen your mind and mind resistance:
- Books and DVDs by Dave Canterbury who teaches survival techniques.
- *Feel the fear and do it anyway* – The phenomenal classic that has changed the lives of millions by Susan Jeffers. In a few words, "Whatever happens to me, given any situation, I can handle it!"

Look into Philosophical tales as a source of inspiration. Here is a list of must reads:
- *The Alchemist* by Paulo Coelho
- *The Little Prince* by Antoine de Saint Exupéry
- *The Way of the Peaceful Warrior* by Dan Millman
- *The Celestine Prophecy* by James Redfield
- *The Monk who Sold his Ferrari,* by Robin Sharma
- *The Prophet* by Kalil Gibran
- *The Go-giver, the story about a powerful business idea* by Bob Burg and John David Mann

Inspiring lectures, conferences, webinars, conventions:
- *Listen to this when you feel lost* – Best inspirational speeches on YouTube
- *It's all within you* – 30 minutes Inspirational speeches compilation YouTube
- *Life at 30.000 feet* by Richard Branson
- *Best Inspirational Speech Ever* Motivational video Amazing YouTube
- *Be Powerful* – By Sandeep Maheshwari on YouTube
- *The Riddle of experience vs. memory* by Daniel Kahneman
- *The power of introvert*s by Susan Cain
- *Finding your why*: Simon Sinek
- Krishnamurti webinars and Anthony Robbins'webinars, and reewebinarwednesdays.com
- Oprah Winfrey's inspiring words
- *What we can learn from Spaghetti Sauce* by Malcolm Gladwell
- *Less Stuff, more happiness* Graham Hill
- Vishen Lakhiani's *Mindvalley Masterclasses,* and *The Unusual advice*
- Watch Brendan Burchard's videos on Youtube
- B*eing an Entrepreneur* by Larry King
- Tim Ferris: listen to his podcast: *http.the four hour work*
- *"Stop wasting time"* a motivational video for success and studying part 1 and 2 on Youtube
- *I wish someone had told me this when I was your age*, Morgan Freeman on Youtube

Inspiring films:
- *The Dead Poet's Society*
- *Riding Giants:* a documentary about surfing
- *The Black Stallion:* the friendship between a boy and his horse competing in major racing.
- *Million Dollar Baby:* a coach reluctantly takes a young female trainee
- *Breaking away*: a movie around bike racing and friendship
- *Hoop Dreams:* making basketball dreams come true

And so on. You get the idea. Find things that inspire you and that launch emotions. Watch, read, listen every day and you will see how they nourish your soul and get you craving for some more. If you are in a sort of rut at the moment and don't really know where you are going or what to do, reading inspiring stories, watching resourceful videos and webinars, meeting interesting people can be just what you need to get you going. When your mind is relentlessly busy going over your daily little problems, all these books, videos, conferences, webinars can become a great source of inspiration. They can give you the willpower to get up and start doing something with your life. If you don't really know what you want in life, just get into the habit of turning to different sources of inspiration and let the words nourish your soul. The next step will come naturally when you least expect it.

Change n°8
YOUR DAILY LOVE

8.

It might seem to be such a simple point, but how many of us actually take the time every day to do something that we are really passionate about? Most of the time we come up with the excuse that we don't have the time.

Why don't you, this week, take at least 15 minutes every day to paint, draw, cook, garden, play basketball, compose or sing, do yoga, meditate, play basketball, you name it! It could be one thing you feel passionate about or lots of different things that simply make you happy. Write a list and this week try to do as many as possible. You deserve it! Doing things you love will make you happier and fill your heart with satisfaction. You will lead a more fulfilling life!

Don't let time be a factor that prevents you from carrying out what makes you happy. Make it a priority and find the time. The best way to ensure that you have sufficient time is to block out, ahead of time, a slot that will be entirely devoted to this goal.

1. Why Should You Do It?

It will make you happy and you will radiate this happiness; in turn, it will benefit everyone that you interact with. Your happiness is contagious. Some people tend to feel guilty about taking a little bit of "self-time", saying that their family or work needs them. Understand that by forgetting yourself, you are slowly burning out that inner flame within which can be sensed by the people who share your life.

With the homeschooling, all the household chores that needed attending, my husband wanting some alone time and so on, I had good excuses not to go out jogging but I would go anyway. Let me tell you this: every occasion I took the time to do something that made me feel good, I returned home happy, excited an energized to tackle what needed to be done and share some time with my family.

To answer the question "Why should you do it?":
- You will actually do more! In order to do the things you love, you will need to organize your day, which will automatically make you more time efficient: you will be working faster, making better decisions in order to go out and have fun!
- Because life is too short to fill it only with obligations. So, ask yourself: if today was your last day, what would you love to do?
- Because pretty soon you will be adding 2, 3 or 4 more fun things to do each day, creating an even happier you.
- Taking care of yourself is good for you. Being happy and laughing has been proven to be beneficial for your health as you will be more relaxed and it boosts your immune system.

2. How to do it?

Look at all the things you do throughout the day that are such a waste of time: a few quick shifts in priorities and what may seem impossible at first, will become enjoyable and require no effort at all.

Read on to find ways to have more time to do what you really love:

- Watch less TV or stop it altogether
- Delegate. Why not ask the kids to do some chores so you have added time for yourself
- Learn to say "no" more often. When people ask you for a hand and you have previously planned your special moment…say "no, sorry I have other plans"
- Reduce your social networking time
- At first schedule only 15 to 30 minutes of "your happy time." You could also do something you love several times a day for short bouts of time
- Let your spouse and kids join in on the fun
- Get some help. If you have kids, find someone to help out: either a babysitter, or do a mommy swap where each mom gets one hour
- Is money the problem? Try service swap, where you help with something in exchange of a service. I used to give English lessons to a boxing coach. One hour of English for one hour of boxing! It was a win-win situation!
- Stop being a perfectionist! The house isn't spic and span? Who cares, you can do it later. Go do more of what makes you HAPPY!

3. Some ideas you might love to do!

To tackle this challenge and do something you love every single day, start by asking yourself the following question: What can I do today that would make me happy? Write your list of happy ideas on a piece of paper and read on to find some other suggestions as well:

- Lie in the grass and read a book
- Spend some time with a special friend who always makes you feel better
- Exercise but do something different, something you don't normally do
- Call mom and dad
- Go shopping
- Declutter: you would be amazed how it can make you happy (once it's done!)
- Draw
- Sing, do a karaoke or take up singing lessons
- Get a massage
- Watch your favorite movie, again
- Organize a dare and train for it
- Get a haircut
- Do that recipe you have been wanting to do
- Buy a book, allow yourself some reading time every day and enjoy
- Go for a walk in nature
- Plan a romantic evening, dress up, get a special dinner ready and relax
- Reach out to someone you haven't spoken to in a long time
- Do something nice for someone
- Take up an activity you have always wanted to try

- If you are good at something, reach out and propose to help others to learn your skill. For example, if you are good at a certain sport or artistically, reach out and help someone who would like to learn. Being in the teacher's position while taking the time for others will definitely help boost your self-esteem and the way you feel about yourself.
- Plan some time for intimacy with your special someone
- Learn to fix your car or dismantle it and then put it back together again
- Get things done: see all of those things that you keep delaying? Do them, it will make you happy and proud
- Go fishing, watch the sunset or sunrise
- Have a girl's or guy's night out
- This week I took the time to have a cup of coffee with my boyfriend. We sat down in the sun and talked for a few hours, with our phones out of the way: we laughed, looked into each other's eyes, recalled memories and made future plans together.

A good idea is to create a poster on the wall with 7 slots, one for each day of the week, in which you can put a photo of you doing various things that you love. And why not design an advent calendar ahead of time with different ideas and open up a window each day to see what positive activity you will be doing for yourself that day!

If you are trying to build your self-esteem, it is essential that you bring some happiness into your life and partake in activities that make you light up inside while smiling to the world around you!

Change n°9
7 RINGS TO LEARN
7 DIFFERENT THINGS

9.

Have you ever been in a conversation where you have no idea what people are talking about or simply have nothing to say? And what about the opposite, have you ever been in a conversation where you spoke confidently about the topic at hand and could simply go on and on?

It's normal not to know everything and have gaps in your knowledge, but certain situations can really affect your self-esteem. Although knowledge isn't everything and it can be really annoying when someone tries to spread everything they know, I believe it's important to constantly strive to learn and understand the world we live in.

So, this week, why don't you decide to learn something new every day. You could either take up one activity, such as learning a new language or improving your special skill or else you could simply decide to read a newspaper every day, for example.

A. The Importance of Lifelong Learning!

Learning shouldn't stop the day you finish high school or University. It should be a Lifelong Process. In fact, the good thing about learning once you have obtained your degree, is that you can learn exactly what *YOU* want to learn. There are no more obligations, whatsoever. Love the process of learning and you will see many different areas of your life improving!

- If you keep learning new skills, you will become more competent. This can improve your financial situation over time. More skills, more knowledge = more qualified = more money!
- People will respect you more and want to listen to what you have to say. Someone who knows how to express himself and is knowledgeable, is someone we can look up to when we need help. This means that your knowledge can help you socially as well
- You will be less gullible. Learning new things every day gives you a certain power and enhances your self-esteem. When you feel comfortable and are able to engage in a variety of different topics, it can help you feel better about yourself
- Improving your knowledge, skills and abilities can help you become autonomous in many different situations: if you know how to fix, create, do things on your own or are curious enough to learn how to, you won't need other people's help: you'll be able to rely on your own self to get things done! Now, how cool is that?
- You won't be labeled as being ignorant: come on let's be honest here, who likes being labeled as anything?
- Becoming more knowledgeable in specific areas such as health and exercise will help you live longer and can set you as an example for your children, friends and family,
- Learning about the world that surrounds you and observing people from different backgrounds, cultures, religions, and their unique rituals, will help you become more open-minded, tolerant and a better person.

B. Tips You might Want To Know That Can Help you with the learning process

- Know that we learn and memorize more and better if the subject interests us
- Getting your hands dirty is part of the process. Ok! It's important to read how to install a new machine or repaint the living room but then you've got to get up and actually do it.
- Understand and accept the fact that failing is part of the learning process: it will take some trial and error before you succeed in getting things right!
- Practice makes perfect: research says that you have to "use" your new knowledge at least 7 times, in order to memorize the process.
- Learn to question yourself frequently, instead of always wanting to be right: When you disagree with someone, do a little research online or read to see whether the facts confirm or repudiate your line of thought… and then if you were wrong, admit it.
- Mimic: ever since you were a child you learned by observing and replicating. If you want to learn how to cook, garden, or play tennis, try to practice with someone who already knows the art and play copycat (You can also watch videos). Chances are key elements will be a lot easier to grasp than if you were only reading about them!

C. Things you might want to learn

Below, is a list of activities to choose from. Some can take as little as a few minutes each day, so why not try bringing more knowledge into your life:

- Enrich your vocabulary by learning new words every day and make sure to use them!
- Spend 30 min every day to improve or learn a language
- Learn a new computer skill (try to progress in Word, Excel, Powerpoint) everyday
- Learn a fact about the history of the world, start from prehistory and work your way up to today. You could also focus on the 90's to today or whatever period that interests you
- If you know your country's history, why not look into a specific historical event
- Learn one fact every day about your country's Geography and then move on to world geography
- If you love gardening, learn, read, watch videos to be even better at it!
- Eat something you have never eaten before every day: discover new flavors!
- Go around the world by making a dish from a different country every day and discovering the world's most famous recipes!
- Learn 7 new techniques (one each day) to improve your photos!
- Decide to learn new things about your sport: new techniques, new warm up and cool down exercises, check out some videos for new tips etc. For example, if you like to jump rope, you could watch videos to improve your technique, or you could learn new tricks or new things to make your jumping look really good!
- Watch 7 movies from a certain period or all the movies with a certain actor/actress
- Walk through a favorite part of your city with a map in hand (this might take more or less time depending of course on the size of your city). Highlight every street you have done with a marker and discover the streets, their names, the neighborhoods, the shops, the parks etc.
- Find out how 7 different things or objects are made (from how do make chocolate to how do you make a phone, you name it, the list is endless)

- Learn 7 different body parts (bones, muscles, vital parts) and find out how they function
- Find 7 facts about something you love, such as baseball, movies, politics, a person you admire or more generally read about something you feel passionate about
- Find out 7 ways to clean stuff (get rid of rust, grind, stains, mold or how to clean the floors, walls, windows, oven, furniture and get your house spic and span clean!
- Read about 7 different inventors and find out how they came up with the idea and how they eventually succeeded. How was Coca-Cola invented, the tin can, the bicycle, the first printer to print books, the camera and so on
- Read 7 biographies about people you admire. It doesn't have to be an entire book, you could read an article and watch a short video online about this specific person
- How about getting to know all the different plants, flowers and endemic animals that you can find where you live? Have a notebook and try to get a photo of each one and create a herbarium in which you collect the ones you found. The best thing is to obtain a book about local plants and animals or have a look online to see how to create a great herbarium. Every time you walk around, try to remember their names and what they are used for. My mother loved doing this and did it with natural curiosity. When you start looking into it, you will discover many interesting facts about plants, herbs, flowers and what they can be used for
- Watch documentaries, have a notebook and write three lines every day about what you learned
- Get a book about general knowledge and read it, one topic a day
- Buy an educative board game that teaches you geography or history or general knowledge such as trivial pursuit, a game in which you learn world flags etc.
- Do a puzzle of 1000 pieces of the world map and try to research about the different continents while you are putting it together
- Meditate and find something new about yourself every day
- Learn 7 things about religions and become more tolerant and understanding toward other people's beliefs
- Do a 7-day makeover in which you create new styles, new makeup, new hairdos
- Write poetry every day about 7 different topics. Start by doing a bit of research about the topic/object. Then do a vocabulary search that has to do with what you want to write about. Finally, write a poem
- Take a photo of yourself every day doing something new and then bind all of them together to create a flip book or get an app that makes them flash one after the other
- Create something different each day: bracelet, flower composition, a new dish, pottery, painting, drawing, finger painting, gardening, hairstyles, origami, table setting, house decorating, towel folding
- Learn 7 things you didn't know about that certain dream you wish to achieve and get seven steps closer to making it come true
- Learn 7 facts about a place / country you would like to visit. If you love Paris for example try to find out different facts about the city, different spots you would like to visit, restaurants you would like to try out. Experience it ahead of time. Buy a travel guide or a book about Paris. Look online for videos or blogs that you can explore

- Make the goal of doing 7 acts of kindness by giving some of your time, energy and strength. You don't have to do something incredible every day but be creative: help a neighbor, friend or a stranger, donate some money, sign up to serve meals to the homeless. Are you good at something? Do it for free just to help out others in need, sign up for a first aids course, propose reading stories to children or the elderly
- Learn the history of your town (visit all local historical points, museums, find out who are the important local people and what your town was like last century)
- Plan to visit as many art expositions, museums, concerts, churches, monuments that you can
- Play the license plate game. I found this game on Amazon. You have a little notebook with the stickers from every single state in America. Every time you see one from a certain state you get to stick it into the notebook. Try to learn a fact about that state that you didn't know about. I played this game with my kids in Florida. It is probably a lot easier to play it there than in any other state of the US due to the number of tourists that flock there on vacation.
- If you don't know America's 50 states, learn them… or learn one new country a day and find it on a map
- Take an imaginary trip around the world this week. Choose 7 countries you would like to visit and each day write a country down with its capital, population, political situation, see where it is and what it is famous for. Stick a photo in your notebook and then watch a short video about it or flip through a tourist guide
- Learn 7 different parts of your car, what they are for, how they work and how to fix or change them
- Have 7 different smoothies/juices this week and find out the benefits of various vegetables or fruits
- Play the TIMELINE game and learn to put historical dates in order. Learn at least 7 dates by heart and what they are relevant to

WORK SPACE

What have you decided to learn this week?

Your answer:_____

D. 7 Rings to learn 7 Different Things - Mapping Out Your New Knowledge

I recommend filling it out in advance and planning what you want to learn/read/watch ahead of time. You are free to improvise on a daily basis and fill it out once you have learned something new!

The idea this week is to enjoy being curious and finding pleasure in the learning process. I propose to learn one new thing a day, but the real goal is to get into the habit of learning new things every time you get the opportunity. When you don't know or don't understand something, simply take the time to research it. Knowledge isn't everything but look around and see how lucky we are to be surrounded by so much technology and information. Make the most of it. Pretty soon you will find it's incredibly fun and so enriching to learn new things every day. My thirst for knowledge makes my life so thrilling and exciting. Perhaps your school years made you feel differently but there truly is *joy in learning*.

7 RINGS to LEARN 7 Different Things

Today, I learned

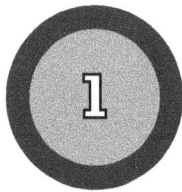

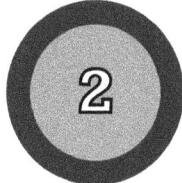

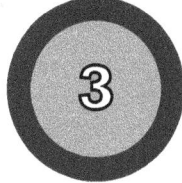

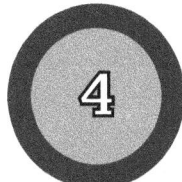

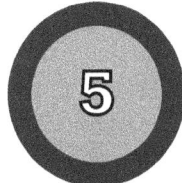

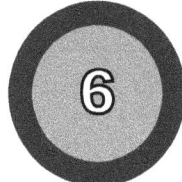

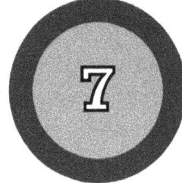

1

2

Today, I learned

Today, I learned

3

4

Today, I learned

Today, I learned

5

6

Today, I learned

Today, I learned

7

Change n°10
RESPECT YOURSELF

10.

At one point my adolescent son was going through a phase where he just didn't care about anything anymore: why bother washing myself? (The smell doesn't bother me!) Why bother cleaning up my room? (That's what artists are like, right?) Who cares about the way I dress? (What really counts is on the inside, isn't it?) Why bother eating healthy? (I'll just grab anything that is within reach when I'm hungry) What the F..ck? (Who cares about the way I speak?).

Every day the list just seemed to be getting longer and he appeared to be sinking in deeper and deeper into his "why bother" phase.

Just like my adolescent son, we all go through difficult phases throughout our life! But if you want to boost your self-esteem, the number one thing to look into is your very own self-respect and everything that it implies. We are often told to respect others: "One can do anything so long as it doesn't bother anybody else". But what about self-respect? Take two minutes to look at yourself in the mirror and ask yourself these questions:

- Do I respect myself?
- Do I eat right so that my body feels strong and healthy?
- Am I getting enough sleep?
- Do I exercise to make my body stronger, more flexible and more resistant?
- What image do I project on the outside? Does my image impose respect? Do I believe that I deserve other peoples' respect?
- Do I take care of myself? Do I dress properly? Do I pamper myself?

Respecting yourself implies a minimum prerequisite: that you dress properly, wash your body, hair and teeth, that your home be clean and orderly, that you nourish your body with healthy foods, that you engage in some form of exercise and that you get enough sleep. It seems pretty basic, but how many of us actually do it? And that's only part of the whole self-respect picture. What about how you think about yourself: do you have thoughts of appreciation or depreciation? Why don't you decide for an entire week to go all the way and everyday do something that shows some kind of respect towards yourself? Take the time to observe and see how you treat yourself, how you act, and think of yourself.

The first part of our exercise will show you different ways to respect yourself on the outside (in other words what's visible). Next, we will focus on respecting the parts that are invisible but equally important.

A. Respect Yourself On The Outside

A good idea to make sure that you do something every day, is to plan things ahead of time. Take your daily planner or calendar and plan your ideas in writing. Some of them might require an appointment, an ingredient, time and so on.

The best way to successfully reach your goal is to plan ahead. Make this week about you, pampering yourself, feeling better and happier. You are worth it! And remember something important: if you are happy, the people around you will benefit from it as well since you will be in a better mood and so much more confident.

a. A List of Ideas To Choose From

To help you prepare your week, you will find below a list of things that will help you feel better about yourself:

- Get your nails done (yes this is for guys as well!), have a friend help or do them yourself! If you don't know how, look online for tutorials and great ideas. No need to get all fancy: just a few clips, getting rid of excess skin and cleaning under the nails, a little bit of Ricin oil or hand cream and for the ladies a little bit of shine and you are good to go.
- Get your hair done or take the time to make it look nice. If you always wear a ponytail, try to see if you can make it look nice and neat. If your hair is the frizzy type, get yourself a hot brush to straighten it out. If your hair looks a little tired, start a vitamin treatment or apply a nourishing mask regularly to bring more vitality. For men, make sure your hair is clean and trimmed nicely.
- Trim your beard and make sure it looks nice
- Do a hair treatment. There are various oils and creams out there to beautify it. If you have dandruff, use a specific medicinal shampoo.
- Do a skin scrub to get rid of dead skin and get your blood circulating.
- Loofah (same benefits as a skin scrub).
- Get a facial or do one (makes your face look younger, makes your skin look radiant and healthy, clears pores, reduces the appearance of fine lines and wrinkles.)
- Get a haircut
- Soak in a nice hot bubble bath
- Get a massage or take turns giving one with husband/wife or a friend. No real need to tout the benefits: improves your overall wellbeing (as if a weight was taken off your shoulders) but it will also improve the quality of your sleep, reduce muscle pain, improve circulation and lymphatic drainage). So, indulge, no restrictions here.
- Get your teeth whitened professionally or buy a product and do it yourself. Start with a whitening toothpaste but there are also mouth pastes or techniques (such as brushing your teeth with baking soda). Nothing can beat a nice smile so make sure you light up every time you do!
- Apply mud or take a mud bath. They are loaded with minerals, soften your skin, make it look younger, relieve stress and detoxify your body. So, go get muddy!
- Get eyelash extensions. Before they were only used by stars, but today eyelash extensions are hot and anyone can get them done.
- Get your eyebrows done by a professional or look online and do it yourself.
- Take a cold shower or a hot/cold shower. (See benefits in the Chapter 3 Change n° 28 – Hot and Cold)
- If you are lucky enough to live by the ocean or the sea, go for a walk in the water, walk in up to your thighs and get your blood circulating.
- Rub your skin with coffee grounds. Try mixing coffee, coconut oil and sugar. Cover up your legs, buttocks and thighs and then wrap with cellophane for 15min. This technique is great for diminishing cellulite and makes your legs silky soft.

- Get your teeth cleaned or brush your teeth for over 5 minutes.
- Apply some cream or oil on your nails, hands, feet, hair, eyelashes, body. Nourish it all.
- Go for a run to get your heart pumping, your blood circulating and your body eliminating. Tonight, you'll sleep better.
- Take the time to dress nicely and see how the attitude people have towards you changes. It might seem unfair and superficial, but your appearance counts whether you like it or not.
- No swear words!!! Stop swearing. Yes! It is disrespectful to yourself and others.
- Be polite and respectful of others. A person who respects himself, respects others as well. Hold the doors, offer help, say "thank you", listen more and see how these little acts of kindness come right back at you and make you feel better about yourself.
- Stand tall: a person with self-respect is comfortable in their own shoes and proud of himself. We are not talking about being boastful but feeling confident. So, breathe deeply, lift your chest, raise your chin, pull your shoulders slightly backwards and SMILE! You are unique and that already is something to be proud of. What are you doing to make yourself a better person today?
- UVA: are you feeling tired in winter or when the weather is bad? Maybe you need a little sun. I am not really an adept, but in winter I'll occasionally enjoy one session. Getting an UVA session to soak up a bit of sun and give your body a little bit of a sunny glow might just be what you need.

**You get the idea:
find things that make you feel good about yourself
and set out to do them.**

7 RINGS to IMPROVE 7 Different Things

Today, I improved

1

Today, I improved

2

Today, I improved

3

Today, I improved

4

Today, I improved

5

Today, I improved

6

Today, I improved

7

B. Respect Yourself on the Inside

- Have a colon cleanse
- Make sure you are hydrated: go drink some water now
- Do a vitamin or a magnesium regimen
- Have a veggie or fruit drink
- Make sure you eliminate every day
- Neti (nasal cleaning)
- Massage your intestines to activate elimination
- Have a meditation session and focus on internal organs. I like to go over one organ after the other starting with the pelvic floor muscles and then working my way up toward the intestines, the stomach, the lungs and the heart. I contract and relax the part I am focusing on while breathing deeply, a bit like Kegel exercises except that I don't hold the contraction and that it feels more like I am internally massaging the part that I am working on. When you reach the heart and lungs let the air you breathe in do the massaging. Feel your lungs and then your heart expand slowly and deeply.
- Quit drinking coffee and alcohol
- Get plenty of Sleep
- Find a diuretic tea. I enjoy drinking Hibiscus. It's a natural diuretic that also prevents the body from getting rid of potassium. I like to buy the variety that has a mixture of dried flowers, seeds and leaves. I will have one tablespoon for one cup (or 3 for a big jug) and contrary to most people, I will pour cold water over it. I will let it infuse 2 or 3 hours or overnight in the fridge. It's a refreshing and actually a natural sweet tasting drink. *Note that I don't pour boiling water over it: I just find that once a food is cooked or heated, it loses part of its nutrients. But this infusion is also delicious hot.*
- Create your very own homemade fruit drink: cut slices of oranges, lemons, apples, strawberries or any fruit that you like and place them in a jug. Add water and place it in the fridge for few hours: you will get a delicious drink that's a change from water with added flavor and vitamins!
- Eat a light and healthy meal
- Close your eyes and pray
- Laugh with a friend (watch a funny movie).
- Spend a little bit of time alone to see what you think about yourself. Are you self-deprecating? Focus on your strenghts. If you find yourself thinking negatively, why not create your very own P.E.T. to help you (check out Change n° 5 *Create Your Very Own P.E.T.* and get back on the positive track of life!

Change n°11
LOVE MORE

11.

What if the answer to your happiness came from giving more and making others happy? What if life wasn't about reaching certain goals like being fit, landing that dream job or being financially secure? What if we had it all wrong and we should only focus on LOVE?

When was the last time you cuddled up with someone or received a real hug? Research has demonstrated that being held for a few seconds relieves stress, brings back confidence, helps you get through painful situations and makes you feel better. When hugging, subtle energy is transferred and gives you an emotional lift. Simply knowing that someone really cares enough to give you a hug can go a long way.
You might be thinking: "But I am not much of a hugger". That's O.K. There are many other ways of bringing love into other people's lives, without necessarily touching them. However, if the opportunity arises, I really recommend giving one. It's one of those things that once you give it a try, you'll usually adopt it! So, this week why don't you decide to engage in altruistic behavior and give more love to those around you.

Give and you shall receive.

How many times have I heard: "The wheel turns: give and you will reap the benefits". Most people firmly believe that if they do good things, eventually, good things will come their way. This quote or belief really got me thinking, and I have a problem with it. I don't give in order to get something in return. I believe that the "giving" in itself *is* the gift. The act of giving makes me feel good about myself: indeed, what a reward to see the other person happy! Giving is a gift because you are making this world a better place. So, give without expecting, because it makes you a better person for it.
In life, we all get our share of joys and hardships. Indeed, life "happens" to all of us, whether good or bad, things come our way but every time there is a lesson to be learnt.

Being nice is no guarantee that nothing bad will happen to us. You might then question the fact that if you won't reap any benefits, what's the point of being kind?
The point is the following: the day will come when you'll live through your last moment on Earth and if you are lucky, you might have a few minutes to reflect and look back upon your entire life. What do you want your last thoughts to be? I know what *I* want *mine* to be. As Ghandi once said: "My life is my message". What message am I leaving behind? Have I tried to make my dreams come true? Have I been there for my loved ones? Was I respectful of others? Did I contribute to bringing happiness to this world? Think about it. What would your last thoughts be? And then, start living accordingly. One thing is certain, I want to live my life to its fullest, learn as much as possible, accomplish many things and also share more love and joy with those that are around me.

A. 35 Ways To Spread More Love

So, all this got me thinking in what ways could one bring more love into other people's lives. Hugs are a good way to start, but there are many other ways of giving. You can:

- Volunteer your time.
- Donate money or give to charities.
- Make someone happy by complimenting them. Call, send a text or say it when the opportunity arises.
- Send a kind text to let someone know you care, tell them to have a nice day and encourage them in their pursuits.
- Leave a little something, a candy, chocolate, a note or a little present for someone.
- Call a friend to see how they are and listen. Be there, give them your undivided attention.
- Give unused items to someone on the streets. A good idea is to have a bag in the trunk of your car with the stuff you no longer use or need and you wish to donate. When you come across someone in need, hand it over and make their day!
- Make love with your special someone. Decide to make love more often, make the time for it and make it special. Or surprise them by making it clear they are desired.
- Give time, attention and compliments to those you love (husband/wife, children, mother, friends). Who do we unload all of our problems on? When we are with certain people we tend to empty our stress on them because we know we can be ourselves in their company. Keep in mind that *they* are your loved ones and that *they* deserve your time, attention and love.
- Listen to others. Be quiet and willingly become all ears: 100% and no judging, please.
- Create your own charity. Is there a way you can do something for your neighborhood or neighbors? Do it. Is there something you have always wanted to do that is kind? Do it today. Is someone in your neighborhood in need or going through difficult times? Offer to help.
- I used to work at a gym in Monte-Carlo and the owner Guy Mierczuk, died from cancer. The day I saw the sign with his name taken down, I was so sad. I remembered how many times I had taken the flight of stairs to access his gym. One day, I noticed that these stairs had no name. I decided to write to City Hall to see if it was possible to have the staircase named after him. Unfortunately, they refused but I am so glad to have, at least, tried. I miss you Guy Mierczuk.
- Create a help or support group. I remember after I had just given birth to my second child, it was a real challenge to go training. We don't have gyms with day care centers where I live, so you basically have to either find a friend who will take care of your child or hire a babysitter. It was challenging to get my training done. And that's how I came up with the idea to create a mother's group that would meet every day for two hours. The first hour, one group of mothers would go workout while the others would take care of the kids and then they would swap the second hour. The training was free, no babysitters required. It was a great idea to get your workout done without the hassle of finding someone to take care of your children.
- Be more forgiving. Forgive someone today that normally you wouldn't.
- Give away something that is valuable to you. I remember when I was at the University, one of my professors told us that when he bought his new car, he decided to place an ad in the paper to *give* his old car away. He actually waited a few days before anyone called. Finally, a student did call and asked: "Are you really giving your car away? What's wrong with it?"

My professor found it very amusing and replied: "Nothing is wrong with it. I can do without the money and I just felt like making someone happy by giving it away." Believe me, I am sure that this kid is still talking about my professor to this day.

- Donate blood, platelets… an organ.
- Designate to donate your organs in writing in case of an accident.
- Give some of your time to entertain the elderly in a home for seniors. Do you have a certain talent? Singing, sewing, reading? Plan to give a bit of your time to make these people happy.
- Make the decision to not interrupt someone today and be fully present. Make sure, when you are listening to them, to turn off your cell phone and to leave it in your bag: make that person feel special, give them your undivided attention. We often feel the need to brag about our own problems…not today. Let this other person have their moment of attention.
- Send a quote to a friend that reflects how this person is feeling or can help, by making them reflect upon their situation.
- Let someone go ahead of you while waiting in line today.
- Set a few minutes aside to relax with the goal to release anger, forgive, give love, receive love, establish peace. What emotion is taking over you? Feel, embrace and release it!
- Next time someone speaks to you in a mean way, breathe and try not to get upset (stay calm and in control).
- Say "hello" more often to the people you meet. You may find this a surprising point but in many cities around the world people completely ignore each other. Try opening up by smiling and saying hello.
- Remember a moment when you were at total peace, shut your eyes and relive that moment NOW.
- Find your inner sanctuary and go there whenever possible. (Inner Sanctuary is that place within you where you come in contact with your inner self!)
- Take the time to forgive someone by writing it down on paper. If there is an apology you never received, take the time to accept that fact: Life becomes easier when you cease to expect an apology you never got.
- If someone near you is sick, offer to accompany them to chemotherapy, radiotherapy, or to the doctors. Let them know you are there.
- Do you feel anger, impatience and pain inside your being? The minute you are aware of it, place your hand on your heart or stomach, or clasp your hands, close your eyes…and ask for inner peace and love.
- Make someone laugh: send a joke, a funny picture, video or comment.
- In India there is a forgiveness day called HOLI. Why don't you have one of your own. Go out and make a little fire and burn all your negative emotions, pains, and mistakes. Use this ritual to forgive and ask forgiveness. Have your HOLI day.
- Identify something that really annoys you with your partner and address it today: either talk them or decide to accept it and deal with it. Is there something they would be willing to do to make things better, why not in another area? The goal is to try and bring a certain balance into your union. As an example: your partner might not feel up to helping you with household chores but is willing to take the kids out, for you to have some free time. Try to find a deal between you two and create a win-win situation.

- Transform your commuting or transportation time into a time to attain more inner peace (listening to a relaxation CD, podcast). If you are on the bus, close your eyes and relax.
- Create a LoveBox: every day write a little love note for someone in your life and place it in the LoveBox. Wish them well, forgive them, say "I love you", wish healing or ask for forgiveness…
- Write a Wish letter and send it off to the Universe. I actually write one, put my address on the envelope, bring it to the Post Office, get it stamped and have it sent. I like the idea that it is being handled, travelling and moving forward. When I find it in my letterbox, it always makes me smile and serves as a reminder.
- Tell yourself: I Love you. Take some time today to nurture yourself. Write down your qualities and what makes you a wonderful person.

B. The Benefits of Giving or Why giving is better than receiving?

In this second part, we are going to see why giving is better than receiving and what are the benefits you get from giving more.

- You will make someone smile and happy
- You will feel happy and better about yourself
- Giving, relieves stress. When taking care of others, you forget about your problems and focus on someone or something else
- When giving to someone you create a special lasting bond with them. Most people don't forget a gesture of kindness especially when it comes without expecting anything in return. Chances are that one day they will be there for you when you need it too.
- If you give more, people will perceive you as being a "Nice" person.
- Being generous boosts your self-esteem because you feel better about yourself.
- Giving has a ripple effect: make someone happy and they will be in a good mood and will in turn communicate their happiness to others. When happy, people tend to give more willingly. Be the first one to start the ripple and watch it ricochet.
- Why don't you decide with your spouse to take turns giving and receiving?
- Did you receive some love, a present, someone's time today? Make plans to give it back.
- When you give, you tend to feel useful and needed, which makes you feel better about yourself.
- Volunteering allows you to learn something new. Learning fills you up. I have always been thirsty for knowledge and seize every opportunity I get to learn something new. It's as if you were watering a plant or a flower and would watch it thrive and grow. Participating in charity events, the Red Cross or other associations allows you to learn new skills, enabling you to put things back into perspective.

- By volunteering in your community, you will get to meet new people, create a bond and a sense that you are part of a family.
- When going through tough times, it often helps to see people who are worse off than you.
- When you are a kind person, others will be motivated to become more like you and will see you as a role model, especially your children.

C. About giving and receiving

Everybody knows it, but I will take the time to remind you of two things in regards to giving and receiving:

- When you are the one receiving learn to be more generous in your return by letting the "giver" feel special and appreciated. We often don't know how to receive a present or a compliment. We downsize it. When someone has taken the time to get you a present or is complimenting you, don't just brush it off. Appreciate it, accept it completely, worship it, be grateful and thank them as they deserve. Receiving properly is an art that often needs to be acquired.
- When giving, don't forget that you want to make someone happy, not yourself. So, when choosing a gift or doing something for someone, keep the other person's tastes and desires in mind (not yours !!!).

D. Try My "Flow" or "Give – Receive – Let it Flow" Meditation!

a. My story

It might not be the case for everyone, but I know that for years I loved to give, never expecting anything in return because that's how it felt right in my heart. But then one day, as I was doing my "Give Love" meditation, a beautiful sensation and a bright light came over me and I realized it was love in return. It dawned on me, at that moment, that I had always shut a certain door. I had seen love going in only one direction, with no possibility to go back. It had always been a one-way street. I thought about that and knew that I was on to something important for my personal growth: love needs to circulate back and forth. Just like my breath. As I inhale, I take and as I exhale, I give. I had to accept to receive love in return. I don't know whether it had come from low self-esteem or if it was just because I hadn't been used to getting anything in return, but I just never expected to get anything. And so, I sat there a little stunned by this discovery. For some of you, this might be and probably is totally evident, but it had never been for me. I understood that I needed to open a certain door, unlatch an invisible valve and that I, too, was allowed to receive.

Just as every child, when I grew up, I had this thirst for recognition: I needed attention, compliments and love to thrive and I desperately tried over and over again to get it. It never came. I got into this habit of always trying to make my mother happy and proud of me, but never succeeded. But today, I wonder, who knows: maybe she was proud. Maybe I was too thirsty or I misread the signs. Maybe my mother just didn't know how to express how she felt. My mother never or only on rare occasions received love when she was a child and having to raise her two daughters, only 10 ½ months apart, on her own in the 1960's – 70's was an everyday struggle and challenge.

So, I don't wish to criticize or downsize what she must have endured to bring us up. I take this opportunity to thank you "Maman", for everything you have done for me. My mother is also a very bright woman and I always found, that it was hard for me, to level up. I always felt as though I was a disappointment and that she was ashamed of me as a daughter. I also felt as though, without me and my sister, she could have had an easier life. Maybe she could have met someone and finally received a bit of love.

As I have mentioned before, we were not a religious family but in one of our numerous moves, we settled down in the town of Sudbury, Canada and rented out a nice house on a lake. My sister and I shared bunk beds. I had the bottom one and I recall a prayer that was stuck on the wall facing me every night as I went to sleep. I still remember most of the words today:

A Child's Bedtime Prayer

Now I lay me down to sleep.
I pray the Lord, my soul to keep.
If I should die before I wake,
I pray to God my soul to take.
If I should live for other days,
I pray the Lord to guide my ways.

Father, unto thee I pray,
Thou hast guarded me all day;
Safe I am while in thy sight,
Safely let me sleep tonight.
Bless my friends, the whole world bless;
Help me learn helpfulness;
Keep me every in thy sight;
So to all I say good night

I recall that I would pray that someone would come and take me away, someone who would want me, someone, who I felt, would be happy to have me. I prayed and prayed but it never happened. Then one night, as I lay there, it dawned on me that I was being selfish: that prayers were not meant to make dreams come true. Praying was an act of Love and I had obviously gotten the whole thing all wrong. A prayer wasn't meant for asking but for spreading love. And so, from then on, I prayed differently asking for my mother to be happy and to finally get the love she deserved. As I look back today, I realize however, that I still had it all wrong, because in doing so, I had denied myself the right to receive love.

b. The Flow Meditation

Today, I enjoy meditating once or several times during the day. Most of the time, it's always the same process: I choose to do, what I call, my "Flow meditation" or "Give, Receive, Flow Meditation."

If you would like to give it a try, it's very simple, anybody can do it and it doesn't require years of practice to reap the benefits.

You can do it sitting or lying down, but it's also interesting doing it while standing up. I find it powerful this way. You might like to do it while out in nature, but you can also do it standing in front of a mirror. It can be done with your eyes open or closed. Breathe in and out quietly and try to relax until your mind and body are calm. Breathe in deeply through the nose, filling up your lungs and exhale through the nose or mouth; whatever feels more comfortable. Remember: no rules.

Phase 1: Give love. Imagine yourself with arms open wide. You can actually stand up and hold your arms wide open, chest open, head slightly tilted back also in an open position. Imagine giving love. Feel the love inside you and give all of it to the world. Continue to breathe slowly and enjoy the act of giving love. Keep spreading out love for a few minutes.

Phase 2: Receive love. This time, imagine that the world, the entire universe, is sending you love. Open up to receive it all. Breathe in, breathe out and, all the while, feel love overcoming you completely. Accept it. Keep taking in love for a few minutes.

Phase 3: Let love flow. Finally, let it all go. Just let love flow. Maybe at first, you will find it easier to go back and forth, alternately giving and receiving. But at one point, just let love be. Feel how love is there, how it is simply everywhere. Remain in this state for a few minutes or as long as you wish.
Slowly come out of the meditation. Try to keep this sensation of "being in love" as long as possible. During the day, to calm down or when in need of comfort, try to reconnect with this feeling and subtle sensation of love.

c. A special Note on Heartbreaks
When I was heartbroken, I found myself with all this love on my hands and in my heart and not being able to give it to that special someone anymore. What does one do, when one has so much love to give and yet no one to give it to? Heartbreaks are painful. I remember my Aunt Tonie telling me, that out of all the pains she had endured, heartbreak and love lost had been the hardest thing to overcome in her life. Let's face it, losing the one you love can feel like the end of the world. It leaves you feeling as though you are dead inside and lost on the outside.
This flow meditation has truly helped me in these times of great pain. One day, as I lay there, crying my heart out, I decided that I wouldn't let this love of mine go to waste. I refused to let it turn into hatred. For me, even while rejected, this feeling of love was beautiful and I didn't want to just "get rid of it." In fact, I realized that the hardest part in breaking up was the idea that I didn't want to let go of something so beautiful. So, at different moments during each day, I would lie down or stand up and give all this overflowing love I had, back to the universe. Sometimes, I would direct it to certain people, including the person who had left me, but most of the time, I just gave it all away freely. It made me happy inside to know that I had spread out my love for him, like seeds to the whole world. I actually have an image that often comes to mind when I do it: it's like blowing on dandelions. Blow and let your love flow. I would always take a few extra minutes to receive love and then to let it go, let it flow back and forth and then just be.If any of you are going through a heartbreak, I truly hope this meditation can help you get past the pain and return peace into your heart again, as it did for me.

Change n°12
YOUR COMMERCIAL

12.

How does a commercial work? Commercials are played over and over again, brainwashing you in order to make you buy a certain product. Whether you believe in it or not, it's proven that it works. For this reason, I came up with the idea of creating my very own commercial; one in which I would try to "sell myself" and after, watch it over and over again.

Since commercials have a proven influential effect over your brain, it might be a good idea to create your own commercial in which you focus on your past: show your successes and all you have achieved, your qualities such as outgoing personality, generosity, your various inventions and specialties. You could also create a second one where you focus on how you see yourself in the future. You are successful, self-confident, going into your dream home or driving your favorite car.

Both these commercials will have the same positive effect on you: They will boost your self-esteem either by reminding you of all your qualities and accomplishments, or letting you imagine your possible future.

A. How to make your commercial?

a. Find out what message you want to bring forth:

First, decide what you want to talk about. Ask yourself: what is it that you wish to put forward and what is the best way of doing it?

- Your accomplishments: your medals, your diplomas,
- What you are good at: drawing, skating, singing, helping others,
- Your story. This can be your incredible life story or a chapter in it that you wish to talk about
- Your personality. Perhaps you love to be around other people or on the contrary you are very private. Maybe you are a fighter, you love to laugh, you are demanding of others and yourself, you are a self-made person or you are very organized,
- Who do you wish to become? This can be anyone from a model, an actor, a successful business man, opening your very business, becoming a life coach, a chef, a writer...

b. Write your Script

The next step is to get it all down in writing. A commercial is relatively short: anywhere from 15, 30 or 60 seconds. It is up to you to decide how long you want your commercial to be. The goal is to have fun. If you don't have any ideas, have a look online as there are millions of tutorials for video ideas or editing. This commercial will not be publicly broadcasted so feel free to copy an idea and use it to your advantage as you don't need to worry about getting permits or asking for authorizations. This is for your sole private use.

Some ideas for getting your script together:
- Watch a few of your favorite commercials to get some ideas
- Lay out your script "comic strip style": in each box you can detail everything: how you are dressed, what is happening, the music, the dialog, how the scene is filmed.
- Remember: the simpler, the better. Don't drown your commercial by putting too much dialog or too many details. Make sure, that the background is not too "crammed" with objects or people as you want to keep the focus on "you" and not on what is going on around or behind you.
- In your script, remember to detail how the scene will be filmed: close up, will the camera be coming in closer or following you?
- Remember to choose your music. Avoid putting your favorite song on; make sure the piece you choose has to do with what you are trying to "sell".
- Try to put some humor or an element of surprise in your commercial.
- The best commercials are the ones that tell a story: try to come up with one.

Below you will find several examples:
Example 1: If you are an athlete and you want to move your "journey" forward, you can flash a few photos of yourself over the years showing how hard you have trained and what you have accomplished. Finish with a few seconds where we can see you training today and showing great athletic skill, camaraderie as well as a moment of exultation. Have a voice-over, instead of a dialog, in which the voice talks about your accomplishments. For example: "Alexia, today 23 years old, has been training consistently since the age of 5 and has participated in numerous competitions in her state and across the country. Her determination and her consistency have allowed her to receive an award in 2014. Her smile and her sense of camaraderie have earned her the esteem of her entire team." You can have one of your teammates say a few words in your favor and then finish it off with a slogan: "I work hard and make my dreams come true!" or "I believe and I succeed!" or "You thought that was cool, wait and see what's coming next!"

Example 2: You can create a sort of "news story": Have a friend be the presenter and have him interview you; you are the guest in a talk show, for example. What's good about doing it this way is that you won't come out as being too boastful since the presenter is the one complementing your hard work and your achievements.
- You can flash images of yourself in action, each photo representing one message you would like to convey about yourself. You can focus on your biggest achievement or goal you are working towards.
- Choose a tag line, punch line or slogan that represents who you are or who you wish to become and say it with conviction.

c. Recording Your Commercial
Try filming the same scene several times from different angles.
Are you going to film indoors or outdoors? Keep in mind weather conditions, sun exposure, light, darkness and noise, such as cars or construction work.
Are you going to film in color or in black and white?
Remember that sound is important. It might be worth the investment to have a small microphone pinned onto your clothing when you are talking.

Lighting is also super important as you can come out looking tired or fantastic. Try filming at different angles and with different lightings and move the light around until you get it right.

If you have the money or are willing to save up for it, you could consider hiring an ad agency. This way you are sure of the quality and you won't have the hassle of organizing, filming or editing it.

d. Editing your commercial

The best way is to use "imovie", "movie maker" or another movie app. Before choosing which one to take, it might be a good idea to watch some tutorials on you tube to see which one suits your needs the most.

The purpose of this commercial is to boost your self-esteem. You are taking the time to acknowledge, promote and highlight your past and present successes - or if you are focusing on the future, the goals you wish to achieve. As we are often hard on ourselves it might be a good idea to have a friend help you with the whole process. Having an opinion and feedback from someone who genuinely admires you, can make a huge impact on the outcome of your commercial. Remember: you are unique! Don't downplay your accomplishments. Be proud of who you are, of your past successes and have faith in your future. Put conviction in what lies ahead and all that has yet to come.

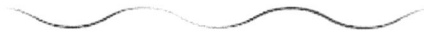

LETTER OF COMMITMENT

By committing in writing what you have decided to accomplish within a predetermined period of time, you increase the likelihood that you will act accordingly. Signing a Letter of Commitment can have a real impact on the outcome of your goal, especially if you have someone close to you sign as a witness.

STEP 1: DECIDE

Week n°_____   Start Date: _____   Finish Date: _____

I, _____, have set out to accomplish
(your name)
Change n°_____

STEP 2: INPUT YOUR PLAN OF ACTION

To increase my chances of success, I agree to make time every single day to **work on Improving** *(input your plan of action)*:
_____
_____

STEP 3: LIST THE BENEFITS

I understand that this binding agreement I have with myself is geared towards helping me focus on _____ and I am confident of its positive outcome.
In one week, I will feel **so much more**_____ and
_____

STEP 4: SIGN AND COMMIT

Rewrite the following *"I have read and fully agree to this Letter of Commitment"* below:

_____

Signature _____ Date _____

Witness _____ Date _____

MY NOTES

_____

_____

_____

_____

_____

_____

_____

_____

_____

_____

_____

_____

_____

_____

_____

_____

IMPROVE YOUR RELATIONSHIP WITH FOOD

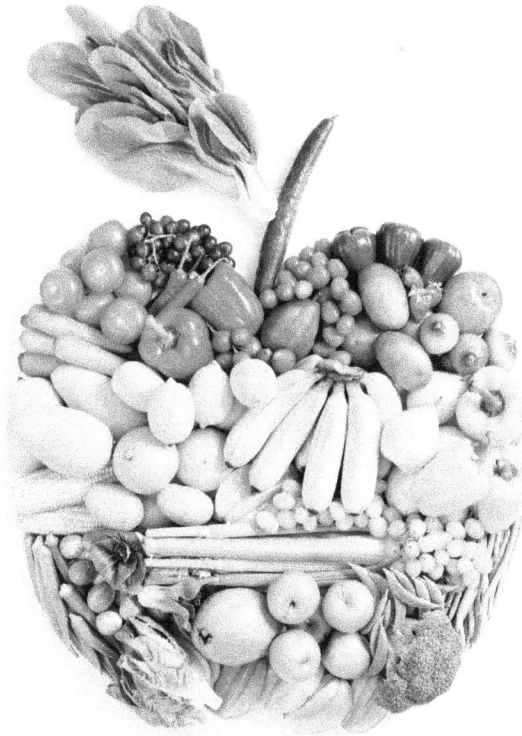

*They were just thoughts
that danced through my little head…
about Relationships.*

Let's play a Japanese psychological game together. I will ask you six questions. Your answers must be as spontaneous as possible. Don't waste your time overthinking any of them. There is no right or wrong answer.

Question n° 1: You are walking in the desert. There is nothing around you but dunes, sand and the sky. You have been walking for a while now when, all of a sudden, you see a cube. Describe this cube? How big or small is it and what is it made of?

Question n°2: You were so busy looking at the cube that you hadn't noticed that there was also a ladder. Can you describe it: what is made of? How long is it? Where is it situated?

Question n°3: You were about to go on your way when you notice a horse. Now, take a moment to describe the horse. What is it doing?

Question n°4: Stop for a second and imagine a flower. Yes, there are flowers in the desert. How many do you see? Where are they?

Question n°5: You have been in the desert for a while now and you are famished. Is it a mirage or reality? I don't know, but there is a table and chair right in front of you with food on it. What food do you see? What do you do?

Question n°6: Final question. You look towards the horizon and you can see a storm coming. It's going to be a huge desert storm. What do you do?

<u>The interpretation of your answers:</u>

Interpretation of question n°1: The cube represents your ego. In other words, seeing a big cube would mean you think highly of yourself or are self-confident, whereas seeing a small one would mean that you are rather shy or maybe lack a little bit of self-confidence.

Interpretation of question n°2: the ladder represents the relationship you have with your friends. Is the ladder against your cube or on its own? It could either mean that you count on their support or are independent. Depending on whether it is over, under or at your level, the ladder could reveal your rapport with your friends: either superior, inferior or your equal.

Interpretation of question n°3: The horse represents your love relationship. Some see a wild horse running freely while others see a horse with a saddle and tied up to a post. It could reveal a lot about how you envision that special someone.

Interpretation of question n°4: the flowers represent your relationship with your children, or the children you might have some day. Are they close to your cube or distant? Are there many flowers? What kind of flowers?

Interpretation of question n°5: *Normally this game doesn't have a question n°5 but since this chapter is about changing our relationship with food, I had the idea that it might be interesting to add it to this game. What will you see on your plate? What kind of food would be readily available? What does the table look like? What are you going to do: will you sit down and eat? Is the table beautifully set? It might bring clues that could reveal your relationship with food.*

Interpretation of question n°6: It tells you how you face fear or problems. Do you climb the ladder and reach out to friends, go on the horse's back and seek the support from your lover? What is your natural reaction?

Years ago, someone asked me these same questions. I won't bore you with all my answers but I wanted to share with you that when I was asked how I would react to the oncoming storm, I replied: "I would duck down, roll into a ball and wait for the storm to pass."
I remember my questioner replied: "But it's a huge sandstorm. You can't just stay there…"
And I answered: "You said to be spontaneous, and if the storm is really huge, I think there is no way that I could run fast enough to get away and avoid it."

I like this game because it makes you stop and think. As I am writing these words, I have just been through a big thunderstorm in my life. All is ok now, but as I look back to see how I tackled the problem, I can't help recalling this game and my answers. You see, after a year and a half of difficult times that included cancer and divorce, I am finally settled in my new home and expect good times ahead.

Instead, I wake up one morning to find a lump in my left breast and I wonder: has that bump been there before? Maybe… but I know deep down inside that it wasn't. Shit! That's the first thing that comes to mind. As I had been through this before, I stood there helpless and wondered: "Could it be happening again?"

First things first, however. I have to go see the doctor. I decide to walk to my doctor's office, it's about a 40min walk. All the while, I am questioning myself: "Should I go? I could turn back. What's the rush?" But somehow my feet seem to move forward and I reach my gynecologist's office. The doctor confirms a lump.

I step outside. The cars. The noise. The people. All is buzzing around me. I am not. I feel like I am floating. I feel like I have to catch a train but it's not stopping to let me get on board. Train, please slow down! I can't run just now. I don't have the strength. Somehow, I reach my office. I tell myself: "No one must know". I put myself in zombie mode and work or do what I can. I am in shock. Colleagues are talking to me, but I am not really listening. I can hear myself talking, laughing. Can they see my distress? Paul Klee said: "One eye sees, the other feels." I guess not. I am thinking that I have to make all these appointments for mammography, scan and so on. And then I will have to wait, wait, wait for the results.

Stop BB. I take a few minutes to question myself: "How do I feel?" My answer: "I am terrorized."

I tell myself: "I'll call a friend. According to the game, it would mean climbing up the ladder or maybe I'll reach out to my boyfriend and choose to "ride my horse". I need to talk. Maybe they can help me climb out of this inferno going on in my mind.

Stop BB. Think.

Why do I want to call them? To help relieve my pain? It hits me that this pain is like a bundle or toxic mass I am holding onto. Talking would be like getting rid of it. I'll just see someone, hand them the bundle and relieve myself from all this pain and fear.

Sure, I will get it off my chest, but then it will be on them. And the more I thought about it, the more it sounded like a cruel choice. In what way will letting them know make it easier for me? In knowing that they care and love me? It will just ruin their day. What's the point of having both of us in pain? If I keep it to myself, there will be only one person suffering: *me*. And then I tell myself that maybe the results will be fine and I would have stressed them all, for nothing.

BB, Stop. Think.

Remember the first time around. When people knew: the concerned looks. Remember those moments when "the thought of cancer" had slipped out of your mind and a sweet text message would arrive saying: "I hope you are ok. I am thinking of you." And "it" would all come back to mind again.

I recall feeling like a ball and chain. I don't want to be that ball and chain again that people feel they have to drag along. I don't want to be dragged. I don't want to be a drag.

Then I start imagining how my death or cancer might affect others. And the negative thoughts start flowing in. Why I am doing this?

Stop. Stop. Stop.

"Why this temptation to feel sorry for myself? Why imagine that the worst is yet to come?"

I guess I need to feel that I matter, that if I left, it would make a difference, that I am loved. Oh, and I must prepare myself: if the results reveal a cancerous tumor, I totally need to be prepared. I don't want to collapse in front of the doctor when she gives me the diagnosis. So, I start thinking negative thoughts again, because I need to be prepared, you see.

"BB, do you really want to do this right now? Is this the way you want to handle the situation? No…You are downright grotesque. Get over yourself BB."

I finally stop.

I remember closing my eyes and leaning back against the wall. Slowly, I let myself slide down to the floor and clasp my legs. My phone rings: it's a friend. A text message chimes: it's my boyfriend. I don't answer and I remember thinking: "I hope you'll understand and excuse me but I think I need to be alone for a while."

The way I see it, storms are not just obstacles that need to be overcome, they also come with a message. Life is constantly sending us lessons but it's up to us to decide whether we want to acknowledge them or not.

For this reason, it's very important to start off by observing yourself to see how you are tackling things. Instead of feeling sorry for yourself, try to constantly keep in mind that now is an opportunity to learn things about yourself and that it's a time to grow.

To help you through this process, question yourself to know why you might have "received this problem." Sometimes, the message will be crystal clear but at other times you will need to repeatedly ask yourself "What's the message behind all of this?" over the course of several days before nailing the right answer.

Self-observation is essential in all aspects of our life and it holds true for your relationship with food as well.
Before reading this second chapter, I would like to share a few words to help you understand how I overcame my struggle with food. Although never overweight, I do understand that eating isn't just "nourishing a body when it's hungry". There is a strong emotional factor involved and this is clearly what needs to be addressed. So, instead of trying the latest diet, why not take the time to slow down, get to know yourself and finally understand the underlying cause of your emotional link towards food.

They were just thoughts
that danced through my little head…
about my relationship with Food

The way I see it, we arrive on Earth with a set of tools: a body, a mind, a heart and it's up to us to decide whether we are the ones to control these tools or whether we are going to let *them* control us. It's one of our most important lessons: our body, mind and heart are like our children and we must learn to love them but also be firm; give them a little bit of tough love.

As I mentioned just above, the very first step to master self-control is to observe yourself.

It's time to eat: Are you going to overeat? Will you be at peace with your plate or will you let greed decide? You choose.
Someone is annoying you: Will you be impatient and become aggressive or will you breathe in deeply and keep your calm? It's up to you.
You see your girlfriend talking to a good-looking guy: you start feeling insecure. Will you see the situation for what it is, just someone talking to your girlfriend or will you let jealousy set in and allow your emotions to completely overwhelm you? You decide.

Take a few minutes to look at your body. Every minute of every day you can decide if you are going to handle it with care: Are you going to feed it properly? Are you going to keep it in shape? Are you going to listen to what it has to say? Normally, each and every one of us is born healthy. Although eating is a necessity – indeed, if we don't eat we die – right from day one, an emotional link is created: you are hungry, you become irritated, you cry, and your mother or father takes you in their arms, offers some food and you immediately feel so much better.

Eating becomes a moment of relief, a moment when you receive food in addition to attention and love. Right from birth this relationship with food is instilled in us. That special bond remains and when we are stressed, sad or in need of love it becomes a reflex to reach out for something to eat: it has worked in the past and we know for sure that it will make us feel better.

Although our parents, our culture and how we feel inside are factors that will influence the way we eat, as we grow up, we must take full responsibility of the way we are. Indeed, if we want to change our relationship with food and our bodies, we must stop blaming the outside world and acknowledge the fact that *we* are the ones to put the food in our mouths, *we* are the ones to choose what and how much we eat, *we* are the ones to decide whether we are going to be active or not. Accepting responsibility is the very first step in this whole process of changing our relationship with food.

Although I have never been fat, I have struggled for many years – a real roller coaster ride – to be at peace with my plate and my eating habits. I knew what food was bad for me, such as chips, wine, candy, chocolate bars, just as I knew the healthier choices. Nevertheless, I spent years bouncing back and forth between a state frustration – because I denied myself the right to eat the food I wanted – or guilt – because I ate some junk. I stayed in this pattern, until one day it occurred to me that frustration was a negative emotion and that forcing myself to do something I didn't want to, was only setting me up for failure. I thought about this: I loved food and really enjoyed eating but it was clear to me that I had an unhealthy relationship with my plate and that I was not tackling this situation the right way. I understood that eating should be a pleasant and peaceful experience. For this reason, I decided to stop fighting and began eating exactly what I wanted, when I wanted, without feeling guilty.

Don't think that I began to eat all day long and shifted to a diet that essentially consisted of eating junk food. Absolutely not, but something had clicked inside my mind and it became absolutely clear to me that a healthy and balanced diet wasn't just the choice of foods I ate... my emotions, obviously, also played an important part in the whole process. It was clear that I had to appreciate the entire experience when I ate and that I had to savor every bite.

Pleasure and joy are necessary ingredients if you wan to succeed in having a healthy relationship with food.

Now, being allowed to eat exactly what I wanted and able to do it totally guilt free turned out to be a big turning point in my life. It marked a 360° shift in my diet and how I envisioned food. The years that followed, were filled with learning, trial and error. I kept pushing forward with confidence, convinced that I was on the right path and that, with time, I would be eating a totally balanced and healthy diet. To strengthen my determination, something became quite clear: I needed to read about nutrition in order to become more conscious about what I was consuming. I started checking labels, reading books and researching.

Indeed, becoming more knowledgeable about food in general, made me aware of certain intolerable facts and there came a point when I could no longer eat certain foods: my conscience just wouldn't allow it. Knowledge has most definitely helped me on my path to a healthier diet. Since my goal was to eat an essentially healthy diet, I knew that I had to make sure I was putting good food into my body. Not an easy task when there is so much tasty, good junk out there! For this reason, I decided, every time I would prepare my meal to ask myself two questions:

Question 1: What do I really feel like eating right now? Often enough, my answer was not something healthy…

Question 2: What can I add to this "unhealthy choice" to make my meal healthier?
Let's say my answer to the first question was "pizza", well then my answer to the second question would be that I could eat one slice of pizza which was exactly what I wanted but I would reduce the quantity. I would make sure that the rest of my meal was healthy by adding some vegetables, fruit, an additional source of protein such as tuna, a hard-boiled egg and so on. This way I could still eat what I wanted, but also felt good because of all the nutritious foods I had eaten.

The choice of food is an important factor, but so is the amount of food that you ingest. Quantity is primordial. For me, at one point, eating had become an obsession and I would constantly go from moments of eating to moments of thinking about food and I knew that it wasn't a healthy state of mind. The problem was, that every time I would sit down to eat, I would have a hard time stopping and often I would leave the table feeling full. Instead of feeling invigorated and ready to tackle the rest of my day, I felt sluggish, drowsy and my stomach would stay bloated for hours. I've always heard that one should finish a meal feeling light. I knew it was just a question of finding the right balance, a midpoint between feeling hungry or full. The ability to stop at that precise moment is easier said than done, right?

One thing became obvious however: if I wanted to eat less I was going to have to listen to my body signals, pay more attention and observe myself…which meant that I absolutely needed to slow down. Paying attention allowed me to realize that I wasn't chewing my food enough. I was just gulping it down without even being aware of what I was doing. It took a little bit of getting used to, but it didn't require any drastic changes.
And then, observing myself helped me recognize that I wasn't grateful for the food in front of me. So many people in the world are hungry and my attitude was disrespectful: Once I had invited gratitude to my table it taught me to give food my undivided attention, I no longer watched TV or used my phone while eating. I savored each and every bite.

So, to conclude, being at peace with one's plate implies that you stop punishing and depriving yourself. Stop seeing certain foods as good or bad. Focus on quantity: reduce portion sizes and make sure that every meal includes a few healthy choices. It means that you have to become more knowledgeable, understanding what you do is a big step towards success. You have to slow down, chew more thoroughly, observe your habits and become grateful for the food that is placed before you.

Change n°13
HYDRATE

Change n°14
DAILY DOSE OF GOODNESS

Change n°15
THE BIG 5 CHALLENGE

Change n°16
ONE SPECIAL MEAL

Change n°17
TRY SOMETHING NEW

Change n°18
VISUALIZE

Change n°19
IN TUNE WITH HUNGER
Meet the FULL-O-METER

Change n°20
SELF-OBSERVATION
My *Mood and Food* Tracker

Change n°21
RULES IN BETWEEN MEALS

Change n°22
EATING MINDFULLY

Change n°23
READ! READ! READ!

Change n°24
ADD VARIETY

Change n°13
HYDRATE

I am sure you're thinking "well that's easy enough!" Although many people often drink lots of liquids during the day, they do not drink a sufficient amount of water. Remember: Not all liquids are alike and although freshly squeezed fruit or vegetable juice or an herbal tea may replace a glass of water, some other drinks, such as alcohol, coffee, soft drinks and certain sports drinks are diuretics. What this means is that they help eliminate water. Hence, if you decide to have such drinks, you have to make sure you drink some water as well because your body's need for more water will increase. Making sure you drink enough good quality water is very important just as getting a sufficient amount of sleep. These are, I feel, the two best goals to begin with.

A. What are the benefits of drinking water?

Here are a few:
- Drinking a sufficient amount of water helps transport nutrients to the entire body, digest foods and flush out toxins
- Although there is no proof that it will make you lose weight, it does make you feel full and curbs your appetite
- It also regulates body temperature: when you are training, your muscles get tired, so making sure you are drinking enough during your workout can help you push through that last set of squats or bicep curls
- Adding fresh orange, lemon or cucumber slices or mint leaves for flavor or consuming herbal tea totally counts as drinking water

Isn't all this reading making you thirsty? Before you continue, go grab a glass of water and learn to enjoy the feeling!

B. How much water should you drink?

Drinking a few glasses a day is a good start but it might be interesting to find out how much water is best suited for you according to your activity level, your height and weight, and season. Do your homework and ask your doctor to make sure you are getting the perfect amount for your needs. A good and easy way is to simply check your urine: if it is clear or slightly yellow throughout the day, then you are probably drinking enough water. Check regularly and adjust accordingly.

C. Going all the way: which water should you choose: tap or bottled?

"Hydration" is this week's goal, remember to go all the way. In other words, take the time to research about it: read, watch programs, look online and find out how water comes to your tap and where it came from originally. Here are a few questions you might want to look into:

- Is your tap water good enough? Ask yourself: Where does *your* tap water come from, what is its source? Why not visit the nearest water company, get a brochure and ask a few questions?
- Should you be drinking tap water or mineral water?
- If you choose tap water, should you filter it? What would be the preferred method to do so?
- If you have decided upon mineral water, which one better suits your needs?

Now, you don't have to know everything before starting: at first, just make sure you hydrate enough and then plan some time during the week to know which system or water works best for you.

Here are just a few points that might help you decide what is a better solution.

Although tap and mineral water are both considered "safe" in the United-States we must take into consideration the ecological consequences of drinking from plastic bottles since most don't end up recycled. If you still choose the bottled option, however, here are a few tips:
- Look for water in high grade containers (glass or PET plastic) This is quite easy since you only need to look for the recycling stamp at the bottom of your plastic water bottle. Number "1" or the letters PET or PETE mean it's "safe". Number "2" or letters HDPE stand for high density polyethylene. Number "4" or the letters "LDPE" stand for low density polyethylene, and Number "5" or the letters "PP" stand for polypropylene. Let's stick to essentials and avoid getting lost in too many details: While all of these types of bottles are allowed for drinking water; the best (that is, other than glass) is PET.
- Always keep bottled water out of bright light and away from heat sources. It's not a good idea to stock up too many bottles for extended periods of time either. Even if you don't find an expiration date, use your common sense.
- If you drink straight from the bottle, you might want to rinse your water bottles before using them: I mean who knows who handled them or what came in contact with them before landing in your hands!
- If you choose a brand because of its taste, check out its label and do a little research to know if it's a good choice.

D. What is pH?
Knowing that the best pH for drinking water is around 9.5, see where your bottle stands and maybe reconsider it if its content is highly acidic. Oh! and if you are wondering what pH is, it stands for "Potential of hydrogen" and refers to the amount of hydrogen present in a substance, in our case in bottled water, which basically allows you to know if your water is acidic or alkaline. There is a scale that runs from 0 to 14, with 0 being very acidic, 7 being a balance between acid and alkaline and 14 being highly alkaline. pH is not regulated in drinking water, however, the US Environmental Protection Agency recommends that public water systems maintain pH levels between 6.5 and 8.5.

E. What are the different filter solutions available?

If you have decided to go with tap water, there are a number of water filters or water purification systems on the market to choose from:

a. Water filter system:

- water filter pitchers: they are basically containers in which you pour tap water that will be filtered into a compartment below.
- faucet mounted filters: directly fixed to the tap. Be sure to take the ones that let you switch between filtered and unfiltered water, as you don't always need to have it filtered.
- You also have countertop water filters, which are installed next to the sink or if space is an issue you might want to opt for an under the sink filter.
- There are many more options to choose from and if you want to have the water filtered in the entire house, that's also a possibility although it will more than likely be costly.

b. Water purification system:

- Reverse osmosis: water is basically filtered of its minerals and certain chemicals.
- Distillation: water is boiled and the steam is taken and turned back into its water form. The water being de-mineralized it is not recommended to use it as drinking water.
- Ozone treatment: destroys bacteria found in the water.

To conclude, make sure you drink a big glass of water first thing in the morning. After a long night of sleep, your body is dehydrated and needs to replenish fluids. Make it a habit for starting your day. Believe me, your body will thank you for it.

Change n°14
A DAILY DOSE
OF GOODNESS

14.

A. Why take up juicing?

- Because one simple glass of fresh juice can really add up and make a great difference in your overall health. Think of it this way: in one snack you can probably incorporate two fruits and three vegetables. I won't go over the benefits of eating enough fruit and vegetables. However, statistics show that most people do not eat the minimum amount of 2 fruit and 3 vegetables a day. So, an easy way to reach your daily goal is to simply drink them.

- You can get 95% of the vitamins and enzymes your body needs by simply juicing raw fruits and vegetables. You could, of course, eat them chopped up on a plate. But believe me if you compare the amount you have to eat to reach the amount of a 16oz bottle of juice you are in for a big surprise. For example, to make an average juice you might use the following ingredients: One big apple (I am no longer hungry), 3 carrots (I am feeling really full), 2 stalks of celery (I can no longer ingest anything), half a cucumber (no thank you…), ½ cup of parsley (please…), ½ a lemon (where are the restrooms?). Whether juicing or eating you would get the same amount of nutrients. However, eating them is a lot of hard work for your digestive system when compared to drinking them: it allows all the vitamins, minerals and enzymes to rapidly enter the bloodstream, with the added bonus of allowing your digestive organs to rest.

- It removes toxins
- It boosts your immune systems
- It reduces your risk of getting cancer, cardiovascular disease and inflammatory diseases.
- You can add vegetables to your juice that you would normally not eat. This is a good way to get a variety of different nutrients.
- Vegetables are naturally alkalizing. Since our diets are often very acidic, making sure our bodies have enough vegetables, sprouts, wheatgrass juice, leafy greens enables it to be at a good pH level, a little over it's neutral pH state of about 7.
- It's a great way to make our kids eat more fruit and vegetables. Just add a few vegetables to their favorite fruit and voilà! They will never know!

B. What do I juice

If you are going to eat or drink vegetables or fruit, make sure, as much as possible, that they are fresh, organic and raw.
Why raw? When cooking your fruit and vegetables you can destroy the good enzymes and alter their nutrients.
Before we continue, a little reminder:
Enzyme: proteins that are produced by cells and act as catalysts in special biochemical reactions.
Nutrient: any substance that can be directly assimilated without having to go through the digestion's degradation process.

If you only have the choice to use canned or frozen food, then use the organic brands. You owe it to yourself to have this juice/smoothie/soup completely healthy. Of course, it's not always possible, in which case buy what is readily available and make sure to peel, or soak and wash thoroughly before juicing or cooking to remove traces of pesticides and other chemicals on the surface.

Note: I recommend spraying your fruit and vegetables with a homemade preparation composed of apple cider, vinegar or lemon and sea salt. Just add a few capfuls of vinegar/ apple cider/ lemon and a few tablespoons of sea salt to a spray bottle containing a few cups of water. Spray your fruit and vegetables and let them sit for a few minutes before rinsing thoroughly.

At any given time try to make the best choice possible: you were planning to have a strawberry and banana smoothie, but there aren't any organic strawberries available. Perhaps they are too expensive, so try the frozen organic variety, or forget about them altogether and go for a less costly organic fruit that is in season.

C. How to get your juice, smoothie or soup:

a. Solution n° 1: Buy it!

You could find a healthy place nearby that makes freshly made juices or smoothies and soups and you could simply buy yourself one, either in the morning, at lunch or before heading home. Some places even deliver. Why not ask if other co-workers are interested in getting their juice as well and each of you take turns in picking them up or maybe the Juice shop might agree to group pricing.

Don't make the mistake of always selecting the same juice/smoothie/soup every time. Many people tend to like one and order it over and over again. Rotate your fruit and vegetables, as well as the leafy greens such as spinach, kale, romaine lettuce, parsley to make sure you are getting a daily variety of different nutrients and vitamins. Also, drinking the same juice day in and day out will end up getting boring. There are numerous options:
• Why not take the "juice of the day"?
• I like to ask the person making the juice to surprise me: I let them choose.
• Or you could turn it into a learning experience by making sure you get only seasonal fruit and vegetables. Watch as your drinks change from one season to the next.

Some of these juices can get pretty expensive but the way I see it: your body is your temple and these juices are your offerings. This is your health we are talking about. Why not turn it into a little ritual and while sipping your juice, tell yourself this juice is healing you. And why not ask "the Universe" for health and longevity.

b. Solution n°2: Make your own!

You can make your freshly squeezed orange, lemon, or grapefruit juice in the morning. Make sure your citrus juicer is ready when you wake up, that way, you only have to cut your fruit in two and squeeze. Here are a few things to keep in mind when having a juice:
• Find time to savor it. In other words, don't gulp it down. Please sip it slowly!
• Don't wait too long before drinking it: if you let it sit and expose it to air, a lot of enzymes, phytochemicals and all the good stuff in the juice will oxidize and degrade. You will be losing many nutrients from your juice and that would be a shame. So, do savor it but to maximize the benefits, drink it as quickly as possible after squeezing.

• Have your juice on an empty stomach approximately 20 min before a meal: mixing your juice with breakfast is not recommended as it will be difficult to digest. Also note that it's best to take your juice on an empty stomach as it increases nutrient absorption.

c. Solution 3: Invest in a juicer or blender.

Now this is not an easy task as there are so many different types of juicers and blenders out there to choose from. There are many different factors involved such as: How much money are you willing to invest? How much time you have? How many times a week you wish to juice or blend? What kind of drink do you want: juices, smoothies or soups?

D. Should you buy a juicer or a blender? What's the difference between juicing and making smoothies ?

They both allow you to drink a great amount of fruit and vegetables in one glass and are both a great option. If you are more of a smoothie drinker, then the blender is the machine you have to buy. If you are more into juices, then opt for a juicer.

a. The Blender

When making a smoothie, you blend the entire fruit and vegetable, thus keeping all the fibers. This creates a much thicker drink. A good idea is to replace your meal with a smoothie turning it into a healthy option that is filling and yet light in calories. If it's too thick, just add some water until you reach the right consistency.

Being rich in fibers, smoothies have to go through the digestive system. This makes it a slower process for the nutrients to reach the bloodstream. But it is in no way a bad thing since these fibers also help clear the digestive system. If you are thinking of buying one, I would recommend one with a glass container.

b. The Juicer

When you are juicing, you are basically eliminating the fiber in the food and ensuring that the nutrients immediately enter your bloodstream. There is no heavy digestion involved.

Before investing in a juicer, it's important to understand the difference between high and slow speed juicers:

• The "high speed" juicers such as the centrifugal juicers:

If a juicer is producing a juice at high speed that means that the machine uses a rotating blade to cut the fruit and vegetables up. The liquid state is obtained thanks to the high-speed spinning and friction usually operating at 1,000 to 30,000 rpm.

Much more affordable than many other juicers and priced as low as $40 USD, this might be your only option. Just make sure that you consume the juice very quickly as storing is not recommended. Another important point about the centrifugal juicers is that they are not very effective with leafy greens, meaning you will get a minimal amount of juice extracted from them. So, if your goal is to make kale, wheat grass, or spinach drinks, this machine might not be the one you are looking for.

However, the positive aspect is that you can have a juice ready very quickly: Most of these centrifugal juicers have a large chute that enable you to put the entire fruit or vegetable inside without having to cut them up into pieces prior to juicing.

These machines are also very easy to manipulate and easy to clean.

What's the debate around centrifugal juicers?

Since these machines spin at high speed, some heat is produced which destroys raw food enzymes. However, some studies say that these machines do not heat to the point of destroying all enzymes. I suggest to place your fruit and vegetables in the fridge before juicing, in this way they will have a cooling effect on the machine.

So, if you can't afford to invest in an expensive juicer and you don't have much time, the centrifugal is the machine for you.

• The " slow speed" juicers, also called "masticating juicers"

They operate between 40 and 200 rpm and are usually more expensive, as they can run from $200 to $1000 USD. Operating at slow speed, they produce no heat or oxidization. You can store your juice between 48 to 72 hours depending on the machine.

The masticating / slow juicers literally "chew", crush and squeeze the fruit and vegetables. The dried-up pulp goes into one bowl and the juice, after having been filtered, goes into another one. With these machines it is recommended that you precut all your fruit and vegetables to prevent clogging. They are quite easy to take apart and wash once you get the hang of it.

A tip: I recommend mixing up the order in which you push your fruit and vegetables through the chute. I like to put leafy greens with a piece of lemon or something soft such as a cucumber to make sure it all goes through easily. If I add ginger or curcuma, or herbs such as mint, basil, parsley, I try to place them between my fruit and vegetables to make sure I get the most out of them.

Note: In case you are wondering: what is "oxidation"?

When you bite into an apple and you set it down for a few minutes, you will notice that your apple, in some parts, has turned brown. It has oxidized. That's a problem because the longer a fruit is exposed to air and light, the less vitamins it will have.

So, oxidation as well as heat and water are the three primary enemies of vitamins and minerals.

c. Questions to ask before investing in a juicer or blender

• Don't forget, when it comes to buying, you have to see what is right for YOU! Not your neighbor, your friends, the reviewer online or the salesman selling you the machine.
• If you wake up at the last minute and barely have time to eat breakfast, go for the centrifugal juicer so you can quickly juice and have the time to enjoy it.
• Do you have to get up early and slip out of the house before anybody else gets up? Then you will need a silent machine. Centrifugal machines can be very noisy whereas the masticating juicers are more quiet and a better option for you.
• Do you have a big family and have to make 5, 6, 7 or more juices? Forget about the chopping; you will want to just quickly push the whole fruit through the chute and serve. Go for the centrifugal juicer. I have many friends in this situation that have invested in a slow masticating machine and it has just ended up boxed away in the cupboard.
• Have you decided to turn your life around and get really serious about juicing and make lots of green juices that involve a lot of leafy greens? Are you a health enthusiast? In this case, go for the slow masticating machines. They are your best option.

Change n°15
THE BIG 5 CHALLENGE

15.

"Eat a minimum of 5 fruit or vegetables every day!" I know this phrase resonates in your mind and that you have heard it time and time again! But do you respect these guidelines or are you the kind of person whose fruit and vegetables are limited to the tomato sauce on the pizza and the sliced apples inside the apple crumble?

First of all, I want to assure you that I am not suggesting a strict fruit and vegetable diet. All you have to do this week is to make sure that you eat the minimum required amount of fruit and vegetables every day. You are not going to drastically change the way you eat or deprive yourself of your favorite foods. The goal here is to find ways to add this food group into your daily lives, not only on a daily but more specifically on a meal basis. Believe me, there are many very simple things that you can do to integrate them and turn your breakfast, snack, lunch and dinner into healthier options. To help you along, let's answer three questions:
Are there any fruit and vegetables that you like?
How do I know if I have reached the Big 5?
How do I reach the Big 5?

A. Question n° 1: Are there any fruit and vegetables that you do like?

If you answered "yes", well, go buy them. I don't care if they're bananas or potatoes, canned or frozen, dried or cooked... just buy them! Of course, if there are fresh varieties you like, make it your priority. It's also a good idea, to stock up on some readily available, such as applesauce, canned beats or green beans, just to make things easier for you. You can also find an assortment of packaged steamed vegetables that simply need to be warmed up.

First, try to clear your mind of all the things you have heard about food, such as:
- Don't eat avocados or bananas because they'll make you fat
- Eat only leafy greens, avoid Iceberg lettuce because it has no nutritional value
- Canned goods contain too much salt
- If you cook your fruit and vegetables, you'll destroy all their vitamins
- The 100% Orange juice you find in supermarkets no longer contains any vitamin C
- Fruit and vegetables are full of pesticides, if you can't get organic then you might as well not buy any
- All the vitamins are in the skin of the produce, if you peel it their nutritional value is lost
- Eat seasonably: if it's not in season, don't eat it
- Avoid the dirty dozen: don't eat apples, strawberries, spinach, baby tomatoes, celery, peaches, cucumbers, potatoes, sweet bell peppers, nectarines, peaches, grapes...
- You should only consume raw fruit and vegetables
- Avoid soups and smoothies because your digestive system needs you to chew your food in order start the digestive process

I am not saying that these are generally untrue, for there *are* good reasons behind these affirmations. My point is, at first, that you try and focus on adding more fruit and vegetables to your diet, *no matter what*. Of course, if you have the opportunity to get fresh, seasonal, locally grown produce, by all means this is the best way to go. But if you are home and only happen to have canned green beans, there is no need to run out and get some fresh ones: it's ok to go for the canned variety.

If you have a hard time digesting raw veggies, have a stir fry! If you can't find organic apples or carrots, well then eat the non-organic variety. You could peel them, or make sure to soak or spray them using a homemade preparation. See soaking and spraying recipe in Change n° 14: *Daily Dose of Goodness*. If you prefer peeled apples then please do peel them! If on your way to work you see a fruit salad that looks yummy, buy it! It's ok, even though you don't know if the fruit are organic or maybe if a little bit of sugar has been added. And don't forget: there will always be someone telling you the way it has to be done, so be prepared! Don't let anyone make you feel guilty. Be proud of yourself. The goal this week is to add more fruit and vegetables, PERIOD. In the weeks to come, you can of course decide to move one step healthier by setting a goal to eat 70%, 80% or 100% organic or raw. Or you may decide to eat 7, 8 or even 10 fruit and vegetables every day! Remember: the secret to success is to take baby steps! If you go all out raw and organic or decide to eat 10 fruit and vegetables each day, you are most likely signing up for failure. So, this week, your only priority is to reach the "BIG 5" every single day.

B. Question n° 2: how do you know when you have reached the BIG 5?

Basically, what you need to know is how much you have to eat to reach ONE portion?
- Normally an average sized apple, orange, pear, banana, tomato, potato, mango, a big tangerine or mandarin or a medium sized grapefruit would be considered one portion
- For smaller sized fruit, it would more likely be 2 apricots, 2 plums, 2 kiwis, 2 small tangerines or mandarins (or similar sized fruit) that would count for one portion
- For large sized fruit, 1 portion would normally be ½ a grapefruit, 1 slice of melon, one thick slice of pineapple
- You would need 2 celery stalks, 2 medium carrots and 2 spears of asparagus to make one portion
- Count 6 strawberries, 6 small broccoli florets and 6 lychees to make one portion
- For smaller berries like blueberries, raspberries, cranberries and grapes, you would need approximately 12 to make a portion

Another easy way to get your portions right, is to count portions in cups:
- 1 cup for chopped fruit and vegetables or canned fruit
- ½ cup if your fruit and vegetables are cooked
- 2 cups for your leafy greens
- One small glass of juice or one small bowl of soup
- About ¼ cup if you are eating dried fruit or nuts

Check out Change n° 17: *Try Something New* for more ideas about how to calculate your portions.

Reaching Your 5 Fruits & Vegetables

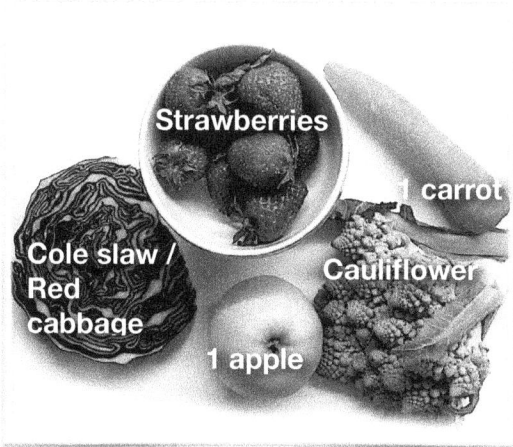

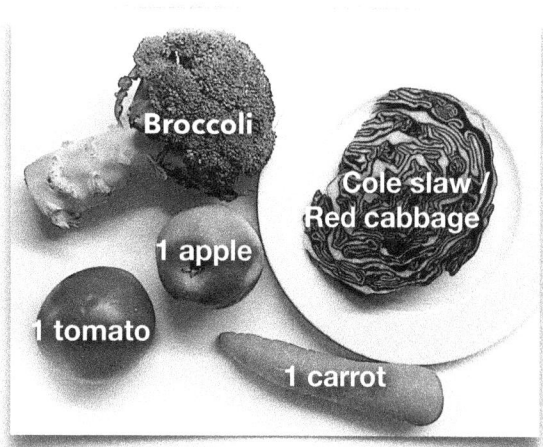

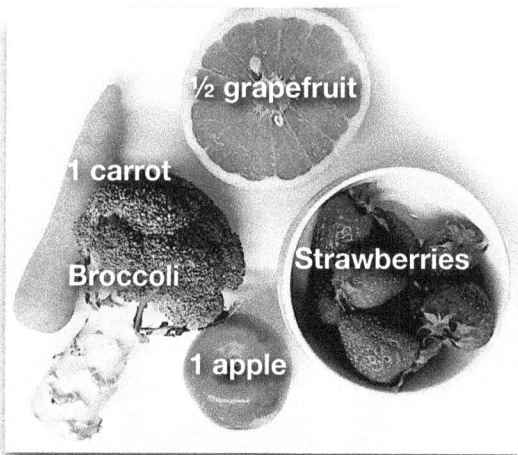

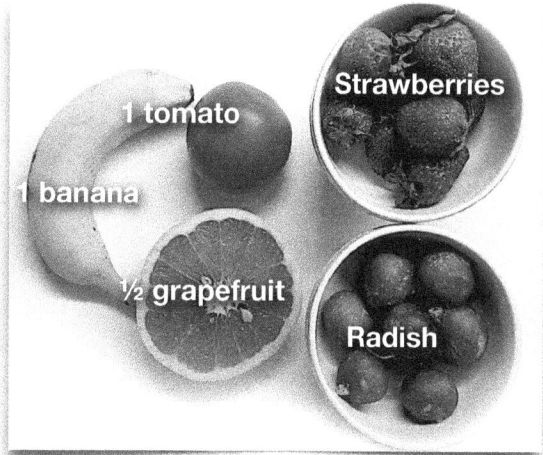

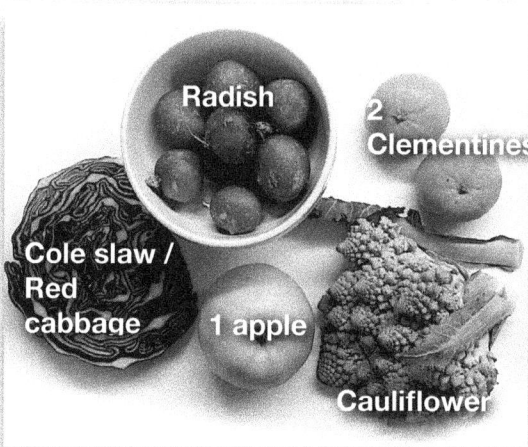

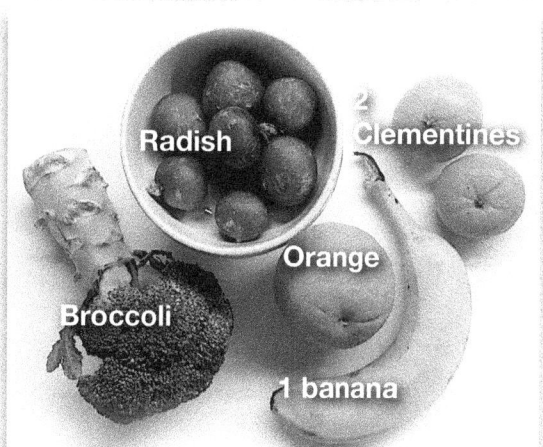

Strawberries

Cole slaw / Red cabbage

1 carrot

Cauliflower

1 apple

Broccoli

Cole slaw / Red cabbage

1 apple

1 tomato

1 carrot

½ grapefruit

1 carrot

Broccoli

Strawberries

1 apple

1 tomato

Strawberries

1 banana

½ grapefruit

Radish

Radish

2 Clementines

Cole slaw / Red cabbage

1 apple

Cauliflower

Radish

2 Clementines

Orange

Broccoli

1 banana

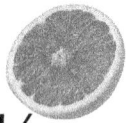

½

Grapefruit

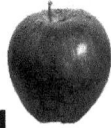

1

Apple

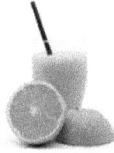

1

Glass of Juice

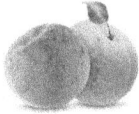

2

Apricots

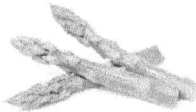

3

Spears of Asparagus

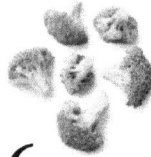

6

Broccoli florets

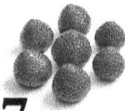

7

Strawberries

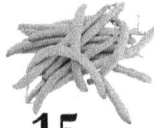

15

Green Beans

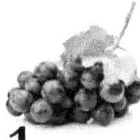

1

Handful Grapes

Mixing healthy food portions

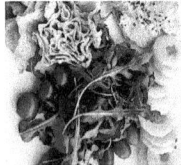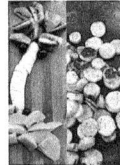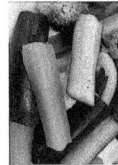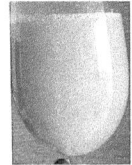
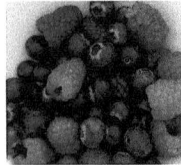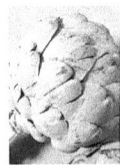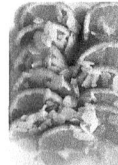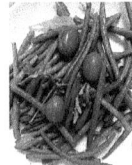
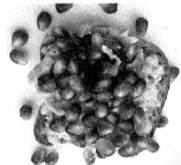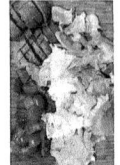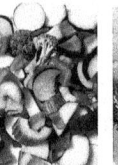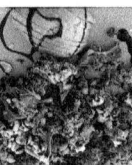
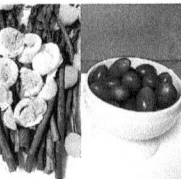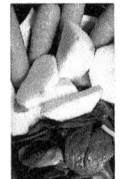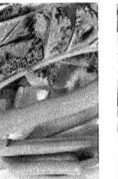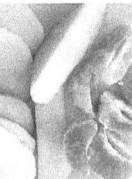

C. Question n° 3: How do I master the BIG 5?

The most important thing to do if you want to reach 5 servings a day is to plan ahead. For example, you could:

- Prepackage your servings: Peal and prepare your fruit and vegetables and store them in plastic packets in the fridge
- Chop one stalk of celery and one carrot into slices and add a small portion of hummus dip
- Prepare an apple and a small portion of peanut butter
- Prepare portions of canned fruit such as pineapple, apricots, mixed fruits and place them in glass containers. Try to go for the ones that don't contain any sugar
- Have a big fruit platter and place it where it is readily available
- Stock up on some freshly pressed juices
- Also stock up on apple sauce. There is a great variety readily available that you can just throw into your bag before going off to work
- Prepackage some bags with fruit and vegetables that you can juice as soon as you get home

The good thing about preparing ahead of time is that you can simply grab a bag or container. No need to start pealing or preparing.

There are many ways to add more fruit and vegetables to your meals. Simply juice more, smoothie more, soup more. Why not have a small bowl of soup before your dinner or lunch?

One sure way of reaching your goal, that I use, is to make sure that each and every snack and meal you have, includes at least one fruit or vegetable, such as a small bowl of salad, a fresh juice, a fresh fruit, green beans on the side...

An easy way to get them all, is by munching on one or two carrots, celery stalks, radishes, or baby tomatoes while getting your dinner ready or by fixing a plate of sliced fruit to eat while watching TV.

Be creative and prepare fruit sticks: chop up a different variety of fruit, add a few marshmallows on a few sticks and enjoy a great snack.

This goal may seem a like a challenge for some of you, but in fact, it's quite easy. Every time you want to eat something, ask yourself: how can I add something healthy to this meal? How can I add one serving of fruit or vegetables to my breakfast, snacks, lunch or dinner? It can be as easy as adding a handful of blueberries to your cereal or French toast, adding half a sliced tomato and three leaves of lettuce to your lunch, drinking a freshly pressed juice for your snack, munching on a few celery and carrot sticks before your dinner. You'll see, it will quickly turn into a habit and soon eating fruit and vegetables will be a part of your lifestyle.

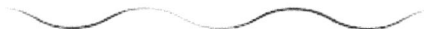

Change n°16
ONE SPECIAL MEAL

16.

When we decide to commit to a balanced and healthy diet, most of us dread the idea and automatically tend to think of everything we are going to have to give up, in other words most of the foods we love. However, because of the frustration it causes, I wonder to what extent it is such a good idea to eliminate any food group at all from our diet. Instead of punishing yourself, why not look at it in terms of *ADDING* as many healthy foods as possible throughout the day or doing your best to make one meal super healthy.

Exclude the frustration factor and see the impact it has on your relationship with food. When I eat, I want to be at peace with myself and what I am eating and so, as much as possible, I try to think in terms of: "How can I make this meal healthier?" I make sure never to express any guilt. You will never catch me thinking: "I really shouldn't be eating this piece of chocolate, pizza or cake." I will never say to myself: "I am really helpless, I will never be able to lose this weight." Deprivation, diet, frustration are words that are totally banned from my mind.

What does this week's goal imply? It implies to have one totally healthy meal during the day with no junk in it at all. The good thing is, depending on your day, you can decide which one of your meals it's going to be: one day, it might be breakfast and another it might either be lunch or dinner. The key here is to make it special: make healthy synonym of fun, creativity, taste and color.

A. What does super healthy mean?

Come on, let's be honest, here. We all know what super healthy means: it means junk free! The good thing is, that no matter which meal we choose to be the healthy one, it helps to know that you can eat as you normally do the rest of the day. With time, it will become second nature and you will be able to add a second and a third totally healthy meal or snack. I found that this technique really worked well for me. I have never been able to go on a diet. The very minute I start thinking about restricting myself, I start feeling frustrated and then… I eat even more.

THE EQUATION TO REACH THE BODY OF YOUR DREAMS

For most people the equation for success looks like this:

RESTRICTION + EXERCISE = DREAM BODY (SUCCESS)

But for me…

RESTRICTION + EXERCISE = FAILURE AND DISAPOINTMENT

The way I see it:

FOCUS ON BRINGING AS MANY POSITIVE CHANGES AS YOU CAN INTO YOUR LIFE THROUGHOUT THE DAY + FOCUS ON PRIDE = SUCCESS

Forget about punishing yourself, restrictions and obligations. Get them out of the equation and out of your mind and start seeing things in a different perspective: throughout the day simply make sure you try to do as many things as possible that are good for you in regards to your diet and your exercise routine. And when you do eat a donut or fries, learn to enjoy them and savor every bite.

Every time you sit down to eat, take the time to step back and ask yourself: what can I do right now to make this meal healthier, to be prouder of myself? And then set out to do it. Are you craving a slice of pizza? Indulge and say "yes". Be happy to treat yourself to a delicious slice of cheesy pizza. And then ask yourself: What can I add to make this meal healthier so I can feel proud of myself? Add a fruit & vegetable juice and a have a leafy green salad on the side.

You feel like having a desert? Say "yes" but save it for a little later perhaps your snack and accompany it with a big glass of water. And why not climb a set of stairs or take an extra-long dog-walk tonight?

LEARN TO FOCUS ON ALL THE POSITIVE FACTORS THAT YOU DO FOR YOURSELF THROUGHOUT THE DAY: IT WILL LEAD YOU TO SUCCESS!

Psychologically it's a lot easier to eat a balanced meal if we know that we can have what we want later on or during the day. Also, keep in mind that pride is an essential component. You have to feel proud of yourself for eating a healthy meal and learn to integrate the idea that healthy eating is fun and delicious. To insure success, make sure to make this healthy meal *extra* special. Why not make your plate look beautiful and colorful? Why not set up the table so that it looks nice? Learn to eat with your eyes, ears, taste buds… let all your senses participate in the eating process.

a. Make a healthy breakfast

If you choose to make your breakfast the healthy meal of the day, go to your local health food store and find foods that you love such as crunchy cereal, fresh bread made from a variety of seeds, fresh fruit, such as blueberries, raspberries, melon, nuts and dried fruit. Decide, ahead of time, what you are going eat. Make sure you have enough time for meal preparation so that is looks nice. The aim is to sit down and enjoy a picture perfect meal. Add a cup of herbal tea. Have you ever tasted nettle herbal tea before? Check its benefits.

Make a point of researching the benefits of all the wholesome foods you have chosen to eat. Be proud of bringing all these essential vitamins and minerals into your body. Be pleased that you are focusing on your health.

Before having breakfast, you could also prepare a cup of freshly squeezed lemon juice. Just add some warm water and drink it first thing in the morning. Check out Change n° 28: *Hot and Cold* to find out the real benefits of drinking fresh lemon juice. Why not create your very own vegetable or fruit juice every day? This way you are sure to benefit from a large amount of vitamins and minerals.

b. Make a healthy lunch

Lunch may be the most challenging meal of the day since for many of us it implies eating at the office, hence preparing and bringing lunch to work or eating out, with all the temptations it implies. It's not easy and let's face it, when we have had a busy and stressful morning many of us just feel like rewarding ourselves with a quick, not necessarily balanced meal. However, there are ways to make your lunch a healthy and enjoyable one.

Why not find a co-worker who has the same goal as you and once in a while go out and eat together. You can both check out all the places close by to your office that prepare healthy meals. Going together will help keep both of you on track. You could do the same thing with a friend. Even if you two can't share your lunch, you could still both become accountable to each other.

Of course, the easiest, surest and cheapest way to have a healthy lunch is to box it up at home. There are thousands of ideas as well as recipes proposing vegetable rolls, healthy salads or sandwiches, mason jar recipes and what not. The key here is to make it really special. Box up food that you love to eat. I like to have lots of little boxes just like the Japanese bento boxes: one with a small mixed ingredient salad, another one with healthy crackers and a piece of cheese, and yet another box with apple slices and peanut butter dip or applesauce and almonds on the side, and one final one with a turkey wrap. I spread a little bit of cream cheese on a slice of turkey. I then add roquette salad, a few slices of carrots, some avocado and finally I will roll and cut it into slices. Delicious! It's like having tapas or snacking but you're actually getting a great lunch with a variety of flavors.

c. Make a healthy dinner

If you choose to have your healthy meal for dinner, then you have many options to choose from such as grilled meat, chicken or fish with a few vegetables, a delicious salad, smoothies, soups, fruit trays, oven baked apples. Make sure, however, that your dinner is as early as possible so you don't go to bed feeling full. I normally eat early and treat myself to a little something during the evening, so I don't feel frustrated.

The key is to make this meal extra special. If you are at home, you can be very creative:
• Set up the table nicely with a tablecloth, candles and dress up a little…
• Present the meal in dishes
• Share your diner with your family which means turning off the TV and all electronic devices. Have your kids come and help in the kitchen and at the table, allow each one of you to talk a few minutes about an event that occurred during the day
• Prolong this family moment by going out for a walk or bike ride for 15 to 20 minutes
• You could also plan a picnic in the park: pack up a healthy meal and play frisbee
I can't express enough that a healthy diner has to be a special and bonding moment.

B. Bring peace to your plate

Starting off with at least one healthy meal each day will get you going on the right track. It's so important to have a healthy relationship with food, to be at peace with it, but also with the act of eating. Sit down and relax, savor every bite whether your food is healthy or not. Don't gulp it down. Learn to embrace each bite you eat and be grateful and happy about eating no matter what you are putting into your mouth: "this donut is so delicious, it was the tastiest thing I ate today" "this apple is so juicy and crunchy."

Slowly, slowly - it might take some time, it might be a long process - but if you persist you *WILL* learn to enjoy eating! You *will* end up eating less while knowing that you are now free to eat whatever it is you want to eat without feeling guilty about it. You *will* also learn to enjoy eating healthy because you will *finally* acknowledge the fact that you are free to eat something "less healthy" as well. Understanding all this was a revelation to me: it has taught me to make peace with my plate. Progressively, I started to eat less and learned to enjoy eating an overall healthier and much more balanced diet. Today, when I sit down, I am at peace with my plate and I thoroughly enjoy every bite.

Change n°17
TRY SOMETHING NEW

17.

This next point should be fun and you should make the most of it while becoming adventurous. There is a huge variety of fruit and vegetables out there, some of which I am sure you have probably never tasted or even heard of. Why not commit to try new things this week. It will be fun so be creative and make the most of it!

A. Why try a new fruit or vegetable every day?

To help you in this commitment I have listed below all the vegetables and fruit you can find. I probably even omitted a few so feel free to add on to the list! At first, try eating it as plain as possible in other words raw or steamed if it needs to be cooked. Next, look online for recipes to see how other people are preparing it. The goal is:

• to discover new flavors
• to integrate new foods into your diet
• Stop the "always eating the same thing" routine
• to become more bodacious!

B. How many fruit and vegetables should I really be eating?

Did you know that is has been estimated that approximately 75% of the population isn't eating enough fruit and vegetables? Are you part of that percentage? The key this week is to discover a new fruit or vegetable every day but it's also a week to do your research! With all that information out there, I am sure that most of you don't even know how many fruit and vegetables you should really be eating. One diet states it should be 7 portions and yet another touts it's 12. So how do we know for sure?

The right amount for you depends on several factors, including age, gender, and physical activity. But to make it easy for you a minimum would be 5 with 3 to 4 vegetables and 1 to 2 fruits. If you can notch it up, 7 would be great with let's say 5 veggies and 2 fruits. Your goal should be simply to eat more and increase the amount until you reach approximately 10 to 12 portions over time.

C. What is a portion?

Turn to Change n°15, *The Big 5 Challenge,* for more details about portion sizes. To make it easy for you, a portion is the palm of your hand. Since your palm is smaller or bigger depending on your age and how big you are, you have a bigger or smaller portion accordingly. You can also use the good old cup system and measure up. There is just a difference when it comes to leafy greens where you would need two cups to reach the equivalent of one regular cup of vegetables and dried fruit such as raisins, apricots, in which case ½ cup would be the equivalent of one cup of fresh fruit. Generally speaking, a large piece of fruit such as a banana, orange, apple, medium tomato or vegetable as in medium potato, large ear of corn, bell pepper, one stalk of celery is the equivalent of a cup.

D. Be prepared

Make fruit and vegetable readily available at home so it's easy to just grab and eat:
- a fruit bowl with 2 bananas, 2 oranges, 2 apples, 2 pears, grapes, cherries, strawberries
- small accessible veggies such as cherry tomatoes, sweet peppers, baby carrots…
- chopped up veggies prepared ahead of time. You can prepare a few packets and place them in the fridge. It will come in handy when you are tired after work
- Canned fruit or fruit cups. Although I highly recommend eating them fresh, canned fruits or fruit cups are better than no fruit
- Homemade or store Applesauce: I recommend the one with no sugar added but if it means you won't eat it then get the sweetened version
- Fruit salad prepared ahead of time. Place it in the fridge, in portion containers, so you already know you are getting one whole portion

E. Find out why different colors are good for you!

Fruits and vegetables come in a variety of different colors. Each one of these colors brings you certain types of nutrients. For example, green fruit and vegetables have a high content in chlorophyll, fiber, lutein, calcium, folate, vitamin C, calcium, and Beta-carotene which means they have specific functions such as reducing risks of cancer, lowering your blood pressure etc. Each different color has its unique health components. Adding variety to your diet is the best way of making sure you are getting all the necessary nutrients your body needs.

The goal here is to eat one different vegetable or fruit every day, but keep in mind that the more you eat from this group, the better. Check out my **Fruit and vegetable lists** and the benefits of each color.

a. Color Benefits

Fruits and vegetables come in an array of beautiful colors that we can classify in 6 different color groups: purple/blue, red, orange, white, green and yellow with each one providing specific health and nutritional benefits. Do you know what they are? I can't insist enough upon the fact that becoming more knowledgeable gets you one step closer to leading a healthy lifestyle. Understanding simple things, such as what the colors of your fruit and vegetables indicate about their nutritional value builds your desire to eat them. Taking the time to understand why certain foods are good but also reading labels to find out why other foods can actually be classified as hazardous for your health will progressively change how you see the food on your plate and make you want to change.

Let's start things off this week by looking into the health benefits of the various colors of our fruits and vegetables. Please note that I have intentionally selected only a few vitamins and minerals for each color group; the idea is to focus only on the essential benefits.

Health benefits of GREEN colored fruit and vegetables

The most popular green fruit and vegetables are:

Celery, cucumber, lettuce, zucchini, kale, endive, brussels sprouts, asparagus, broccoli and broccolini, artichokes, avocado, green beans, rocket, green peppers, cabbage, spinach, snow peas, sugar snap peas, arugula, leeks, bok-choy, green lemons, kiwis, green apples, grapes, honeydew melon, pears.

MY VEGETABLE LIST

- [ ] Alfalfa Sprouts
- [ ] Amaranth
- [ ] Artichoke
- [ ] Arugula
- [ ] Asparagus
- [ ] Aubergine / Eggplant
- [ ] Azuki Beans
- [ ] Basil
- [ ] Bean Sprouts
- [ ] Black Eyed Peas
- [ ] Black radish
- [ ] Borlotti Bean
- [ ] Broad Bean
- [ ] Beet
- [ ] Bok Choy
- [ ] Broad Beans
- [ ] Broccoflower
- [ ] Broccoli
- [ ] Broccolini
- [ ] Brussels Sprouts
- [ ] Cabbage
- [ ] Calabrese
- [ ] Carrots
- [ ] Cauliflower
- [ ] Celery
- [ ] Celery Root
- [ ] Chanterelles
- [ ] Chard
- [ ] Chickpeas
- [ ] (Garbanzo Beans)
- [ ] Chives
- [ ] Collard Greens
- [ ] Corn
- [ ] Corn Salad
- [ ] Courgettes
- [ ] Cucumber
- [ ] Eggplant
- [ ] Endive

- [ ] Frisee Lettuce
- [ ] Fennel
- [ ] Garlic
- [ ] Ginger
- [ ] Green Beans
- [ ] Herbs and Spices *(anise, basil, caraway, cilantro, parsley, dill, fennel, lavender lemon grass, marjoram oregano, rosemary, sage and thyme)*
- [ ] Horseradish
- [ ] Kale
- [ ] Kidney Beans
- [ ] Kohlrabi
- [ ] Jerusalem Artichoke Jicama
- [ ] Leek
- [ ] Lentils
- [ ] Lettuce
- [ ] Lima Beans
- [ ] Mangetout
- [ ] Mung Beans
- [ ] Mushrooms
- [ ] Mustard Greens
- [ ] Navy Beans
- [ ] Nettles
- [ ] New Zealand Spinach
- [ ] Okra
- [ ] Onion and Green Onion
- [ ] Parsley
- [ ] Parsnip
- [ ] Pearl Onions
- [ ] Peas
- [ ] Peppers (green, red or yellow)

- [ ] Pinto Beans
- [ ] Potato
- [ ] Pumpkin
- [ ] Radicchio
- [ ] Rhubarb
- [ ] Radish
- [ ] Rocket
- [ ] Runner Beans
- [ ] Rutabaga
- [ ] Salad Savoy
- [ ] Salsify
- [ ] Shallot
- [ ] Skirret Snap Peas
- [ ] Snow Peas
- [ ] Soy Beans
- [ ] Spinach
- [ ] Split Peas
- [ ] Spring Onion
- [ ] Sweet Corn
- [ ] Sweet Peppers
- [ ] Sweet Potato
- [ ] Topinambur
- [ ] Turnip
- [ ] Squashes
- [ ] Sweetcorn
- [ ] Taro (Hawaii and Australia)
- [ ] Tomato
- [ ] Tubers
- [ ] Turnip Greens
- [ ] Wasabi
- [ ] Water Chestnut
- [ ] Watercress
- [ ] Watermelon
- [ ] Yam
- [ ] Zucchini
- [ ] Other_____

MY FRUIT LIST

- [ ] Apple
- [ ] Apricot
      or Dried Apricot
- [ ] Avocado
- [ ] Banana
- [ ] Bilberry
- [ ] Blackberry
- [ ] Blackcurrant
- [ ] Blueberry
- [ ] Boysenberry
- [ ] Cantaloupe
- [ ] Champagne
  Grapes
- [ ] Clementine
- [ ] Currant
- [ ] Cherry
- [ ] Cherimoya
- [ ] Cloudberry
- [ ] Coconut
- [ ] Cranberry
      or Dried Cranberry
- [ ] Custard Apple
- [ ] Damson
- [ ] Date
- [ ] Dragonfruit
- [ ] Durian
- [ ] Elderberry
- [ ] Fig
- [ ] Goji Berry
- [ ] Gooseberry
- [ ] Grape
- [ ] Raisin
- [ ] Grapefruit
- [ ] Guava
- [ ] Honey Berry

- [ ] Huckleberry
- [ ] Jabuticaba
- [ ] Jackfruit
- [ ] Jambul Jujube
- [ ] Juniper Berry
- [ ] Kiwi
- [ ] Kumquat
- [ ] Lemon
- [ ] Lime
- [ ] Loquat
- [ ] Longan
- [ ] Lychee
- [ ] Mandarine
- [ ] Mango
- [ ] Marion-berry
- [ ] Melon
- [ ] Miracle Fruit
- [ ] Mulberry
- [ ] Nectarine
- [ ] Nergi or Mini Kiwi
- [ ] Nance
- [ ] Olive
- [ ] Orange
- [ ] Papaya
- [ ] Passionfruit
- [ ] Peach
- [ ] Pear
- [ ] Persimon
- [ ] Physalis
- [ ] Plantain
- [ ] Plum
- [ ] Pineapple

- [ ] Plummet (1/4
  Apricot and ¾ Plum)
- [ ] Pomegranate
- [ ] Pomelo
- [ ] Purple
- [ ] Mangosteen
- [ ] Quince
- [ ] Raspberry
- [ ] Rambutan
- [ ] Redcurrant
- [ ] Satsuma
- [ ] Star Fruit
- [ ] Strawberry
- [ ] Tamarillo
- [ ] Tamarind
- [ ] Tomato
- [ ] Tangerine
- [ ] Ugli Fruit
- [ ] Yuzu
- [ ] Other_____

What do they contain and what are they good for?

Most Dark, leafy greens are jam packed with nutrients that are important for your health and help prevent cancer as they contain:

- **Fiber:** helps soften your stools and maintains bowel health. It is also associated with weight loss or maintaining a healthy weight since you feel full for a longer period of time and it slows down the emptying of the stomach.
- **Vitamin C**: is a strong antioxidant that can strengthen your body's natural defenses.

Definition: **ANTIOXIDANTS**

They are molecules that boost the immune system. They do so by protecting cells from harmful molecules called free radicals. The different kinds of antioxidants are Vitamin C, Vitamin E, Selenium, Beta Carotene, Glutathione, Polyphenols and Zinc.

- **Vitamin K:** *a fat-soluble vitamin helps with vision and with maintaining strong bones and teeth.*

Definition: **FAT-SOLUBLE VITAMINS**
& WATER-SOLUBLE VITAMINS
also known as non-soluble vitamins
Vitamins A, D, E and K are fat-soluble vitamins. They can dissolve/are soluble in lipids (fats), which means they are much better absorbed into your bloodstream when you eat it with fat. Water-soluble vitamins, Vitamins B and C, dissolve in water and are not stored by the body contrary to fat-soluble vitamins that are.

- **Chlorophyll**: it's a pigment that gives plants their green color. It is touted to boost energy level, fight illnesses and even to help reduce facial acne.
- **Calcium**: important for optimal bone health.
- **Iron**: Your body can't produce iron on its own and needs iron-rich foods to produce red blood cells that transport essential nutrients and oxygen to the various organs around the body. Most people turn to red meat for iron but many vegetables and legumes are high in it as well. Good sources are green leafy vegetables, spinach, peas, collard greens and lima beans.

Health benefits of RED colored fruits and vegetables

The most popular red fruit and vegetables are:

Radishes, red pepper, radicchio, cabbage, red onions, beets, red skinned potatoes, cranberries, cherries, red apples, red grapes, rhubarb, blood oranges, pink grapefruits, strawberries, watermelon, pomegranate, goji berries.

What do they contain and what are they good for?

Most red fruits are said to help memory function and help to keep your heart healthy.

- **Lycopene:** is the main ingredient that gives fruit and vegetables their red color. It is a powerful antioxidant that has been linked to preventing cancer, heart disease, prostate problems and that reduces the skin damage from the sun but also your risk of getting cancer, diabetes and Alzheimer's.

• **Vitamin C**: is a strong antioxidant that helps limit cell damage from free radicals, heal wounds, keeps your gums and teeth healthy, repairs body tissue and can strengthen your body's natural defenses.

Interesting fact about Vitamin C and something to think about

If we compare a red bell pepper and an orange we will see that ½ a cup of red bell peppers provides 95 milligrams of vitamin C, whereas an orange only 25 milligrams. And this gets me thinking: just like coffee, some of my friends refuse to drink cofeww or eat an orange in the evening, fearing insomnia. Never, however, have I heard them say "Last time I had red bell peppers and spinach for dinner and had a sleepless night: I tossed and turned for hours!". Which gets me thinking about all this information we receive and on how it affects our brain to the point that it influences how we feel and even perturbs us in our bedrooms where we should be fast asleep.

Vitamin A: is a fat-soluble vitamin. There are two different forms of vitamin A in food:
-Vitamin A or Retinol present in animal products such as dairy, liver or fish
-Provitamin A or Carotenoids present in plant foods such as fruit, vegetables and oils. Carotenoids fight free radicals.

Definition: FREE RADICALS
Free radicals are highly reactive molecules that can harm your body by creating oxidative stress.
To simplify they harm your body by damaging cells, causing wrinkles, aging, cancer, and other diseases.
Carotenoids are good for you since they fight free radicals.

• **Vitamin A:** improves night vision, contributes to a healthier skin (namely if you have eczema, stretch marks, wrinkles or acne), helps in the formation of bone and teeth, helps maintain memory function, fights off infections and can help lower high blood pressure.
• **Fiber:** read above for details

Health benefits of ORANGE colored fruit and vegetables
The most popular orange fruit and vegetables are:
carrots, pumpkin, squash, sweet potatoes, oranges, tangerines, nectarines, apricots, peaches, cantaloupe, mango, papaya, orange peppers, turmeric.

What do they contain and what are they good for?
Orange fruit and vegetables contain carotenoids…
• **Vitamin C:** read above for details
• **Vitamin A:** read above for details

Important fact about Vitamins and Minerals
Let's say you have high blood pressure and you read that vitamin A helps to lower its levels. Will eating more ingredients rich in Vitamin A make your cholesterol go down even more? The answer is "no".

Overdosing on vitamin A, or any other vitamin for that matter, can be toxic and have serious health effects. Some symptoms of toxicity include fatigue, headache, stomach pain, lack of appetite, skin problems and so on. It is not to be taken lightly. So, if you have any questions or before using any product or making any drastic changes to your diet, consult your health care professional.

• **Potassium:** counteracts the adverse effects of sodium on blood pressure and is especially important for nerve and muscle proper functioning (including the heart).

Health benefits of YELLOW colored fruit and vegetables

The most popular yellow fruit and vegetables are:

yellow peppers, corn, yellow tomatoes, lemons, grapefruit, squash, pineapple, pears, yellow figs, yellow apples,

What do they contain and what are they good for?

• **Lutein:** is especially important for eye health and recommended for the elderly as it prevents age related macular degeneration.
• **Vitamin C:** read above for details

Health benefits of WHITE & BROWN colored fruit and vegetables

The most popular white & brown fruit and vegetables are:

Mushrooms, cauliflower, onions, potatoes, garlic, ginger, parsnips, turnip, pear, nectarine, white peaches, bananas, coconut, dates, fennel, horseradish, leeks, lychee, white corn, shallots.

What do they contain and what are they good for?

Although they are white or brown, these fruit and vegetables can be highly nutritious.

• **Allicin**: contained in Garlic, onions, leeks, scallions and chives is said to help lower your risk for high blood pressure, high cholesterol, cancer, heart disease and reduce risk of heart attacks.
• **Polyphenols**: Plant polyphenols are rich in antioxidants, which, as said beforehand, protect cells from harmful molecules called free radicals. They are touted for reducing blood clot formation.
• **Potassium:** read above for details
• **Niacin:** Niacin is water-soluble and one of the eight B vitamins also know as vitamin B3. It is said to lower bad cholesterol (LDL)and increase good cholesterol (HDL). Your brain needs it to get energy and function properly and studies are starting to show that they have a role in reducing symptoms of arthritis.
• **Vitamin C:** read above
• **Folate:** read below for details

Health benefits of PURPLE & BLUE colored fruit and vegetables

The most popular purple & blue fruit and vegetables are:

Eggplant, cabbage, purple pepper, prunes, figs, purple grapes, black currants, blueberries, blackberries, plums, mulberry, purple onions, plums, raisins.

What do they contain and what are they good for?
The color is due to the fruit's content in anthocyanin

- **Anthocyanin**: has antioxidant properties that help limit damage caused to your cells by free radicals. It is also said to improve memory and mineral absorption, reduce inflammation as well as your risk of getting a stroke, cancer and heart disease. Especially found in blueberries, eggplant, pomegranates, blackberries, prunes, plums and more.
- **Vitamin A**: Read above for details
- **Folate**: Also known as Vitamin B9 helps produce and maintain new cells and is needed for the formation of DNA. It also prevents anemia and cancer development. It has been shown to foster positive mood.
- **Vitamin C**: Read above for details

F. Find out what's in season!

If you have chosen to discover new fruits and vegetables this week, it might be interesting to get to know more about them in general. So why not go all the way by, first of all, finding out which ones are in season right now and second, researching the benefits of the ones you have picked today. I will not put a **Seasonal Fruit and Vegetable Chart** since it is really dependent on where you live. Indeed, seasonal fruit and vegetable at this very moment in Australia and New-York are not be the same. So, do your homework and research what's in season where you live at this period of the year.

Change n°18
VISUALIZE

18.

A. WHAT IS VISUALIZATION?

When it comes to reaching your goals, numerous techniques are proposed to help you move forward and achieve them. For your goal to be clear, it's important to take the time, sit down and actually write what it is you want. You can also share this with your friends which will make you accountable (*"I told my friend about my goal, she will now expect to see results. If I don't get any or if I quit, I will be seen as a failure. I want my friends to see that I am an achiever, so I will do my utmost to succeed"*).

You could also visualize. It's an intricate part of old techniques of meditation. But what is visualization exactly? According to the dictionary, *"to visualize is to form a mental picture of something that is invisible or abstract."*

B. VISUALIZATION MADE SIMPLE

Just for a second, close your eyes and visualize a chocolate covered strawberry. See it's beautiful bright red color! Just look at it for a few moments. Then imagine grabbing this chocolate covered strawberry with your hands and feel its firmness. Now smell the mixture of both smells: the chocolate and the strawberry. Take your time. Feel how your mouth starts to water before you finally put it in your mouth and take a big bite. Feel the firmness of the strawberry, it's perfume filling your nose. Feel how the chocolate starts to melt and how both flavors are now blending perfectly in your mouth.

C. ADDING COMPONENTS

This whole process is called visualizing. Why visualize something to eat? Because it's simple and easy to do. You will begin to practice with easy things such as something to eat or an object. What's really important is to have all your senses participating in the process to make it as real as possible. Once you get used to it, extend the experience to something broader such as sitting on the beach while looking and listening to the waves and everything that surrounds you: feeling the sand beneath your hands and feet, seeing the waves and hearing them crash in front of you, smelling the salty air and, for activating the sense of taste, you could imagine yourself drinking a refreshing lemonade. Take the time to savor the moment and truly live the experience. And then explore some other happy, pleasurable, relaxing experiences. Remember to breathe slowly and be totally in the moment.

D. A DIFFERENT APPROACH: GOING THROUGH THE ENTIRE PROCESS

Once you have mastered the basics of visualization, then you are on your way to *creative visualization,* in other words to *visualize* something you would like to *create* in your life, such as reaching your goals or having a dream come true. I must make a point here that you won't find in most visualizing books. Usually when you visualize, you are asked to see yourself as already having accomplished what you desire.

Most authors will say that the key to success is the "ending": see yourself slim, see yourself succeed, see yourself rich and you will become slim, successful and rich.

How's that been working for you? I am not saying it doesn't work. What I would like you to do is question this technique, regarding yourself. The way I see it: make it a rule to find out things on your own and then stand by what you discovered. Don't depend on anybody. I can't help but think that we all are different, and that our needs vary. If visualizing yourself succeeding has not convinced you or has not reaped the results you were expecting, maybe it's worth trying a different approach.

A few years ago, I was reading about visualization and something bothered me, something clicked in my mind and came in the form of a question. Let me explain what happened:

The very first time I thoroughly looked into visualizing was when I was studying to become a personal trainer. Visualizing was a tool to help athletes reach their goals. However, they were not only asked to simply visualize the end result like holding the trophy or jumping up for joy at the moment of victory. No! Visualizing athletes were asked to view and analyze every detail of their every move: they were asked to see the entire process.
For example, if a tennis player wanted to improve his serve, then he would visualize each and every step: from the moment he would take the ball in his hand, make it bounce three times on the ground, bend the knees, throw the ball up in the air, swing the racket and hit it. It was important that the athlete actually saw himself playing, kind of like in slow motion, repeating the same movement over and over again in his mind before seeing himself succeed. This method of preparation is known to be highly effective for athletes.
For this reason, I questioned myself whether it was enough to simply see yourself at final destination…would it have been enough for an athlete to simply see himself up on the podium? I pause and wonder. Maybe, I am just saying maybe, a little more action needs to be involved into the equation for it to really work.

a. Example n° 01: *My goal is… to publish my book*
Let's take the example of getting my book published. I could see myself signing a contract with a publisher or buying my book in a bookstore and focus only on the end result. Or... I could start by seeing myself working hard and fully concentrating at my desk; I could see myself typing away and feeling inspired and creative. I could imagine the number of pages increasing, I could envision myself smiling and feeling satisfied with the whole process. And then, I could visualize myself sending my book to different publishers and succeeding. Just like the athlete, I will see myself going through each and every step in slow motion and feel how inspired and enthusiastic I am during the whole process.

b. Example n° 02: *Visualize yourself telling your whole story to a crowd of people while being on stage*
Personally, this is my favorite way to visualize: I visualize myself telling a crowd of people the different challenges I have had to tackle. I believe it's important to be specific. I share with them my daily struggles: the fact that I just didn't seem to have enough time, that I tended to put the blame on others or on exterior factors for not getting my writing done, that there were days of doubt and discouragement and so on. But then, still facing the crowd, I continue telling them how I managed to push past these obstacles.

What were *your* challenges? Was it the fact that you were overweight and found it too challenging to go out and exercise because everyone could see you? Was it due to your low self-esteem? Were you in a routine rut? Face the crowd and tell them how you conquered and managed to go past your fears to finally succeed! Although it's important for you to visualize your success, I believe it's also important to acknowledge the challenges you will have to go through to reach that final destination. It's NOT going to be easy, but you WILL tackle all the obstacles, jumping one hurdle at a time. To be armed for success it might be worthwhile to prepare yourself ahead of time by facing various challenges, first by imagining what they could be and then by finding ways to overcome them.

Everyone knows, the path to success, isn't always easy but you *can* succeed, and you *will*. As the saying goes: *"You must climb before you can enjoy the view."*

What this means is that it's going to require some work, some action on your behalf. The way I see it: You can't simply visualize, sit back and expect wonderful things to happen to you. That equation just doesn't sound right or even fair.

> *"Destiny is not a matter of chance; it is a matter of choice.*
> *It is not a thing to be waited for; it is a thing to be achieved."*
> *W.J. Bryant*

c. Example n° 03: *See the challenges and obstacles*

• Why not see yourself participating in some sort of race or challenge, such as a marathon, an obstacle course, climbing up a mountain or even a boxing match or any other sport challenge. The focus here is not on your specific goal but to see yourself getting out there, fighting and succeeding. You could start off by seeing yourself as confident and feeling great. At first this challenge is easy for you. Then progressively, see yourself getting a little discouraged, feeling tired. Other participants are overtaking you. Hear yourself questioning the whole process: Why are you doing this anyway? What have you got to prove? And then at one point say "I'm doing this because….! I am succeeding! I am finishing this challenge!" Then, envision yourself with rage in your heart, your eyes full of determination, you can even yell. See yourself overtaking those participants that had previously overtaken you. See yourself smiling. And finally see yourself as you cross the finish line full of pride!

> **Successful people are not gifted,**
> **they just work hard, then succeed on purpose.**

If your goal is to exercise more frequently at the gym, follow the same idea: imagine you are at the movies and that you see a projection of what you went through: see yourself walking into the gym enthusiastically, then exercising and feeling strong. After a while, see how you start feeling a little self-conscious or tired, even discouraged wanting to quit. Then the image stops and a few questions appear: "What's the purpose of all this? Do I really want this?" See yourself saying out loud: "YES! I really, really, want this!". Then, the images start again and you can see yourself getting back on track even more determined, with a big smile on your face! The last images show you pushing past the gym doors feeling fantastic, full of pride to have kept on going. Try it!

To conclude…

If classic visualization works for you, no need to change anything. However, if something seems to be missing or if you have tried it in the past and don't seem to be getting results, it's time to contest what you have read, to think things through and try things differently, while creating your own path. I was raised to believe that I live in a land of opportunity where anyone can succeed if they work for it. However, it has always been clear to me to never expect anything to be given to me on a silver platter. Sure, once in a while, it happens: life sends you a present, you find a 10$ bill, you win playing at game but most of the time, success comes from hard work. And when you receive the reward, you feel so much prouder after all the hard work you have put into it because *YOU* earned it! So, apply the same principle to visualization: first see yourself striving towards your goal…. and then, see yourself succeed!

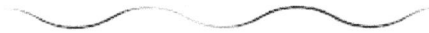

Change n°19
IN TUNE WITH HUNGER
Meet the FULL-O-METER

19.

How do you feel when you leave the table? Do you feel just right? Slightly full? Completely stuffed? For many of you reading this book there is even the possibility that you don't know how you feel anymore because you have lost track of your inner sensory guide. Yes, your inner sensory guide. You know, it's that little voice inside your tummy telling you that you are hungry or that you have had enough. Normally if we are about to eat something it should be because we are hungry. But let's face it, in our busy and hectic lives it seems as though we are no longer in tune with something as basic as our eating habits.

A. Why do we eat?

Many people just eat because it's breakfast, lunch or dinner time. Sometimes people eat simply because it looks or smells good, whether they are hungry or not. Other times people eat because they have to fill an emotional void. I, for example, often eat when I am tired or stressed out. I don't know why I tend to think that if I eat something it will relieve my symptoms of stress or sluggishness. Another good reason to eat is when you are happy and socializing or when you are sad and feeling sorry for yourself. And then, what about those times when you are just plain bored?

It just seems that there is always a good reason to be eating and it's rarely synonymous of hunger. And the fact that food is readily available, just begging to be grabbed by you, anywhere you go, whether it's at the gas station, in a bookstore, or while paying for a prescription or a magazine, doesn't make things easier, does it?

It's good to be aware of this and decide that it's time to be a little more mindful when you eat. So, this week, why not slow down the pace and practice being more in touch with yourself and your inner senses?

Every time you think about food and feel the urge to eat, learn to stop and breathe deeply. Listen to what both your body and mind have to say. Your mind may claim "I want food!" but is your body really hungry? Many people have, unfortunately, lost complete contact with their inner sensory guide and have become incapable of recognizing the emotion they are experiencing. Whether they are bored, frustrated, stressed or sad they classify their emotion as "uncomfortable" and directly reach for food in order to feel better.

If you want to find peace with your plate, it is essential that you listen to yourself and that you become capable of naming and expressing each and every emotion that you feel. "I am bored." "I am stressed." "I am sad." Once you can put a name on how you feel, you can then address it. Indeed, you wouldn't necessarily treat boredom the same way you would treat anger or sadness. Be prepared. Why not make a list of things you can do depending on the emotion you are experiencing. For example, if you are bored, find things that you can do that make you happy and feel good such as pampering yourself, going for a walk, reading a book, taking a bath, listening to music, singing, watching an online motivational video or a funny sequence from a movie that you loved.

Create a list for each and every emotion you have a tendency to experience and next time it occurs, review it and start doing something about it: learn to change the way you feel.
Check out the organizational chart that I have created. It has helped me in the past to assess whether I was hungry or not, what emotion I was undergoing, and what I could do to avoid reaching out for comfort food.

B. Being in tune with what I call your "inner sensory guide"?

Just like everything else, it takes practice. One of the most important things is to slow down and be more mindful while you eat. At every single meal sit down with intent and tell yourself "OK, I am going to eat this meal with intent and total awareness. I will take my time and be in tune with my inner signals and what they are telling me." A good idea is to place something – such as a small piece of paper with written word "slow" or a special object such as a mini Buddha right in front of your plate as a reminder because there is a big chance you might forget to be mindful very very quickly. You will see that even with the best of intentions, you may start off by eating mindfully and then suddenly it will hit you that you have finished your meal and have forgotten all about paying attention.

Don't be too hard on yourself: it takes practice, lots of practice to slow down and be in tune with yourself.

An important thing to understand in this whole process is that it takes approximately 20 minutes for your brain to receive the fullness signals transmitted from your stomach. So, if you eat too fast or are not concentrating on your meal because you are distracted by conversation, electronic devices, or are stressed because of time, it's easy to miss the signal telling you that you have reached satiety and have eaten enough.

The area in the brain that regulates hunger and fullness is called the hypothalamus. Once your stomach has had enough food, it sends signals to the hypothalamus, which in turn sends you a warning signal that you are full.
At one point in my life my nickname could have been Speedy Gonzales given the way I would gulp down my food. Today, I really enjoy taking my time and savor every bite. Often, when I go out with my friends, I notice that I still have three quarters of my plate left while my friends have already finished and are patiently waiting for a desert.

For my part, I seldom order desert as I usually feel that I have eaten enough after the main course. But that doesn't mean I can't have my desert a few hours later. That way I am not frustrated or missing out on something: and when I eat my desert, I am usually hungry again and I can really enjoy every bite.

I WANT FOOD, I ASK: "AM I HUNGRY?"

YES

Where do I situate myself on the hunger scale?

Ask yourself 2 questions:

1° What do I feel like eating?

2° What can I do to make my meal healthier?

I AM NOT SURE

I drink water and determine how I feel?

Why do I want to eat?
1° I am bored
2° I am stressed, it relieves my stress
3° I am sad or depressed, it comforts me
4° I am tempted (satisfying my sweet tooth)
5° I am eating out and there is a lot of food

NO

I drink water

Still craving for food?
Set a timer and commit to not eating anything for another 1 or 1 1/2 hours

EAT

Prepare with love
Set a nice table
Sit down
Take your time
Breathe
Be aware
Enjoy
Savor every bite
Be grateful

See what can I do to make my meal healthier.

STOP

TAKE A BREAK OR GET BUSY

Isolate yourself to really get in tune with what you are feeling
Listen to a P.E.T. (refer to Change n°05)
Call a friend
Do some breathing exercises
Exercise or stretch
Go for a walk
Listen to relaxing music
Watch a funny video or something that makes you laugh
Read
Take a cold shower

C. The technique: 4 Simple Steps

Knowing that it takes about 20 min to reach satiety, it's important:

- To sit down every time you eat. You can't be focused if you are eating on the go. Sitting and eating in the car doesn't count! You have to actually be seated at the table with the option to put your fork down and see the visual cues: the "slow" note, the Buddha or whatever object you have chosen.
- Start eating: put tiny bitefulls in your mouth and chew slowly. Swallow only when your food is completely chewed. We are looking for totally mushy or liquid here!
- Enjoy the process. Be happy that you are doing this for yourself. Smile!
- Regularly STOP and take a breather in between bites and listen: Is your stomach starting to tell you something? Sit back in your chair, relax and listen again.

At first this may all seem like a bit much but once you get used to it, you are going to love it. The first thing you will notice is how relaxed and calm you feel when you leave the table and then you will get a great feeling of lightness inside. You will leave feeling satisfied, and your energy level will be high. No more feeling sluggish, no need to take a nap and you will be ready to tackle whatever it is you have to do.

D. What are the different phases of hunger and fullness?
The FULL-O-METER.
Meet the FULL-O-METER, your hunger specialist as she takes you through the different hunger stages that range between 0 and 10.

Most of the time we tend to overeat simply due to a lack of awareness, lack of attention or what some of you might call "busyness". Hence the necessity to be more in tune with your inner guide. So, with the help of the FULL-O-METER learn to pay closer attention to all the signs and symptoms you are experiencing.

What are the different phases of hunger and fullness?

Meet the FULL-O-METER, your hunger map that guides you through the different hunger stages that range between 0 and 10.

FULL-O-METTER

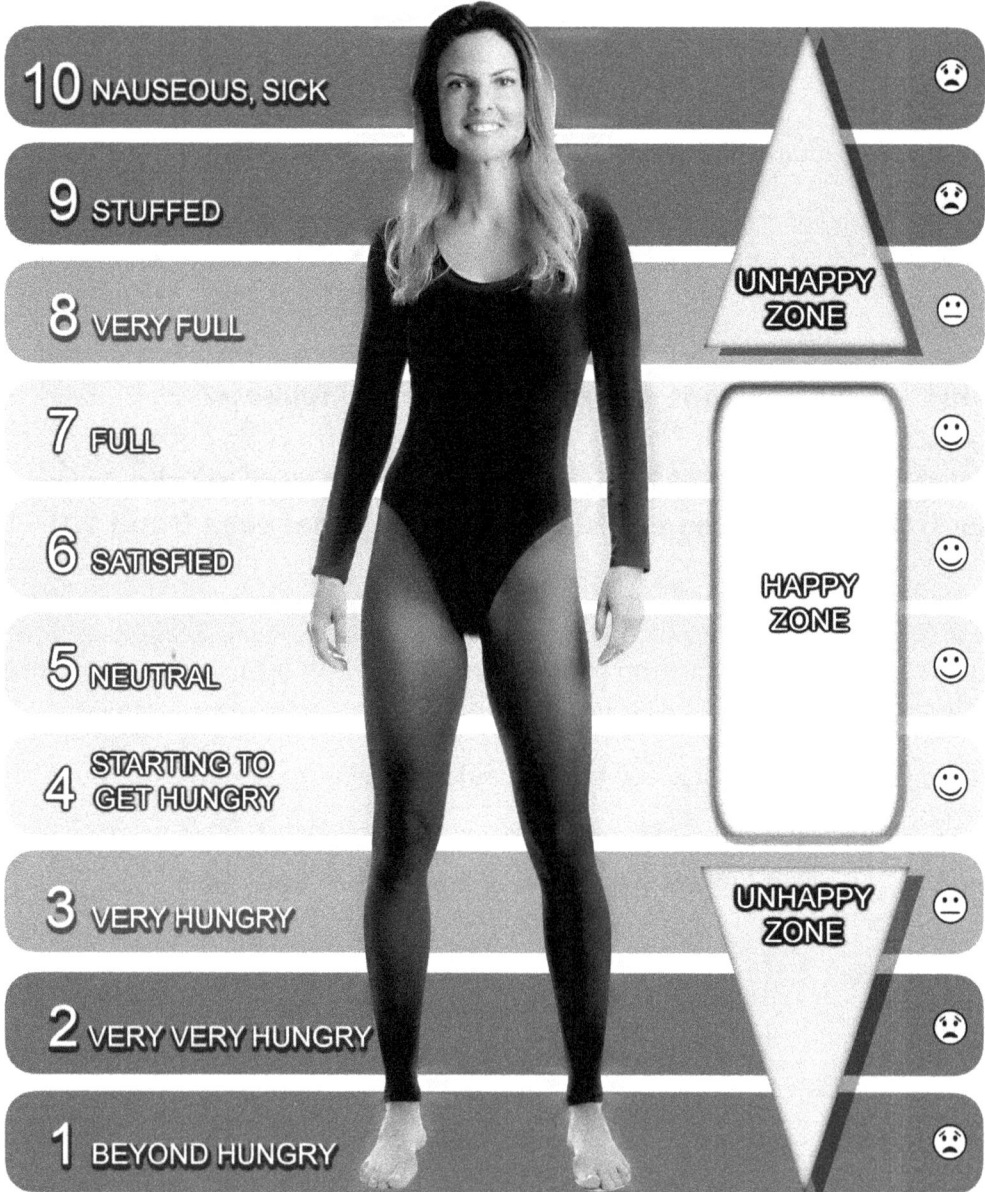

10 NAUSEOUS, SICK

9 STUFFED

8 VERY FULL

UNHAPPY ZONE

7 FULL

6 SATISFIED

HAPPY ZONE

5 NEUTRAL

4 STARTING TO GET HUNGRY

3 VERY HUNGRY

UNHAPPY ZONE

2 VERY VERY HUNGRY

1 BEYOND HUNGRY

Zone 1: You are beyond hungry. Expressions: Having stomach in heels, could gobble anything down, feel like you could eat a horse. Synonymous of ravenous, famished, starving. In Zone 1, you will be feeling grouchy, aggressive, irritable, light headed, no energy at all. Don't ever let yourself get into this zone as you will most likely overeat when in presence of food again.

Zone 2: You are feeling very uncomfortable, it's difficult for you to focus clearly. Symptoms: lightheaded, shaky, loss of focus.

Zone 3: You are very hungry and have hunger pangs, your stomach might be growling. You will want to make sure that you start eating and that you don't get past this point.

Zone 4: You feel a little hungry. Your thoughts tend to drift toward food. Some will say they have the munchies. You are slightly hungry but are not yet uncomfortable. Avoid going grocery shopping when in this zone or below as you will tend to buy a lot more and will not make reasonable choices.

Zone 5: In this zone you are neither hungry nor full. You are in a neutral state. Eating is pleasurable. If you are at peace with your plate you enjoy and savor every bite, taking in all the flavors and textures of what you are eating. Now is the time to really slow down, by making sure you chew your food as much as possible, which will also help with digestion, and by putting your knife and fork down regularly. If you are busy doing something such as watching TV, checking social network or working, I would recommend you stop to focus on your inner sensations and learn to be in tune with your inner satiety level.

Zone 6: You feel satisfied, content. You can sense the food inside your stomach. At this point, you feel like you could eat a little more. **You should STOP eating at this point.** If you haven't finished your plate or haven't yet had your desert, get into the habit of boxing it up and/or saving the rest for later: enjoy those leftovers or that desert in a few hours when you are back in Zone 4 or 5. This way, you leave the table feeling just right and are not frustrated: the moment to savor the rest or that desert is simply delayed.

Zone 7: In this zone, you don't need to eat anymore. You are full, replete, satiated, completely satisfied. Your stomach is starting to feel comfortably full. You will have a tendency to eat slowly or to slow things down naturally. Avoid ever going beyond this point.

Zone 8: You're feeling very full. You are feeling uncomfortable with a need to unfasten your belt. You know you have overdone it. Your stomach is upset.

Zone 9: You're stuffed. Your stomach is in distress. There is no room left for food. You are feeling very uncomfortable. Your stomach is starting to stretch. You feel the need to lie down.

Zone 10: You have eaten way too much and are feeling nauseous and your stomach is very painful. You could be sick or even throwing up.

What would be good, for the next 7 days, is to write down the number where you situate yourself on the FULL-O-METER at the end of each meal. It might be interesting to write down how you feel immediately after your meal as well 20 minutes later. Sometimes we leave the table feeling content but as the digestion starts to settle in, we realize that we should have eaten just a little less.

a. A few pointers that might help you reach your goal this month:

- Eating alone as much as possible! Indeed, in order to be more aware, you need to get as many distractions out of the way as possible. By distractions I mean: people, electronic devices, books or magazines etc. You don't have to eat alone at every meal but whenever the opportunity arises, especially at the beginning of this goal, seize it and turn it into an awareness meal.
- If it's really not possible for you to eat alone, at least try having your snacks in a quiet place. And, when eating in the company of others, focus your attention on listening. While listening, you can quietly chew your food.
- Try to put your fork and knife down regularly and lean back in your chair to take a break.

Remember, in order to get through all of these goals there will be a lot of trial and error. Just keep trying, trying and trying again. When babies learn how to walk, they don't say "Ah forget it, it's not for me." They get up and try again. And when I recall some of the falls and flops my boys went through, you can only call it "determination". Find that inner determination; it's still in you and just keep on trying!

Remember:

> ### FAILURE is not the opposite of success.
> ### It is PART of success!

b. How do I use the Full-O-Meter?
Frequently monitor yourself and ask questions

When you are in a situation where food is available, stop and ask yourself:

"Am I hungry right now? If yes, then how hungry am I?" If you are at stage 1 (starving), 2 (very very hungry) and 3 (very hungry) then it's time to eat. Normally it's not recommended to let yourself get so hungry that you reach stage 1 or 2 as you most certainly will eat more than you really need to. When starving, many people tend to reach for rich, processed foods to calm their ravenous state.

Try as much as possible to eat when at stage 3, which means your stomach is growling and you are uncomfortably hungry. If you are starting to get hungry (stage 4) then try drinking a big glass of water and get busy again. See how you feel in another 15 minutes. If you are just bored or if the food is only tempting, chances are your craving will diminish. If you really want it but are not hungry yet, consider buying/bringing it and keeping it for later. That way you won't feel the frustration of having to turn it down and you will be able to reward yourself with it later while being in tune with your "inner sensory guide".

What are the signs to be in tune with, while eating?

While eating, and this is probably the most challenging part for most of you, it's really important to listen to your inner signals. At one point, you will notice that you tend to slow down. That's an important cue to catch. By then, depending on how fast you ate, you are probably already at a stage 6 or 7. It's very important to put your fork down, breathe and see how you feel. Is your stomach starting to feel a little full? Do you feel less pleasure when eating? Are you just eating because you have to finish your plate? Do you really want the rest of the food? Are your belt or clothes starting to feel a little tight around the tummy? Do you feel your stomach stretching? These are all signs that you have to stop.

For some of you it's just not possible to waste food, or it's impossible to have a meal without having a desert. We are not throwing out the food and you *can* have a desert! All you have to do is put the rest of the food aside for later and you can have desert in an hour or two when you are hungry again. By delaying the moment you eat your desert, you will actually have something to look forward to and will appreciate it even more when you are hungry again in a couple of hours.

Try to aim for that feeling when you **could** eat more, but you know that if you do, you would feel bloated or would regret it. Think of it: these few extra minutes of eating or these 5 or 10 extra bites could make a huge difference on how you are going to feel the next couple of hours and how much you are going to weigh on that scale. Or let's put it another way: what's more important for you: those extra bites you are not even really hungry for, or feeling really great all afternoon?

*Remember the **LAW OF THE FORK**:*
***You** are the one*
placing the fork in your mouth!
AND
***You** are the one*
choosing when to put that fork down!

*In other words: **You are fully RESPONSIBLE***
for where you are right now with your weight
***You CAN change things**!*

Endorse full responsibility and move from there. You can change. You really truly can.

c. What if I can't detect hunger or fullness signals in my body?
It is important to note that there are a number of reasons why people can't detect hunger or have lost touch with their hunger and fullness signals. To name only a few:
- If you have been dieting for long periods of time
- If you have an eating disorder
- If you have been raised with certain habits: parents already overeating or made you always finish your plate etc.

- If you have emotional issues linked to food
- If you are on some kind of treatment that might alter how you perceive certain sensations (some treatments stimulate or cut your appetite)
- If you are depressed

In all of these cases, it can still be a goal, but as always, I recommend that you consult and seek help from a specialist or a medical professional.

I personally had emotional issues with food: as soon as I felt sad or not in control of my life, I would overeat and it would often be junk. But these issues today are a thing of the past: I have managed to overcome them on my own through self-observation and trial and error. I have learnt not to feel guilty about anything I eat and to put my fork down and eat slowly. That was a big step forward for me. Food has become a friend. I know that for many of you it's a worst enemy. Today I share a generally healthy relationship with food. I can look you in the eye and affirm that I am totally at peace with my plate. What about you, are you at peace with yours?

Change n°20
SELF~OBSERVATION
My Mood and Food Tracker

20.

Why don't you become a self-observer? Self-observation can be one of the most interesting things a person can do for himself. Most of us simply breeze through our days without taking the time to step back and look at what we are doing, how we are behaving, how we are interacting with others, when and why we are eating, what our posture is like and so on.

Why not decide to become an observer this week? As with everything, it will take a little getting used to. At first it will be quite a challenge to observe yourself. It might be a good idea to buy a funny little ring or cut a piece of string and place it on your finger, in order to remind yourself to pay closer attention to what you are doing and how you are reacting to the situation you are in. You may want to spend as much time as possible observing yourself throughout the day or you might simply decide to be fully present every time you are eating a meal.

A. What are your "Where, When, Why, What and How's" of eating?

The goal this week is to try to see:
- What you eat: what kind of foods are you eating? Do you eat a variety of different foods or do you stick to one or two food groups only?
- Where you eat: Is it at the table, standing up, in a busy or quiet environment, alone or with someone…
- When you eat: Try to see if there are any patterns, when do you tend to eat more/less or binge…
- Try to understand why you eat, for what reason you have chosen to eat: are you hungry, bored, stressed, sad, tired and so on
- Assess how you feel after you have eaten, whether you feel light, bloated, stuffed, sluggish, tired, energized, satisfied, content…

B. Journaling the "Where, When, Why, What and How's" of eating

It is well established that people self-regulate their moods by eating or engaging in physical activity. We often overeat when we feel down, are tired or under pressure. Eating appears to be the easiest way to boost our mood up again. I don't know about you, but when I am tired or stressed out I tend to go directly to the kitchen cabinet and grab something to eat.

It's important to know when these moments occur because it's at this specific moment that one tends to sabotage their diet. By observing yourself you will be able to note how your moods influence your attitude towards food.

For this reason, it would be a good idea to buy yourself a notepad or a food journal to write the "Where, When, Why, What and Hows" concerning your eating habits.

My "MOOD & FOOD" Tracker

I remember, before each meal, to start off by asking myself what it is that I really feel like eating. I have one or two small portions of what I am craving for but then I make sure that the rest of my meal is super healthy. I accompany my craving with fruits and vegetables, whole grains, a source of proteins and lots of water.

Then, throughout the meal, I observe myself and take the time to ask the following "Where, When, Why, What and How" questions:

1° Where am I eating?

☐ I am eating at home
☐ I am eating out

☐ I am eating at work

☐ Other_____

☐ I am alone

☐ I am in company of_____

2° When am I eating? *Place the hands on the clock.*

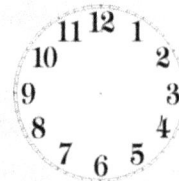

3° Why am I eating? *Take a moment to reflect and then select the real reason*

☐ I am hungry

☐ I am under stress

☐ I am sad

☐ I am in good company / convivial atmosphere

☐ I am feeling uncomfortable

☐ Other_____

☐ I am bored

☐ I am angry

☐ Because it's time to eat

☐ Because it smells or looks good (I feel tempted)

4° What am I eating and drinking? *(Taking a good look at my plate)*

I write down what I am eating and drinking:

_____
_____
_____
_____

I assess my meal:

☐ I am eating a healthy meal or made sure there is something healthy to accompany it

☐ I am eating only junk. (I then reduce my portion and add a healthy component)

☐ I am eating something I love and that makes me happy

☐ I am drinking alcohol or unnecessary drinks. (I then make sure to drink a big glass of water)

☐ I am having fruits and vegetables

☐ I feel proud of myself because I am one step closer to leading a healthy lifestyle

5a° How am I eating?

☐ I am eating slowly   ☐ I am eating fast

☐ I am chewing my food   ☐ I am swallowing without chewing

☐ I am eating in a quiet environment   ☐ I am eating in a noisy environment

☐ I am seated   ☐ I am standing / on the go

☐ I am eating with awareness   ☐ I am eating unconsciously

☐ I feel in control   ☐ I am eating compulsively

☐ I am only eating   ☐ I am doing something else while eating (such as reading, texting etc.)

☐ Other_____

                                ☐ Other_____

5b° How do I feel after my meal?

☐ I am still hungry   ☐ I feel slightly full or full

☐ I feel fine, light   ☐ My stomach is painful or I feel bloated

☐ I feel proud of myself   ☐ I feel guilty - I regret what or the quantity I ate

☐ I feel energized

☐ Other_____   ☐ I feel sluggish, lethargic

To Conclude *(I write what I am proud of and what measures I can take to improve my next meal)*:

_____

_____

Take the time to stop a few minutes and observe yourself. Get in the habit of keeping track of where, when, what and how you eat. Ask yourself for what reason you are really eating and throughout the meal assess how you feel.

C. Why use a food journal or your Mood and Food Tracker?

The goal here is to try to recognize your recurring patterns such as specific times when you tend to overeat or on the contrary not to eat, times during the day when you feel the most energized, drowsy or stressed. You could even add other important information such as when you most enjoy exercising and when not. By learning to track these patterns you will be able to act accordingly.

If, for example, you notice that around a specific time during the day, you tend to feel stressed, be prepared: try to see what you can do to enhance your mood ahead of time:

- Could you shut everything out for 5 minutes by taking a break or finding a place where you can be alone?
- How about drinking a big glass of water or splashing some cold water on your face?
- Or maybe you could treat yourself to something you like to eat? If this is the case, make sure you make this moment special and savor every bite.
- Or, would taking a 5 minute brisk walk offer a solution?

Let's press the "pause" button here. I don't know about you, but when I read this type of information, it literally makes me stop in my footsteps. Does the type of exercise and the intensity at which I train really affect my mood and how I eat?

Once the information has been planted in my brain, it's a thing with me... I just have to go and try it myself to see whether it's true or not, and find out what this information can reveal about myself regarding my relationship toward exercise and food. Research says:

"Moderate exercise raises energy". It's written on paper, you read it, and you tell yourself, it must be true. I would like you to go one step further and try it!

Go for a 15 minute walk and see for yourself how you feel. I know. I tried it and I felt a real boost of energy every time. For having read it *and* tried it, I can affirm that moderate exercise raises my energy level.

"More intense exercise reduces tension". Once again, I would like you to question this fact and try it! Today I had an intense leg workout at the gym and as I walked out, I noticed how calm I was. My boyfriend and I started joking about it saying that if you wanted to get someone to do something, just make sure you ask them after a leg workout! Neither him, nor I were up for any discussion or dispute. We were feeling totally Zen. For having read *and* tried it, I can affirm that "more intense exercise reduces tension."

"Both moderate and intense exercise improves mood." After these two tests, I can also affirm that it is true, however in different ways. Moderate exercise energized me to feel ready to tackle work, chores, the kids and so on.

More intense exercise, however, put me in a more quiet mood and in need of maintaining a state of inner calmness. After this kind of workout, I could write my book with improved concentration, spend some quiet time with kids, while reading them a story, meditatating and so on.

Finally, **"moderate exercise can temporarily reduce appetite."** We are all different and so it is important that you observe yourself to see how you feel after moderate or intense exercise. Do you feel ravenous? Did the training cut your appetite? Being a regular exerciser and also a self-observer, I know for a fact, that exercising totally suppresses my appetite for about 40 minutes to an hour. Now it's your turn to find out how the intensity or type of exercise, has an affect over you and how much you eat.

This is all a trial and error process to get to know yourself. Remember what works or is true for one, might not work or be true for another.

D. Being prepared allows you to *RE-act*

Knowing that it is normal for our moods to go through these ups and downs will help you take control of them. It's important to understand and be aware of the entire process. "Oh! It's almost 5 pm, I am going to have that crash I normally go through. I am quickly going to run up and down several flights of stairs and then I will go to the restroom to splash some cold water on my face. If I still crave for something I will make sure I drink a big glass of fresh water and eat that apple I brought with me."

What, how much, and when you eat will greatly affect your mood and how you feel in the next couple of hours. For this reason, I must add I have often found that self-observation has helped me become aware of certain patterns and habits. Once I started seeing myself doing the same thing over and over again, there came a point when I felt annoyed with my attitude.

It was like: "Here I go again." Or "I can't believe I just did that again. It's been 10 days in a row. When will I learn?" The next phase, usually, is to anticipate the moment, in other words, know that it's coming. You might still succumb to your bad habit, but you are doing it fully aware. Eventually, there will come a point when you will say: "No, I am not doing it anymore."

Keeping track of these patterns by writing them down in a notebook will help you on your path to self-observation. Keep in mind that awareness is half of the job.

E. First, write things down and then, step back and observe

If you want to reach a goal, it's important to write it down on paper. It creates intent and, whether you realize or not, it helps create intent, and begins a whole process that will enable you to achieve it. Taking the time to write down how you feel when you are eating is, in a way, very similar. It will allow you to become more aware of what you are doing and why you are doing it. In a sense, you are stepping back to observe the situation, taking a little bit of time to understand why you are eating.

I love to read Krishnamurti's books as they always give me material to think about. In *The Kingdom of Happiness,* he talks about habits and takes the example of a smoker. Have you ever observed a smoker and how it becomes a habit for them to smoke.

Although they lose part of their freedom and must go outside several times a day to have a cigarette and repeat this same ritual 365 days a year, they can't help it, they are slaves to this habit. But, what would happen if a smoker became really conscious of their habit? What if, every single time they engaged in this ritual, they were fully attentive to what they are doing, without ever emitting any judgment whatsoever and without ever saying that it's bad to smoke? You would see that when you start doing things consciously, you progressively stop reinforcing this specific habit.

Being in awareness, being fully present while engaging in an unhealthy activity, is already one step toward cutting that bad habit for good. And, once you manage to be in this state of self-observation, you can start digging a little deeper by questioning yourself: why did you start this bad habit in the first place and why do you spend your time living and doing things without paying any attention? Reflect upon Krishnamurti's words as well: "It is of utmost importance to understand, in detail, the reason why your spirit lets itself wander away and not be fully attentive." Repeat the question to yourself several times. Plant the seed. Stir the ground by coming back to the question several times in the next few days and pay attention to the answers that come your way.

I would like to add the necessity for slowing down. With our jam-packed days, we no longer have the time to pay attention. If we want to create an ideal atmosphere in which we can observe ourselves, it is of the utmost importance that we learn to slow down.

Many times, eating is in fact an emotional reaction: we eat for comfort to relieve pain, stress, anger, or boredom. Junk is often called comfort food. I like to make the analogy between food and motherly love. Indeed, food can be like a loving mother that brings you comfort, makes you feel better, brings relief at a moment when you are feeling down, stressed or in need of a little attention. It's important to be aware of this. Maybe all you need right now is just a little bit of love or maybe it's something else…*something that you have to figure out.*

Have you ever taken the time to sit down and ask yourself why you reach out for food, why you accept and constantly repeat any destructive pattern you have towards yourself in regards to food? I am not asking you whether you have occasionally asked yourself a question here and there. What I want to know is whether you have actually taken 20, 45 or even 60 minutes to really understand what is going on inside of you? Try it. Sit down, maybe grab a pen and paper and persist until you get some answers. Think it through, thoroughly. There is a high probability that you might cry your heart out and that's ok. I feel like saying it's even a good sign, because you are onto something.

We keep so many things bottled up or even bury them completely and simply assume that if we keep ourselves busy, we will end up forgetting. It doesn't work that way. You need to know why. Once you understand the underlying cause, accept it. You might not be able to do anything about it, since you can't change the past, but if you choose to see these painful events as lessons, you might learn something positive after all. What have you learned? Has the pain transformed you? Don't start going down the path of hatred and self-pity. It won't get you anywhere. Let these negative emotions go down another path.

What you want, is to see how these events have allowed you to grow. Were you heartbroken? Maybe you were basing your happiness only on your relationship with this person. The lesson might be that true happiness never comes from someone else… you have to learn to be happy on your own. The same holds true for your parents. Do you feel you were never loved enough? Stop craving for love you will never receive and start focusing on the greatest love of all: yourself. If you have two minutes and 30 seconds, listen to Whitney Houston's song *The Greatest Love of All*. It says: "I found the greatest love of all inside of me…Learning to love yourself it is the greatest love of all." And then get up, start doing things for yourself, start taking extra special care of *you* and put a smile on your face because you are on your way to CHANGE.

To conclude: knowing *when* you tend to eat more, but also *why* you are doing it, is getting you one step closer to healing your relationship with food. This week decide to make peace and become friends with your plate. Start applying self-observation to your life and see yourself one step closer to gaining control over your eating habits!

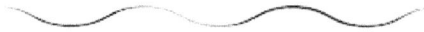

Change n°21
RULES BETWEEN MEALS

21.

This week why not give your digestive system a break by eating at regular intervals and doing a 10 hour fast every night by not eating anything between 8 p.m. and 6 a.m. (or 9 p.m. and 7 a.m.)

• Become a detective, take your magnifying glass and hunt for hidden clues

Have you tried, time and time again, to lose weight without ever succeeding? Whether you are severely overweight or are simply carrying around a few extra pounds, there could be any number of reasons to explain why you have failed. But what if you decided this week to get rid of those sneaky snacks that you tend to grab in between meals? You know when you say you are just going to grab a coffee – 2 calories - but then you add two lumps of sugar – 100 calories – and 2 tbsp of cream – for a total of 204 calories! Or, how about that handful of peanuts you grabbed before your meal - 125 calories! Oh and that extra glass of vino – between 80 and 150 calories depending on the brand. And what about when you ate that bun while waiting to be served at the restaurant – 49 calories – or tasted the dinner 5 or 6 times while it was cooking, just to make sure it was cooked?

Indeed, we tend to think "Oh I haven't eaten that much" but then we forget all those hidden calories taken in "hic e illic", that is latin for "here and there". And what about those late-night snacks you eat while watching TV? Those are all caloric numbers that add up as well.

So, why not give your body a break for ten hours every day this week by refraining from eating anything after 8 or 8:30 pm and see if you feel any different? And why not let your digestive system work at regular intervals during the day by stopping those in-between meal munchies? So, beginning tonight, at 8 pm decide to put up a "Sorry we're closed" sign on the kitchen door! This way you will make sure you are going to bed feeling light and won't fall asleep with a heartburn. Now it's important not to change anything else and you mustn't see this as a diet. You can go on eating everything you usually do, your only goal being to let your digestive system take a break. Many people tend to go through an "eat – think about eating" pattern, in which food has become a real obsession throughout the entire day. If they are not eating then they are most likely thinking about food or doing their best to refrain from eating.

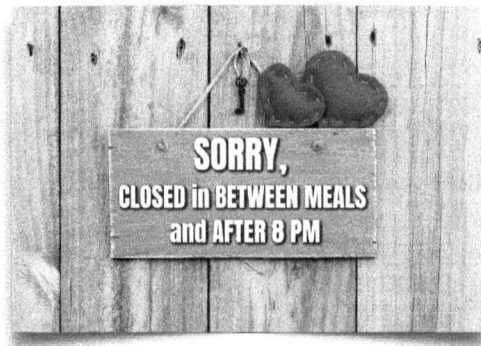

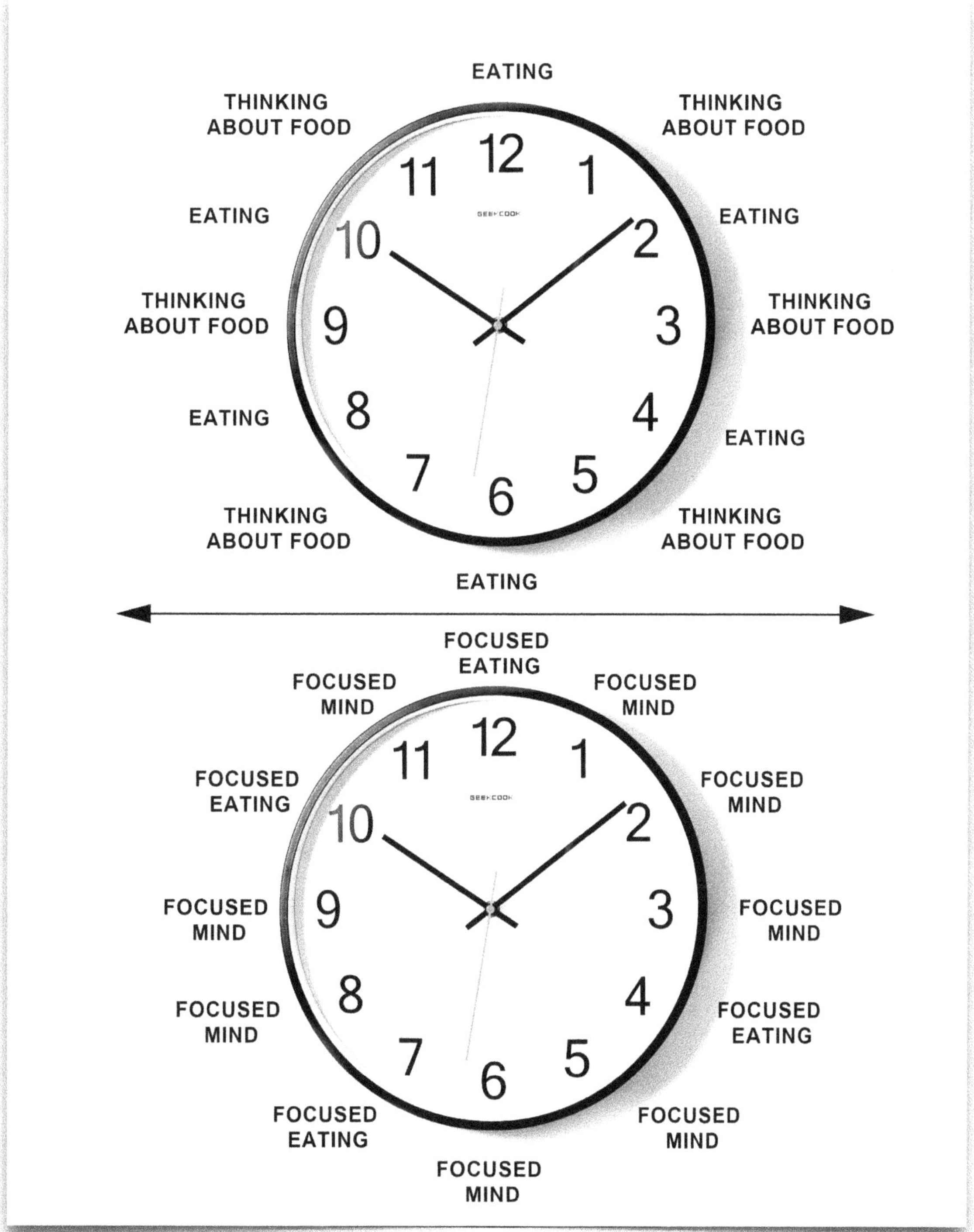
EATING
THINKING ABOUT FOOD
EATING
THINKING ABOUT FOOD
EATING
THINKING ABOUT FOOD
EATING
THINKING ABOUT FOOD
EATING
THINKING ABOUT FOOD
EATING
THINKING ABOUT FOOD
12 1 2 3 4 5 6 7 8 9 10 11
FOCUSED EATING
FOCUSED MIND
FOCUSED MIND
FOCUSED MIND
FOCUSED EATING
FOCUSED MIND
FOCUSED MIND
FOCUSED EATING
FOCUSED MIND
FOCUSED MIND
FOCUSED EATING
FOCUSED MIND
12 1 2 3 4 5 6 7 8 9 10 11

- **Why take up this challenge and what are the benefits of letting your digestive system rest?**

  - The very first reason why you should tackle this change is because statistics show that most people ingest the biggest amount of calories once they are at home, at first to unwind at the end of the day and later because it has become a habit and a pleasure to eat while watching TV. If you knew that an 8 ounce bag of chips has 1300 calories, a big bowl of buttered popcorn over 1000 calories and 40g of fat, a 5 Ounce bag of gummy bears 660 calories, and a big 7 ounce bar of chocolate contains 1064 calories it would seem obvious that by cutting these out in the evening, you will lose weight. Don't change anything else throughout the day and see what happens. If you stop ingesting calories after 8 pm, chances are you will be cutting out approximately 500 calories and 500 calories less on a daily basis is 3500 calories less a week, in other words one pound less every week. This reason alone should motivate you to try!

  - You will learn to be more in tune with your body. Take the time to hear its signals. At different moments throughout the day ask yourself: "How do I feel? Am I hungry? Am I satisfied? Do I feel uncomfortable because I ate too much? Am I drowsy?" Most importantly, listen to the answers. Reconnect with your digestive system. Having this dialog frequently will get you one step closer to having a better relationship with your plate and body.

  - You might rediscover what hunger feels like. Many people tend to eat throughout the day never allowing their digestive system any rest. This was the case at one point in my life: I never knew what it felt like to be hungry as I always tended to eat before any symptoms occurred.

  - You will feel like you are the one controlling your mind. I have always had this strong belief, deep down inside, that at birth, we were given a certain number of "tools": a body, a mind, a heart and a temper, to name only a few. It is up to each and every one of us to decide whether we will be the ones controlling these tools or whether we are going to let *them* control us. Are you going to overeat at dinner tonight and let greed decide, or will you take the time to be grateful, to savor every bite and stop when you are no longer hungry? Next time you are under stress, will you let impatience or anger control you or will you step back, breathe and try to calm your overall state? You're in charge. I truly believe this to be our biggest mission on Earth.

  - You will sleep better if you are not feeling too full. As with any type of pain, trying to sleep with a heartburn is very difficult. Why not get in the habit of massaging your stomach (intestines). Check out   Change n° 29 the Physical Assessment Checklist (P.A.C.), that proposes an entire section on digestion as well as different techniques to improve your digestion.

  - You won't overeat. Many people consume a big portion of their calories between 8 and 11pm. By not ingesting anything after 8 pm, you will definitely cut down on the amount of food you eat.

- You could very well create a positive lifestyle change for your entire family. Often kids tend to imitate their parents, especially if they see positive results.

Additional tip: I have found that brushing your teeth, going for a walk after dinner, meditating or going to bed earlier can really help.

• An easy and yet challenging goal

• An easy goal

On the one hand, this is a fairly easy goal since you are not really required to do anything aside from:
- making sure that you are only eating at mealtimes,
- no longer eating after a predetermined time at night.

• A challenging goal

On the other hand, however, this goal may be very challenging for some of you. A number of jobs make this goal seem almost like an impossible task. Let me give you a random example:

My hairdresser: She works from 9 am to 6 pm every day and has no lunch break. Basically, this is how her day goes: she will have to stand on her feet all day long and take care of a never-ending procession of clients, she will have to put up with them, chat and smile, forgetting the pain in her back and the swelling of her legs, as well as ignoring the fact that she would love to have a little peace and quiet, at a certain point. She is expected to gulp down her meal in between two clients or while a color is setting. Her dining space is a tiny cubicle where she can sit but is seen by all. Her lunch breaks should actually be called "fast feeds" since they are taken in a stressful and unfavorable environment. She will most probably have several of these "fast feeds" throughout the day, never really consciously participating or enjoying her meal.

According to Marc David in his book *The Slow Down Diet*, which is a reference book to learn how to be at peace with your plate, the author explains that your tummy and taste buds are not the only ones to experience pleasure: your mind plays an active part as well. Your brain can actually "taste", find pleasure and feel satisfied. But how can you expect your brain to experience "taste, pleasure and satisfaction" when it is busy doing something else such as working, reading, talking and so on. If your mind is focused on a specific task while you are eating, it can actually zap out the fact that you have eaten anything at all and will then have you claiming for more food to be able to experience the pleasurable sensation it gets when you eat mindfully.

• To guarantee success!

• Break your schedule down and get organized

It is a good idea to stick with the traditional three meals, as in breakfast lunch and dinner and two snacks. It's up to you to decide when to have these meals and snacks according to the type of job you have, your work shifts and what works best for you. So, plan it and stick with it!

Everybody is different and there is no way I can lay out a "one fit for all" schedule. If you have doubts, of course, I recommend you see your dietician. What's important here is:

- find a rhythm that works for you and you are comfortable with,
- adapt your lifestyle as best as you can to make sure you're enjoying these mealtimes in awareness and with as little stress as possible.

Let's come back to my hairdresser…

There is always a solution, using your common sense, to get yourself organized!

If we look at my hairdresser's situation, there a few little things she could have tried to implement to make her meals a real break:

- For one thing, she and the other hairdressers could have asked for a 15 or 20 min break and adjusted the schedule by crossing out a time slot in red: no appointments can be taken at that time.

- Right across the street from the hair salon is a little park. Although in rainy or too cold weather it might not be an option, on other days of the year, however, my hairdresser could grab her little lunch bag and take that 15 min break at the park sitting on a bench. This would allow her to physically get out of the salon, breathe some air and eat quietly. It may seem like nothing but even such a short break can help a great deal in recharging your batteries and being in connection with your food.

- If the 15/20 min break is not an option, the hairdressers could try to make the small cubicle more comfortable. They could concert each other to see in what way it could be redecorated to turn it into a more relaxing environment by adding a little color, some pictures, a plant, a mirror, a small water fountain and to ensure that each one of them could eat without being disturbed and seen by the customers they could install some saloon doors.

- **Applying the principle when at the office**

If you are working in a stressful environment and there is no other possibility but to eat at your desk in the midst of noise and phone calls, well then, so be it. Don't try to fight against an impossible situation. Accept it. What you *can* do in this case, however, is to try as much as possible to eat at a regular time before becoming too ravenous and to eat and chew mindfully. *Bring awareness into your eating.* Take one bite at a time, put your fork or sandwich down and chew. It won't be easy at first but, as they say, practice makes perfect. You might wonder what this has got to do with eating at regular intervals. I have explained this point before but I will insist upon it again: eating without awareness, for your mind, is almost the same as not eating at all. If you don't let your mind partake in the joy of eating, it will feel left out and frustrated. It's of utmost importance that you try to enjoy the moment so your mind can register this fact and feel the satisfaction as well…. Because if your mind doesn't get that "high", it will want to have it later even if you are full. Pay attention and it will not claim any more food until your next programmed break.

And, if it's really impossible to change your meal situation at work, well try your best to change your other meals. There is no need to bring additional stress into your life.

• The night fast

• Walking or meditating

If you have decided to focus on the nighttime goal, one thing that can help is to engage in some stress-reducing activities such as walking or meditating. They will help combat your urge to snack. While writing this book, I made the decision to no longer watch TV in the evenings in order to get more reading done. Sometimes I read but at other times I would also head outdoors for a nice long walk and meditation. Both of these activities, I find, are always relaxing and tend to bring all that pressure built up during the day, all the way back down.

If you are worried about missing out on a TV Series, you can always walk or meditate three, four or five evenings every week. It doesn't have to be an all or nothing option. Keep the things you really enjoy while gradually adding new little changes. The thing to remember here is that it is far more tempting to munch on something while watching TV then when you are walking or meditating.

• Going to bed a little earlier

A nice shower after that walk or meditation and then head straight to bed before you get tempted to eat anything else. Believe me your body is going to yell: "Thank you". A little bit of exercise, a relaxing meditation, a shower and more sleep! Your body will thank you for it and your mind will be more at peace.

• Drink an herbal tea

Another good idea could be to make yourself a huge jug of herbal tea. Discover the benefits behind different herbs and try as many new varieties as possible: try chamomile tea to soothe the stomach and relieve bloating and indigestion, lavender tea to soothe your mind and body and induce sleep, Rosemary tea to help your muscles relax, or lemongrass tea - commonly called after-dinner tea - to aid with digestion. There are many more options to choose from.

This week's goal is to commit to letting your body adapt to its natural rhythm. Listen your body's language and what it has to say. And remember, the reason behind this change is not really weight loss... you are trying to learn to be more in tune with your body and are seeking to create a peaceful relationship with food.

Change n°22
EATING MINDFULLY

22.

I like to compare eating to a conversation. In both cases we are taking something in. If you are in a casual conversation with someone, you are either talking or listening in a relaxed manner. You let the other person's words flow into you: there is no stress involved and your body is calm. If your dialogist starts saying something hurtful or that you disagree with, those harsh words will come in and make your body tense up, it will bring anger inside of you, your stomach will contract. The list of symptoms are numerous depending on how virulent your interlocutor is. Words affect us not only emotionally but also physically.

Think about it. The same holds true for food. If you eat quietly and in a peaceful environment, your food will be welcome and will be easily digested. However, if you eat while you are stressed, your body will no longer be in an optimal state to welcome that food since you feel tense, your stomach is in a knot and your attention is focused on something else. So, when eating, try to keep these questions in mind:

How are you having your meals? Are you enjoying them in a nice relaxed setting or are you always distracted and busy? Are your meals synonymous of peace or chaos? How long does it take you to eat your meals?

• Why should you chew your food?
- It keeps your teeth, gums and tongue healthy
- By chewing thoroughly, you are being "stomach friendly" since you are helping with digestion and also allowing nutrients to be extracted in a maximal way. The goal is to swallow your food when it's as mushy or liquid as possible. Remember it takes time and requires practice.
- When you chew your food, it triggers the production of substances such as hydrochloric acid, that help speed up the digestive process.
- When eating fast, you don't give your body enough time to realize when it is no longer hungry and so you end up eating more. By simply slowing down you will avoid overeating.
- Giving your body a chance to digest food properly will do wonders for how you feel after the meal: chances are you will have fewer indigestions and heartburns, you will be going to the bathroom to eliminate more often and feel empowered and energized!

• How many times should you chew every bite?
I am not into counting how many times you chew. I think it's important to relax and simply enjoy your meal. Out of curiosity, I thought I would research this question anyway: it is recommended that you chew your food approximately 30 times. Ok. Let's be realistic here and use our common sense: one should chew according to the foods one eats.

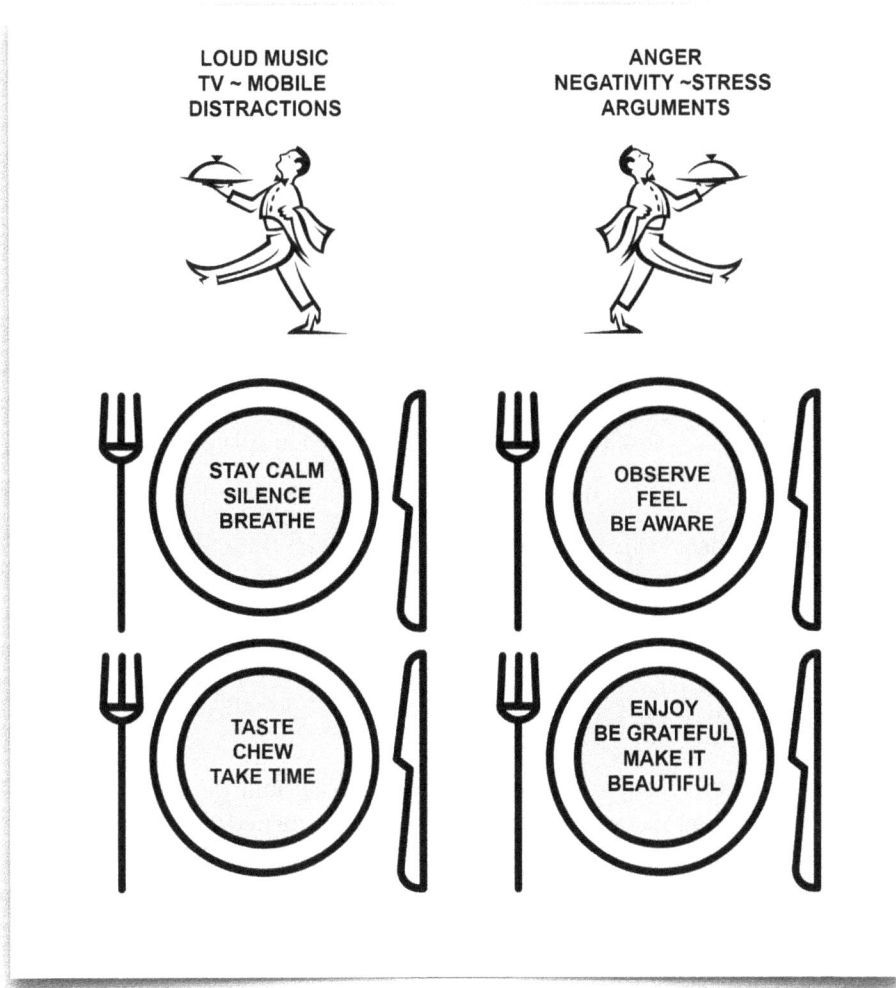

LOUD MUSIC TV ~ MOBILE DISTRACTIONS

ANGER NEGATIVITY ~STRESS ARGUMENTS

STAY CALM
SILENCE
BREATHE

OBSERVE
FEEL
BE AWARE

TASTE
CHEW
TAKE TIME

ENJOY
BE GRATEFUL
MAKE IT
BEAUTIFUL

You don't need to chew a green bean as much as a piece of steak! So, how do we know? Observe the consistency of the food you are eating: some will need approximately 10 chews such as a soft peach or a bite of watermelon and others around 25-30 such as hard vegetable or meat.

Make use of your knife and keep your fork light

It is best to make sure that what you put into your mouth is already tiny. Make use of your knife by "chop, chop, chopping" it all up and keep your fork light! Note that if your bites are tiny, you will probably have to chew fewer times.

Once the food is in your mouth, place your fork and knife down as a reminder that you have to slow down and chew.

> ***It's as important to space your bites***
> ***as it is to chew them completely***

When do we know if it's OK to swallow your food? If you can still feel parts or little chunks of food in your mouth then you haven't chewed enough. As I said before, we're aiming for a totally mushy, almost liquid texture here!

• Let's share a meal and eat mindfully

Eating mindfully implies being totally aware of the whole process. Ideally, it means to:

- Close your eyes and take a few moments to sit in silence and breathe quietly and deeply just before taking your first bite.

- Open your eyes and observe the food that's on your plate: the colors, the shapes, take in the smells.

- Once the food is in your mouth, take the time to really taste and savor it: feel the texture on your tongue. How do you like it? Is it hot or cold? Is it spicy or sweet? Is it smooth or crunchy? What's the flavor like?

- Enjoy your meal and the company that is with you. It should be a moment of sharing, meaning that TVs and all electronic devices should be turned off. Why not have your kids come and help you in the kitchen. When at the table, let each one of you talk a few minutes about an event of their day. This isn't the right time to talk about homework, grades or be reproachful about things that haven't been done about the house. It's a moment to share, to be happy.

- Take your time. Chew thoroughly.

- Pay attention to your body and what it is saying. How are you feeling right now? If you are stressed, place down your utensils and breathe deeply. Relax. Breathe again. If you are calm, how do you feel? Are you ravenous and feeling empty inside or are you starting to feel satisfied? Are certain signs starting to tell you that you are full or have you passed that point and your stomach is already beginning to feel painful? Gradually learn to be more aware, take notice of how you feel and listen to the different signs. Include them in your meal process.

- Leave the table feeling just right: that would be ideal! In other words, you are no longer hungry, you have energy and you feel invigorated and ready to handle what you have to do after your meal whether it be to get back to work, giving a bath to the kids or walking the dog.

Change n°23
READ! READ! READ!

23.

I don't know if you are like me, but I LOVE books and reading them! I actually find great pleasure flipping through one, simply holding it in my hands and smelling its pages: it's all part of the buying process. But maybe I am just old school.

The way I see it, each book is a mine full of glittering ideas and sparkling facts from which you can learn and that will help you grow. Every time I grab a new book I am excited, and every time I finish one I am grateful for what it has brought me and for what I have learned. Of course, not all books are interesting but today with internet we are lucky to be able to get a lot of feedback from most books before buying them.

The idea this week is to read and learn as much as possible about health and nutrition. You could decide to read the entire chapter two and three of this book or you could go to a bookstore and choose to read about a specific topic of interest that is related to health and nutrition such as eating habits, psychology of eating, new ways to prepare your food or the benefits of eating organic.

A. Enjoy learning again!

The real goal is to become more knowledgeable. That way, you will not only understand how your body functions, you will also discover what it needs as well as the benefits you will get from the food you eat. So, become a child again and enjoy the process of learning:

- Feel free to underline
- Take notes
- Research, research, research! Research online whenever you have any questions that pop up. Research in a dictionary or go to your local library and research there too!
- Put sticky notes up on your wall with the important stuff that you have learned!
- Get in the habit of writing down on a piece of paper or on the "notes" app of your phone any question you might have as soon as it pops up *and look it up later!*
- Take an online or a home study course and why not consider attending college? Just be excited about the whole process, have fun and be proud that you are learning something new that is putting you one step closer to becoming a healthier person!

Even if you are tested at the end there is no need to stress and remember *everything*. This is something you are doing for yourself. The great thing about this change is that there is nothing to prove to anyone. There might be grades and deadlines but they won't be life-threatening: you are simply there to **ENJOY LEARNING about health and nutrition!** The purpose of this goal is to feed your mind, become more knowledgeable.

Stay clear from diet books, the focus is on having a *HEALTHY LIFESTYLE!*

As I said before: don't start punishing yourself by refraining from certain foods. You must focus solely on the positive side: what can I bring to this meal to make it healthier? There aren't enough fruit and vegetables? I could add a delicious fruit and veggie drink or a green salad on the side and some apple slices for desert. I feel like having some chips? I could eat some organic tortilla chips and make a delicious guacamole. I would be adding avocado, tomatoes and onions to this snack and make it a lot healthier.

Many healthy nutrition books have a tendency to push you towards a specific diet which is the exact opposite of what I am encouraging you to do. The goal here is not to try out a new diet. Absolutely not! You are looking to develop your knowledge about the foods you are eating, trying to understand what nutrition really is and finding out simple ways to improve it. Some books might encourage you to stay clear from meat, gluten or other types of foods. Others will encourage you to eat a big amount of a certain type of food, such as protein. I am not judging their validity here, I just want you to focus on the basics of nutrition. Just remember to focus on how you can change the way you eat in a positive way. Concentrate on books and passages that:

- Give general facts and information about different foods
- Detail the vitamins, minerals of each food and what it is good for (skin, eyes etc.)
- Teach you how to add variety to your diet
- Bring new ideas and recipes
- Suggest healthy and delicious snacks that are quick and easy to prepare
- Focus on your specific goals or needs. Some of you, for example, might want to lose weight or bulk up while others might have cholesterol, are anemic, have a hard time sleeping at night, are athletes or breastfeeding moms. We are all the same but we each have specific needs. Try to see what foods and what type of nutrients could be beneficial for you. Make a list of them and what they are important for. Be curious, research, research, research.

> ***Before using any product or making any drastic changes to your diet, always consult your health care professional.***

How to research?
An example with a fruit: The Pomegranate

1. Why is it good for me?

For example, if you read about pomegranates, you would see that this fruit is "rich in vitamin C and antioxidants. It contains a large amount of vitamin B9 but also vitamins B5 and B6, potassium and copper."

What do you think about this information? I now know which vitamins and minerals it contains, however, I don't have a clue what I need these vitamins and minerals for.

So, let's take this research a step further.

Let's have a closer look at Vitamin C: why do I need it? How much should I be taking every day?

• **Why do I need Vitamin C?**

Vitamin C, also known as Ascorbic Acid, has many health benefits, including:

• prevention and treatment of scurvy
• treatment of the common cold
• boosting the immune system
• lowering hyper tension
• curing cataracts
• treatment of cancer
• combating stroke
• maintaining elasticity of the skin
• helps to heal wounds
• and controls asthma symptoms

So, for example, if you have a cold right now, vitamin C might help you get back on track.

• **What other foods contain Vitamin C?**

The important sources of Vitamin C are all citrus fruits but also grapes, strawberries, raspberries, cabbages, cauliflower, leafy vegetables, red peppers, potatoes, broccoli, watercress, parsley, brussels sprouts, cantaloupes, kiwi...

• **How much Vitamin C should I be taking every day?**

Normally you need 0.00282 ounces (= 80 mg) per day which you can obtain by eating 2.5 ounces (= 70 g) of red peppers, 5.3 ounces (= 150 g or 2 ½ kiwis) of kiwis and 7.76 ounces (= 220 g) of broccoli.

However, it's not because it's good for you or recommended for a specific ailment that you can or should ingest more. Indeed, a large dose of vitamin C can cause many unwanted side effects such headaches, nausea, diarrhea, vomiting, abdominal cramps to name a few. Simply make sure your diet includes foods that are rich in vitamin C.

An example with a vegetable: green beans

1. Why is it good for me?

They are a great source of fiber and they also act as an easy source for acquiring vitamins like vitamin A, C, K, B6, and folic acid. In terms of minerals, green beans are a good source of calcium, silicon, iron, manganese, potassium, and copper.

You see where I am getting at. It's up to you now, to research why you need vitamin B6 or iron? What other foods contain vitamin B6 or iron? How much Vitamin B6 / Iron should you be taking every day and how can you reach that quantity?

2. Ask questions

Learn to be curious and to enjoy the process of learning. Be a three year old again and start questioning "Why?" things are the way they are, "what?" words mean exactly, "how?" it works.

Before using any product or making any drastic changes to your diet always consult your health care professional.

3. And please, no need to be ashamed

We tend to think that, as adults, we should know it all and that it is shameful to ask for an explanation or to show that we do not understand. But I will let you in on a secret: a lot people out there are just like you and have become experts at hiding the fact that they don't know everything either. Although it is true that some people have extensive knowledge in multiple areas, many of us know a lot in one or two domains. We are all different. If it ever happens that someone does make fun of you, SHAME ON THEM! Don't let it stop you. Unfortunately, there will always be people out there that need to put others down to show there self-worth! Just think about it for a second: if they need to put you down, it's proof enough to show how low their self-esteem must be. Just move forward and forget the incident.

Look ahead and think about it this way: if you start questioning today, imagine how many answers you will have 5, 10, 20, 30 years from now. You have to start somewhere: so, START RIGHT NOW!

When choosing several books about nutrition, don't forget to choose one that details the health and benefits of each food you eat. You have many options to choose from. Check out a few suggestions at the back of the book for references.

What's in my Plate?

Once you have these books start reading information on how to buy, prepare and store food and what nutrients are on your plate. And why not, every time you prepare your meal, open them to look up the different ingredients that are on your plate or, if it's too fastidious, to at least find the main ones. Get yourself a notebook and take the time to write down all the information and start learning to understand what you are putting into your mouth.

I find it incredible that we eat maybe 3 to 4 times a day and that most of us have absolutely no clue about what we are eating: we have no idea what the benefits or risks, for that matter, are. At this point, I would like you to focus only on the benefits, to stick with a positive vibe.
After one week, you will see that you won't need to look the ingredients up as much: pretty soon you will master your plate.

As I have mentioned before, it's important to read, but action is important as well. At times, try to integrate some new tips you have learned into your diet. We are not talking about drastic changes here. The goal is to be aware of what you are eating, to try new foods and add a few positive changes into your daily eating routine.

It could go from learning how to wash your fruit and vegetables, looking at the labels on the foods that you buy, discovering new places to shop, such as a farmer's market, preparing meals in a new way or integrating more healthy juices and vegetables at certain meals… the list is endless. Remember, the key is to focus on positive changes and not on diet or restriction.

Change n°24
ADD VARIETY

24.

Do the 11 Essential Vitamins and Minerals Challenge

Are you one of those people who tends to eat the same things day in and day out? Is this week's shopping list a carbon-copy of last week's and is your shopping cart always hauling along the same items, the same fruit and vegetables? Do you tend to choose between 10 to 15 quick and easy dishes every night and call it variety?

> ## To fulfill your body's needs,
> ## you must eat a variety of different foods!

Maybe you are thinking: "I eat pretty healthy". Remember, however, that no matter how healthy any food is, it was not meant to be eaten every day. Your body has needs that must be satisfied in order to be in good health and they come in the form of 11 essential vitamins and minerals. This means you must vary and diversify the foods you eat in order to bring your body all of these good nutrients. Many people choose to take a multivitamin pill just to make sure they are not missing out on any one of them. Whenever possible, however, it is a wiser choice to stick to the real deal by eating nutrients that come from a natural source.

I take this opportunity to ask: Do you even know what these 11 essential vitamins and minerals are? Let's have a quick look at them. They range from vitamin A to Z or Zinc: Vitamin A, vitamin B, Vitamin C, Vitamin D, Vitamin E, Vitamin K, Folic Acid, Calcium, Chromium, Iron and Zinc. Why not take the time this month to have a look in what foods they can be found. Variety is not always an easy task when you have such a busy lifestyle; it can really be a challenge. It's so convenient to simply prepare and eat your usual food and cook it the same way. But why not take the time to think about your diet and have a look at your plate: is it boring? If it's limited to one set of food and a specific way of cooking it, chances are, it probably is. You don't necessarily have to eat lentils, sardines or sauerkraut, or force yourself to try eating liver and brussels sprouts again? There is a huge array of different foods out there that are really worth trying and that are also easy to prepare.

Let's also have a look at where you shop: when was the last time you went to a farmer's market or a real farm? Once again, this week, I am going to ask you to go all the way: we aren't just looking to change what we put in our plates here, we are also looking for variety when we buy our food, variety when we prepare our food and variety when we eat and taste it. So, let's get started!

The goal this week is to push yourself out of your comfort zone by finding ways to change how and what you eat. Remember to take baby steps and start off with small changes. There are many little things that you can do and here are a few tips to help you get started:

A. Bring variety to the way you shop

This week why don't you change grocery stores? If you are used to going to the same supermarket, why not try a different one! Another idea is to look online to see if there are any markets or farms nearby. Bring the kids along and turn it into family fun! Program your grocery shopping so that you can take your time: instead of rushing through the aisles grabbing the usual products, why not schedule ahead of time at least one hour to have enough time to look at what you are buying. This way you can review the labels, the prices, where the produce is from and so on. There is pleasure in taking your time to choose what you are going to eat. Look at the colors, find out what's in season, and try something new!

Why not be bodacious and every time you go grocery shopping, decide to buy one or two foods (no more) that you are not accustomed to eating. Be careful however not to get carried away: bring these little changes in progressively.

B. Bring variety into your meals

It is beneficial to open up to new ideas and new sources. A good way to do this is to look at new recipes. Flip through magazines, recipe books or go have a look on internet. If you see a picture and your mouth starts watering: make a list of the ingredients and do it!

Another good idea would be to take a cooking course. It's fun and you actually have someone there to help you in the process. And as much as possible, make it a pleasurable moment: if you are not much of a cook or are a bit shy at first, take along a friend or your husband.

Learn to relax and enjoy making your meals; by doing so, you are adding a special ingredient that is often left out: *LOVE*.

At first, it might be a good idea to maintain the same meals you usually prepare but to simply switch a few ingredients you normally use. Here are a few examples:

- *For Breakfast*: if you have an omelet, make sure you add a different vegetable every time. If you have cereal, change brands and try different varieties, or change the toppings you put on it. Try bananas, berries, canned fruit, mangos, dried fruit or nuts. If you press your own juice, vary at least one of the veggies and fruit you put into it.
- *For lunch/dinner*: If you have salad, change its composition: add one vegetable you don't usually have, add nuts and seeds, vary the seasoning by adding different spices, herbs or flavors. If you are having pasta, try a variety of shapes, colors and sizes and vary the toppings. Tomato and basil one day, celery and tuna the next or salmon and zucchini.
- *Bring a bit of change to the proteins you usually eat*: do you consume enough eggs? Do you eat enough organic red meat? And what about getting your protein from other sources than meat such as fish, Greek yogurt, tofu, beans, nuts, soya milk, spinach.

Please note that I am aware that there is a huge tendency toward Veganism or Vegetarianism and my goal is certainly not to encourage people to start eating more meat. But we all have different needs: some of you need red meat to function in a healthy way while others don't and have chosen not to consume any for the time being. We all go through experimental phases and that's fine. I just want to point out that it's important, to be aware of what your body needs.

- **For you Vegans and Vegetarians: Are any of you up to trying my breakfast challenge!** Every morning I prepare myself a small plate composed of 2 slices of fresh organic curcuma, 2 slices of fresh organic ginger, 2 slices of fresh organic lemon, 10 to 15 pepper grinds and half a teaspoon of organic coconut oil. Makes two bites. The very first time my boyfriend asked me to share his breakfast this is what he placed before me. Instead of backing off, I looked at the food that was place before and thought: "It's all fresh and I will be getting the nutrients directly from the food source instead of supplementing. This is the real deal and can only be good for me. I have to try this!" Today, I truly look forward to eating it: My mouth is a little on fire at first but the coconut is quick at soothing things up and I especially love the fact that it clears my nose every morning, so make sure you have a kleenex handy.

- *What kind of carbs do you eat?* Have you ever tried quinoa, wild rice, coucous, Ebly (also known as Ebly wheat)? Why not also try new varieties of bread: have you ever eaten sourdough bread? It is made through a fermentation process that makes it easier to digest. What about oat or sprouted bread? if you usually eat white bread try 100% whole wheat or breads that contain seeds. Have you tried gluten free bread? Why not try it for a week or two and see if you feel any different? Without being celiac or gluten intolerant, you might feel that it takes a load of your digestive system and leaves you feeling lighter than when eating regular bread. I know I feel a great difference!

And why not decide to make an entire meal from scratch: homemade bread, yogurt, lemonade, spaghetti, spaghetti sauce and fruit salad? Have fun preparing it. This way you are sure to be sprinkling some love into as well. So, this week, step out of the box, think different and question what you eat!

C. Change the way you cook your food

Eat your vegetables raw with a homemade dip or eat them cooked but vary the way you prepare them. Stir fried, steamed, using a slow cooker or a pressure cooker. You could also have your food oven grilled.

Last time, I had my friend's son over for dinner, I served carrots. The next day, my friend called me up wanting to know how I had managed to make her son eat carrots; she wanted me to give her my secret recipe. They were just plain whole carrots, which I had peeled and rinsed, and placed in a pressure cooker. I told her that cooking them this way keeps the flavor and makes them almost melt in your mouth.

Do you always eat your eggs the same way? Change the way you prepare them: omelet, sunny side up, poached, soft or hard boiled. One way I like to have them is by mixing one or two soft-boiled eggs into the seasoning and drizzle it on top of a green salad: it's a great way to reduce the amount of oil you put in your seasoning and it's also a real treat!

Vegetarian option

For those of you that stay away from foods that come from animal sources, why don't you have some fun with one specific fruit and vegetable? Choose one and research every single different way of cooking or preparing it. For example: Zucchini. I eat them raw. I simply chop them up and add them to my salad. Whenever possible, I feel it's important to eat my vegetables in their natural form to preserve all of their nutrients. But I also enjoy making zucchini spaghetti. There is a cooking device, called the Veggetti, that can transform your zucchini into long spaghetti strands. Put them to boil a few minutes only and simply add homemade tomato sauce. What about zucchini bread and chocolate zucchini pudding? Ever tasted these? Next week, let's have an apple and carrot week!

What about meat? if you like it breaded, why not try grilling, broiling or stir frying them?

D. Vary the way you cut your veggies and fruit. You can slice them into little cubes or sticks. You can shred them. There is a very convenient fruit and vegetable cutter called the Nice Dicer that allows you to cut them into a multitude of shapes and sizes. Try to completely peel your vegetables into long strips with a peeler or as mentioned above using a Veggetti. This way your vegetables turn into a sort of pasta. You can either cook them or eat them raw, both are delicious.

E. Bring variety to the way you present your food. Why not try to make your plate look beautiful? Why don't you do the cooking and ask the kids to lay the table and prepare the plates: make happy faces, garnish them with colorful vegetables or set a beautiful table with candles. Turn off the TV and share a special time with your family.

F. Make your plate colorful. By adding lots of different colors to it. Mix your greens like spinach, cucumbers, broccoli with a few reds such as beets, tomatoes, strawberries add a bit of orange like peppers, carrots, oranges and a little bit of white by adding radish, turnips, onions. Fruit and vegetables come in a rainbow of different colors. You also have yellow such as pineapple, grapefruit, lemons and apples and purple/blue beauties like eggplants, plums and blueberries.
Start things off by eating with your eyes: next time you go shopping, keep in your mind the rainbow and pick one fruit and vegetable coming from each of the 6 rainbow colors!

G. Vary the flavors.   This is also a great way to enhance a dish. Find some new seasonings, try out new vinaigrette recipes that include different herbs and spices or make it tangy by adding some fruit and fruit rinds. Try to drizzle new oils and vinegars or sprinkle some herbs over your meat or fish.

H. Last but not least, vary your food textures:
By going crunchy or crispy: Have you ever tried to bake your vegetables in the oven? Cut them into thin slices, drizzle a little olive oil over them, add a dash of Provence herbs and bake. They will be a little crispy and simply delicious! Or you could try all your fruit and vegetables raw for the crunchiest of meals!
By going smooth: check magazines, recipe books and online to discover and create new dips you can dip your veggies into, or how to make delicious purées.
By going liquid: try juicing or making a smoothie! And what about nice homemade soups, when was the last time you enjoyed one?
By learning to vary the origins, colors, flavors, textures, shapes, food temperatures and the way you shop and prepare your meals, you will turn them into a whole new experience!

The 11 Essential Vitamins and Minerals Challenge

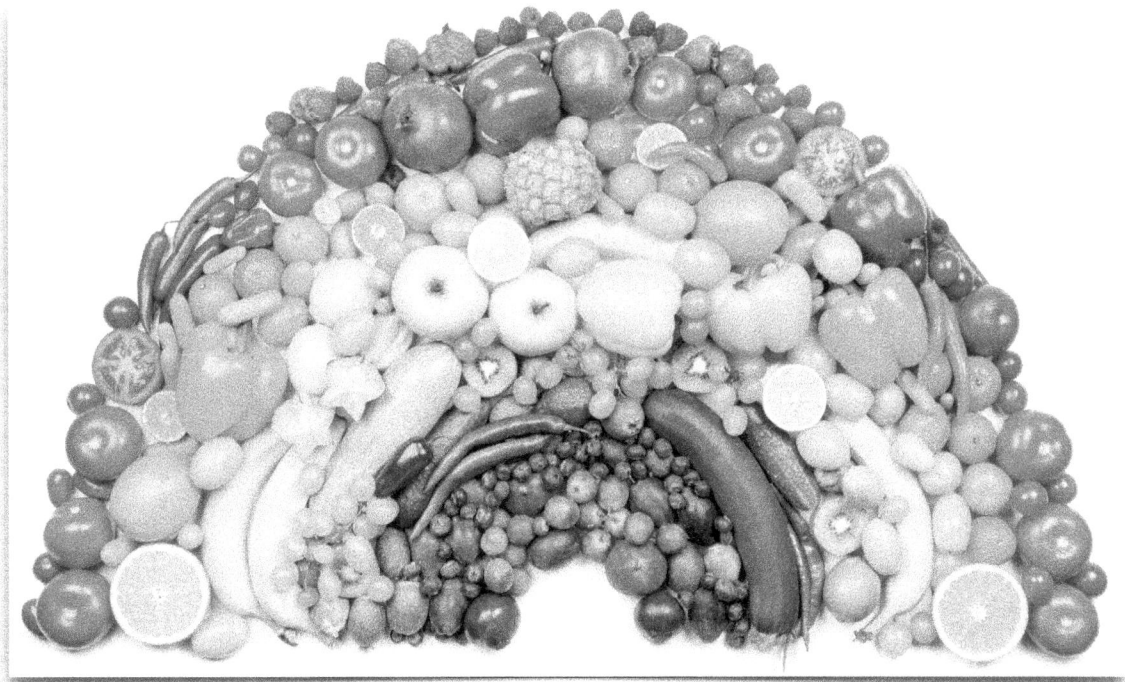

To make sure you are getting all your vitamins and minerals, why not try the "11 Essential Vitamins & Minerals Challenge"? As a reminder: the 11 essential vitamins and minerals are: Vitamin A, Vitamin B, Vitamin C, Vitamin D, Vitamin E, vitamin K, Folic Acid, Calcium, Chromium, Iron and Zinc. To make things easier for you, I have listed these essential vitamins and minerals below, with their main food sources as well as their benefits.

Vitamin A sources (Retinol beta-carotene)

☐ Carrots	☐ Sweet potatoes	☐ Melons
☐ Romaine Lettuce	☐ Leafy Greens (Kale)	☐ Squash
☐ Red Peppers	☐ Dried Apricots	☐ Tuna and other Oily Fish
☐ Butter	☐ Mangoes	☐ Liver
☐ Other…………..		

Why eat vitamin A? Found in most orange colored foods, it's good for your eyes (namely fights cataract and essential if your eyes tend to be dry), good for your gums (gingivitis), fights infections, helps to heal skin wounds and is essential for the skin in general, fights certain cancers (prostate, lung and cervix).

Vitamin B sources

☐ Brown Rice	☐ Citrus Fruits	☐ Bananas
☐ Red Meat	☐ Barley	☐ Other Whole Grain
☐ Eggs	☐ Poultry	☐ Fish Especially Salmon
☐ Avocados	☐ Chickpeas	☐ Green Peas
☐ Sunflower seeds	☐ Almonds	☐ Broccoli
☐ Romaine Lettuce	☐ Collard Greens	☐ Cheese
☐ Dark, Leafy Vegetables	☐ Kale	☐ Spinach
☐ Edamame	☐ Back Beans	☐ Beans
☐ Yogurt	☐ Milk	☐ Molasses Anyone?
☐ Potatoes	☐ Chili Peppers	☐ Other……..

Why eat vitamin B? *Note: there are 8 different B vitamins: B1 (thiamine), B2 (riboflavin), B3 (niacin), B5 (pantothenic acid), B6 (pyridoxine), B7(folate), B12 (cobalamin).* It helps to maintain a healthy scalp and stops hair loss, B2 (gingivitis), B3 (gingivitis)B6 (irritability). Depression, fatigue, lack of energy, problems with memory can be linked to a lack of vitamin B. strengthens the nervous and immune system.

Vitamin C sources

☐ Oranges	☐ Guava	☐ Red and Green Peppers
☐ Kiwi	☐ Kale	☐ Broccoli
☐ Grapefruits	☐ Strawberries	☐ Brussels sprouts
☐ Cantaloupe	☐ Tomatoes	☐ Peas (Mange Tout)
☐ Potatoes	☐ Papaya	☐ Other………………

Why eat vitamin C? Used to make collagen; depression has been linked to a lack of vitamin C; helps to heal wounds; antioxidant; increases the absorption of iron from plant foods.

Vitamin D sources

☐ Eggs	☐ Oily Fish (sardines, salmon, tuna)	☐ Red and Green Peppers
☐ Oysters	☐ Shrimp	☐ Tofu
☐ Soy Yogurts	☐ Pork	☐ Mushrooms
☐ Dark Chocolate	☐ Milk	☐ Other

Why eat vitamin D? 30 minutes of sun a day and you will receive most of the daily vitamin D needed to build and maintain bones and teeth. It strengthens the nervous and immune system, helps metabolize calcium and phosphorus.

Vitamin E Sources

☐ Wheat Germ	☐ Almonds	☐ Hazelnuts
☐ Pine Nuts	☐ Peanuts	☐ Brazil nuts
☐ Sunflower Seeds	☐ Spinach	☐ Tomatoes
☐ Avocado	☐ Shrimp	☐ Fish (Salmon and Trout)
☐ Olive oil	☐ Broccoli	☐ Squash
☐ Pumpkin	☐ Kiwis	☐ Mangos
☐ Other …………	☐ Other………….	☐ Other……..

Why eat vitamin E? Helps to maintain healthy skin and eyes, it fights against skin dryness and scratching (namely when you have eczema). Is an antioxidant: protects cell membranes and red blood cells from oxidation damage.

Vitamin K Sources

☐ Kale	☐ Spinach	☐ Cauliflower
☐ Cabbage	☐ Brussels Sprouts	☐ Broccoli
☐ Turnip Greens	☐ Parsley	☐ Romaine Lettuce
☐ Most Leafy Greens	☐ Liver	☐ Meat
☐ Eggs	☐ Fish	☐ Cereal
☐ Other …………	☐ Other………….	☐ Other……..

Why eat Vitamin K? It is needed for blood clotting (helps wounds heal properly) and needed for the building of bones.

Calcium sources

☐ dark, leafy vegetables	☐ Collard Greens	☐ Spinach
☐ Kale	☐ Watercress	☐ Bok choy
☐ Low Fat Cheese (mozzarella)	☐ Milk	☐ Most Dairy Products
☐ Yogurt	☐ Cheese (Especially Parmesan)	☐ Tofu
☐ Edemame	☐ Other Soy Products	☐ Okra
☐ Broccoli	☐ Dark Green Vegetables	☐ Snap Beans
☐ Lentils	☐ Black Molasses	☐ Figs
☐ Rhubarb	☐ Poppy Seeds	☐ Sesame Seeds
☐ Celery Sticks	☐ Chia Seeds	☐ Other ....

Why eat Calcium? Calcium has a soothing effect on the nervous system and can help with insomnia and depression, bone development and blood clotting.

Chromium sources

☐ Seafoods (Mussels)	☐ Oats	☐ Whole Grains (English Muffin)
☐ Broccoli	☐ Green Beans	☐ Potatoes
☐ Tomatoes	☐ Romaine Lettuce	☐ Herbs (namely Basil)
☐ Nuts	☐ Wheat Germ	☐ Beef
☐ Turkey	☐ Orange Juice	☐ Grape Juice
☐ Apples	☐ Bananas	☐ Brown Rice
☐ Eggs	☐ Other............	☐ Other............

Why eat Chromium? It assists with muscle function and glucose regulation.

Iron Sources

☐ Pumpkin Seeds	☐ Most Nuts	☐ Cashews
☐ Pine Nuts	☐ Peanuts	☐ Almonds
☐ Clams	☐ Oysters	☐ Liver
☐ Beef	☐ Lamb	☐ Turkey
☐ Beans	☐ Pulses	☐ Whole Grain
☐ Bran	☐ Leafy Greens	☐ Spinach
☐ Broccoli	☐ Dark Chocolate	☐ Egg Yolk
☐ Tofu	☐ Other	☐ Other ....

Why eat Iron? It is needed as it helps make red blood cells.

Zinc Sources

☐ Seafood (Oyster)	☐ Wheat Germ	☐ Oatmeal
☐ Quinoa	☐ Beef	☐ Lamb
☐ Pork	☐ Liver	☐ Spinach
☐ Legumes	☐ Beans	☐ Lentils
☐ Chickpeas	☐ Peas	☐ Soybeans
☐ Cashews	☐ Pumpkin Seeds	☐ Dark Chocolate
☐ Cocoa	☐ Mushrooms	☐ Tofu
☐ Low-Fat Yogurt	☐ Other	☐ Other ....

Why eat zinc? It helps make new cells and process carbohydrates, fat and protein found in food. It is also essential in the healing of wounds.

All you have to do is make sure you choose one ingredient from each of the eleven groups in order to reach 11 essential vitamins and minerals needed each day. Try as much as possible to vary the sources daily, or at least regularly. So just start ticking, it's that easy!

MY LITTLE RITUAL

Grab a simple piece of paper or a scented one, and a pencil.
Write down what it is that you wish for yourself or for someone else.
Strike a match and place it in the bowl.
Place your wish over the flame.
Observe your wish as it flows all around you and dissipates.
Take a moment to close your eyes…..

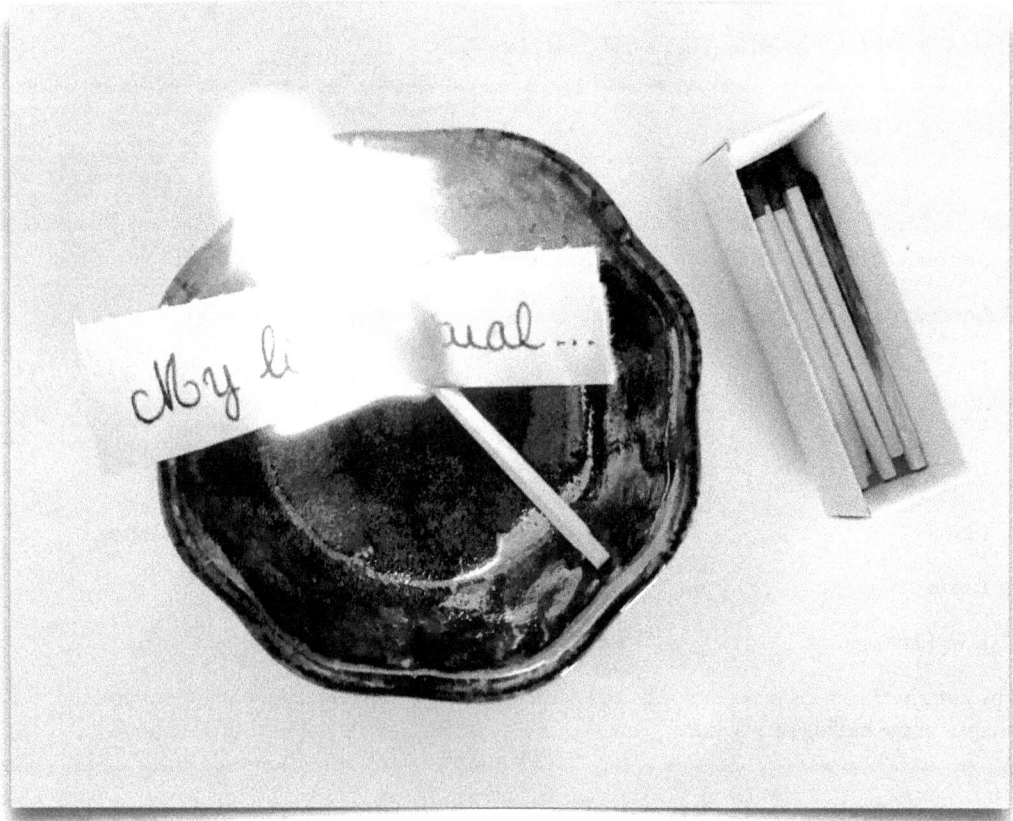

MY NOTES

CHAPTER THREE

ON THE PATH TO PHYSICAL TRANSFORMATION

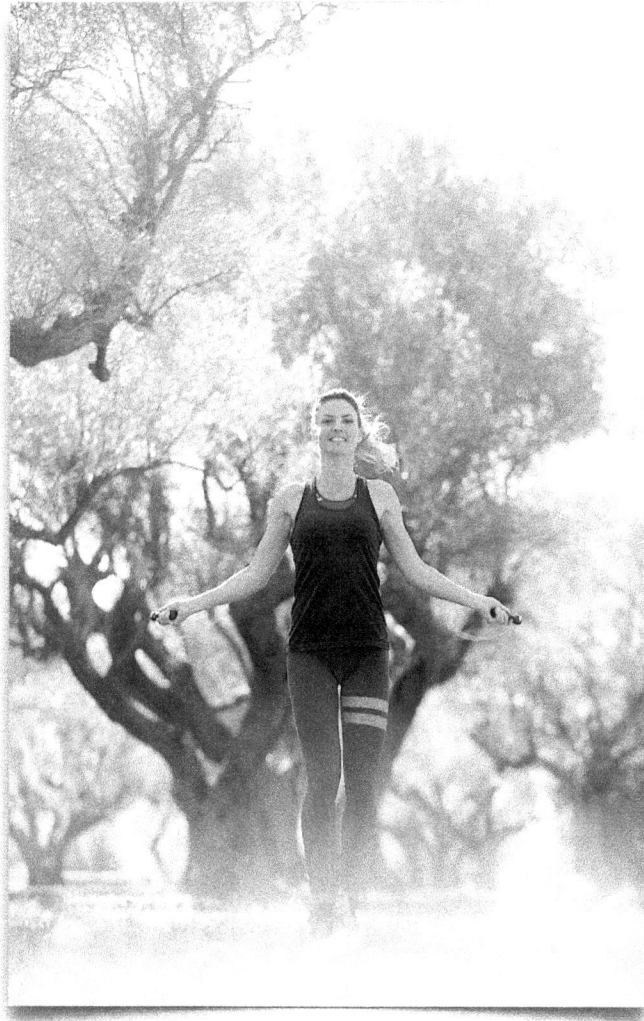

They were just thoughts
that danced through my little head…
words have wings.

Ever since I can remember I always enjoyed running. Today, after over 25 years of regular jogging I can't help looking back and wondering: When, exactly, did I start? Did I enjoy it the first time? What got me started? And especially, what inspired me to continue?
I can't really say for sure. All I know is that running has accompanied me throughout my life, during the happy but also the difficult times. It has been there, just like a faithful friend, holding my hand through thick and thin.

Come to think of it, I do recall something that happened one day. As I was in my last year of high school, my gym teacher told me that when I ran I looked so radiant and happy. I remember this clearly. It lies vivid in my mind as if it were yesterday. Is it possible that a single compliment triggered it all? That my whole life changed around because of it? As George Eliot said: "Words have wings." Did that gym teacher, with his kind words, give me wings? The wings that I needed to get going? It's funny, when I think of it, that he had no idea how much his compliment would spin my whole life around. Teenage years can be such a challenge. It's a moment when we search who we are and are expected to know who we want to become, but don't necessarily have all the answers. Educators do not realize the impact they have and how a brutal remark or a compliment can go such a long way.

And so, right now, I can't help but look back on my life, somewhat horrified, knowing how much I just love running, and wonder: what would my life have been without my regular jogs? Because, throughout the years, it has been with certainty my lifeline and my moment of meditation.

Indeed, when I would shut my front door, I would often leave feeling down, angry, hurt, tired or frustrated about something that was going on in my life… But as I ran, I couldn't help but notice how, with each step, I would sweat out part of my sadness, anger or pain and it felt as if the soles of my shoes had pounded them down into the ground. I couldn't help but notice as I accelerated, how with each breath I took, I felt more empowered and STRONGER. It was as if all these emotions that were taking up so much space in my mind, clinging onto each one of my thoughts, couldn't handle the speed anymore… and as I exhaled, they had no choice but to let go, losing all control they had over me. As I would get closer to home, the mess in my mind would clear up and everything would magically sort out. Finally, as I would reach my front door, I would feel totally energized and in total control again.

Words will never be forgotten, so choose them wisely. Knowing how much of a difference they can make in people's lives, make sure it's in a good way.

Your goal is to finally get back into shape: you have decided that it's time to lead a healthy lifestyle and attain the physique of your dreams! If you are in search of long lasting results then you had better stay clear from drastic diets and excessive exercise. Focus on feeling good and doing activities that are fun and make you happy. Before you start reading the 12 changes that I propose, keep in mind the following:

• Take baby steps: it's not an "all or nothing" strategy, on the contrary it's all about gradual improvement

• Embrace change: start seeing change as something positive and get into the habit of bringing little changes into your life

• Mentally focus on achieving your goal which means diving towards it 200%. Engage both your mind and body100%, for a 200% implication

• Ask yourself 10, 20, 30 times a day: what can I do right now to improve my physique – whether it's simply drinking a glass of water, watching a motivational video or going for a walk and set out to do it, right now!

• Find any opportunity to move and be more active

Check out the list of changes you can do this week. Pick one, and stick to it! Remember to stay focused on your goal: think about it, read about it, dream about it! It's the best way to make your dream come true.

Change n°25
YOUR
TRANSFORMATIONAL JOURNAL

25.

Keeping a journal in which you write down everything you do every day regarding your fitness journey should be your very first step. Most studies show that keeping track of your progress is not only a great motivational tool, it's also the best way to make sure you reach your goals.

This chapter is about exercise so the goal here is to keep track of your journey, your struggles, and your success on your way to fitness. Buy a nice notebook in which you write everything you do each day to improve your level of fitness. Every little bout of exercise counts during the day so, note each and every one of them.

A. Write everything down in a journal *My Daily Positive Fitness Checklist*

I have created "My Daily Positive Fitness checklist" with lots of ideas on how to increase the amount of exercise you do each day. The idea is to tick as many boxes from the checklist you possibly can, over time and throughout the day. Remember that this is a gradual process. At first you will only tick a few boxes, but quickly you will see how fun it becomes and you will be trying to tick as much as possible. So, stick it in your notebook, on your fridge, in your agenda…and see how motivating it is to increase your number of points!

Remember that your goal is not so much to force yourself to exercise, but to focus on bringing positive elements into your life, such as bouts of exercise, learning about being healthy, partaking in fun activities, increasing the amount of time or the number of times you exercise… Focus on having fun and on embracing change.

Remember to constantly ask yourself throughout the day:

> *What positive element can I bring into my life TODAY*
> *to be more active,*
> *and include more exercise into my life?*

My Daily Positive "Fitness" Checklist

Here are 25 different ways to improve your relationship with your body.
Set a goal to tick at least 5 boxes every day. Your ultimate goal: ticking at least 15!

☐ I Wrote in my journal and kept track of my activity:_____

☐ I Read a book about exercise, on how to include more_____

☐ I Walked today:_____ *(number of steps or time)*

☐ I Practiced walking more mindfully

☐ I Visualized myself on my path to success

☐ I Went to bed earlier

☐ I Tried a new exercise or activity today: _____

☐ I Created or took 5 minutes to go over my vision board today

☐ I Exercised with someone today_____

☐ I Learned something new _____

☐ I Trained for a programmed event such as a race, competition _____

☐ I Did something I love today _____

☐ I Worked on improving myself or becoming more competent _____

☐ I Did the Barbara Ratkoff B.E.S.T.^{2} Workout!

- **B^2**: **B**rain and **B**ody invested in a 200% workout
- **E^2**: **E**ndurance and **E**quilibrium for a stronger heart and improved balance
- **S^2**: **S**tretch and **S**trengthen for toned muscles and reformed posture
- **T^2**: **T**echnique and **T**ranquility: train with perfect form and unwind

☐ I finally succeeded in doing _____

☐ I Was active several times during the day _____

List activities:

( ) I Took the stairs instead of the elevator

( ) I Walked instead of taking the bus or car

( ) I Took a break from work to stretch, go up and down the stairs or other

( ) I Did an extra 5, 10 or 15 minutes at my workout

( ) I Participated in a recreational activity with the children, my dog or a friend such as shooting hoops, relays, throwing frisbee or football, hula hoop, racing the dog etc.

( ) Other Activity : _____

☐ I Did a challenge such as a squat, pushup or pull-up challenge _____

☐ I Hired a personal trainer and did _____

☐ I Took a cold shower or went swimming in cold water

☐ I Stood tall today and did my best to correct posture

☐ I Had fun while training

☐ I Put some music, got crazy and danced

☐ I Had a yoga session

☐ I Drank 8 glasses of water

☐ Other Positive factor_____

The idea is to tick as many boxes from the checklist you possibly can, throughout the day. Remember that this is a gradual process. At first you will only tick in a few boxes, but quickly you will see how fun it becomes and you will be trying to tick as many as possible. So, stick it in your notebook, on your fridge, in your agenda…and see how motivating it can be to increase your number of check marks!

Remember that your goal is not so much to force yourself to exercise but to focus on bringing positive elements such as bouts of exercise, learning about being healthy, partaking in fun activities, increasing the amount of time or the number of times you exercise into your life. Focus on having fun and on embracing change.

B. Everything counts: 20 Ways to bring more activity into your life

Probably the most important aspect to consider, if you wish to succeed, is to make sure you have fun and that the whole process seems easy. Don't listen to what people tell you, such as: walking is for the elderly, playing with your kids is not exercise, climbing two flights of stairs won't change anything, exercising for 5 minutes is of no use… I have heard so many people make these remarks. IGNORE THEM! Everything counts! So, get moving throughout the day and start seeing changes in your life!

There are lots of fun ways to increase the amount exercise you do:
- Instead of going out for a coffee with a friend, go for a long walk
- Make your dog happy and take it out for a long walk/run, or play ball catch
- Shoot a few hoops with family or friends at a nearby park
- Go for a 10 minute bike ride
- Plan weekends ahead of time and get away: take a hike and get in contact with mother nature! Organize a walk and picnic (bring a frisbee or some jump ropes),
- Put on some music and go crazy for 10/15 minutes alone or with family or friends. They will love it! This definitely counts as exercise!
- Get off the bus a little before your usual stop and walk the rest of the way
- From now on take the stairs instead of the elevator
- During 5 minute breaks at work, start the habit to go up and down 2 or 3 flights of stairs
- Do some stretching exercises the first 15 minutes of your TV program
- Find a hill and walk up and down 10 times
- Go for a walk and jog workout: walk one minute and then jog for one minute. Start doing it for 15 minutes and then gradually add one or two minutes every workout
- Organize a relay race. Create two or three teams. Place two cones and start running. You could walk the first time, go as fast as you can the second time, jump in bags the third time, go backwards the forth time, do sideway straddles the fifth time, juggle and walk the 6th time
- Play kid games such as hopscotch, hula-hoop, jump rope, tag, monkey bars, cartwheels, hand stands, somersaults, jumping jacks
- Go walk in the water at hip level whether it's the pool, the lake, or the ocean
- Organize a walk. No need to walk the whole Pacific coast like Cheryl Strayed did – as she described in her book entitled "Wild"- but why not decide to walk between two towns or around a lake. My boyfriend and I are from two different cities (Toulon and Monaco) and we decided to walk from Toulon to Monaco for a three day walk with back packs and all.
- Is there an activity you have always wanted to try such as Zumba, Aqua gym, spinning, yoga, Pilates, kayaking, paddle boarding, indoor or outdoor rock climbing, cross fit, indoor or outdoor roller skating, trampoline park? Why not sign up and do a class today! Why not tackle a new activity this week? Decide to step out of your comfort zone and try new things. Decide which activities you liked best, or better yet, keep varying your workouts.
- Start a challenge with push-up, squats, jumping jacks, burpees
- If you live in or nearby a big city, decide to find the highest building and climb all the way up using the steps. Time how long it took you to reach the top and then do it again next month to compare!

- Create a YouTube channel in which you share your fitness journey. Every day film yourself and what you're doing to get one step closer to being fit! Film yourself exercising, being more active, shopping and eating healthy! Also talk about your struggles, lack of motivation, slip outs. Be authentic and real.

The goal here is to find anything that will get your heart pumping even if just for 30 seconds. Choose to be more active every time the occasion pops up and keep track of it by writing it down.

C. Keeping track of the "Before and After"

It's a good idea to keep track of your evolution:
- Take sporadic before and after pictures, (front, back, sideways). Make sure you do it with a neutral background and with the same clothes and lighting. You could get it done professionally every month, this way you are sure that it is done correctly and your results are the real deal!
- Write down your statistics such as your weight and measurements. Why not get a watch to keep track of your workouts. There are many different watches on the market today that enable you to keep track of your activities distances, calories etc. Why not create a yearly chart to see your progression at a glance.
- Fill out your "Daily Positive Fitness Checklist".
- Create an Instagram account on which you log your progression: include photos of yourself also while exercising and fun pictures of the food you eat. Make it beautiful, have fun, be creative! Look at other peoples' accounts and try to bring your very own personal touch. What do you do differently?

D. Make your notebook a fun and colorful companion!

As I have already developed this aspect in Chapter 1, Change n° 1: Your Daily Positive Checklist, I will not go into too much detail here. But I definitely encourage you to read it to become more creative and make it personal. Try to turn your time with this notebook into a special moment, one that you look forward to. You could make it motivating by adding for example:
- lots of colors: use a variety of colors to write
- pictures: stick in some motivational pictures but also some fun shots of yourself exercising or being active
- some motivational quotes and stickers

You get the idea: write down everything positive that you have done for yourself today – in regards to exercise…but also feel free to write about any other positive aspect that happened today that has to do with your diet, how you feel, what you have done for yourself to increase happiness. For years, I have had many different kinds of journals and I have to say that fitness journals have often been a great source of motivation for me. Writing down my goals, keeping track of my progress, taking the time to flip through magazines to find motivational photos and inspiring quotes, charting my monthly result, but also noting the nutritional value of the different foods I eat, have all really helped me in succeeding on my path to a fitter lifestyle. So, go get yourself a nice notebook and start your transformational and motivational journal today!

Change n°26
GET OUT AND WALK

26.

Every once in a while, I would go out for walk with my son after dinner. He would take his scooter and I would tag along. We discovered many different spots in our city and took a lot of pleasure in chatting about our day or about topics of interest. Sometimes we laughed our heads off and other times we didn't talk at all, but it was just nice to know that we were there together. OK, I'll be totally honest here: and sometimes we argued. But then, that's just a part of life and getting to know each other and our limits. I honestly believe that these walks helped me bond with him and made our relationship grow stronger and deeper. As the months went by, I found myself looking forward to these walks more and more and so decided to make them a priority. When the homework, dinner, and cleaning up were done, we would head outdoors for our evening walk. I thought this would be challenging as it meant no more TV. Well, you know what? I had no regrets and I never looked back.

To get you motivated, let's take a closer look at what's in it for you, if you decide to take up walking.

A. Recommended amount of exercise or walking?

According to the standards of the American Heart Association, the current recommendations for overall cardiovascular health is to do:
• at least 30 minutes of moderate-intensity aerobic activity at least 5 days per week for a total of 150 minutes.

OR

• at least 25 minutes of vigorous aerobic activity at least 3 days per week for a total of 75 minutes. You can also combine moderate and vigorous- intensity aerobic activity.

AND

• Moderate to high-intensity muscle-strengthening activity at least 2 days per week for additional health benefits.

Note for those of you that need to lower Blood Pressure and Cholesterol:
An average 40 minutes of moderate to vigorous-intensity aerobic activity 3 or 4 times per week.

IMPORTANT REMINDER
Consult your health care professional before using any product or making any drastic changes to your exercise or diet regimen.

One of the easiest and best ways to achieve this goal is simply by walking. So, I know that when we say the word "work out", we automatically see someone training hard and sweating a lot. And for this reason, we tend to downsize certain activities, including walking but also dancing or other recreational activities such as playing basketball, walking the dog, going out for a bike ride. All these activities are exercise and are beneficial to your health. They truly don't get the respect they deserve. The most important thing is that you are out there moving and having fun! You don't have to kill yourself to start reaping the benefits. It's very important to understand that SOMETHING IS BETTER THAN NOTHING! And if you actually have fun during the process it will be even more beneficial for you as it will also boost your mood and self-confidence. Who says that putting on your favorite music, turning up the volume and dancing your heart out isn't exercise? Start out with something easy that you will stick to. For this reason, walking is a great choice. Just about anyone can do it, anytime, anywhere! No equipment is needed, no training, instructions or skills are required and there is a very low risk of getting injured. You can walk indoors on a treadmill or outdoors, alone or with a friend, at home or when travelling and you can't beat the price: it's totally free!

B. What are the benefits of walking?

a. You will burn calories

By simply walking you can actually **lose weight**. Although there are many factors involved to calculate exactly how many calories you have burned, the chart below can give you a relative estimate. Of course, your weight and the speed at which you walk will determine how many calories your burn.

Calories Burned Per Mile By Walking According To Weight				
Pound / Speed	2.0 mph	3.0 mph	4.0 mph	5.0 mph
100 lb	57	53	57	73
120 lb	68	64	68	87
140 lb	80	74	80	102
150 lb	85.5	79.5	85.5	109
160 lb	91	85	91	116
180 lb	102	95	102	131
200 lb	114	106	114	145
220 lb	125	117	125	160
250 lb	142	133	142	182
275 lb	156	146	156	200
300 lb	170	159	170	218

How do you know at what pace you are walking?

If you count the number of steps you take in one minute, you can estimate in what range your pace is:

• 80 steps per minute corresponds to a leisurely pace
• 100 steps per minute corresponds to a brisk pace
• 120 steps per minute corresponds to a fast pace

As we age, we tend to progressively gain weight, between 1 to 2 pounds a year. Although it doesn't seem to amount to a lot, it can lead to obesity over a certain number of years. Walking is one of the best ways to stop this accumulation of weight.

b. Walking tones your legs, your bum and your abs!

When walking, not only do you burn calories, you also **tone your muscles**. When you know that you lose as much as 3 to 5 percent of your total muscle mass each decade after your turn 30, it's important to keep those muscles working. To get the most benefits from your walk, try to vary the terrain by hill walking or taking the stairs, but also by walking on sand, earth or grass instead of always opting for concrete.

A good idea would be to vary your circuit whenever possible. Why not try to get out of the city on weekends or explore a different park or area altogether to enjoy new sceneries and avoid getting into a routine rut. I can't insist enough about the importance of connecting with nature. The benefits are huge. Bring your dog, your kids, a friend and enjoy the great outdoors. Look around you at the simple beauty of life such as a squirrel, the clouds, birds chirping, the smell of pine trees. Take it all in and notice how you wind up getting a sense of total freedom.

c. Walking lifts your spirits!

Try this:

Go for a 10 minute walk. Beforehand however, write down on a piece of paper how you feel on a scale between 0 and 10. Are you stressed? Tired? Angry? Is your head foggy? Do you have a headache? Are you overwhelmed with all the things you have to do? Write it all down. Then when you come back from your walk, pick up the paper and see how you feel. Chances are you will feel a lot better. Why? Because walking is the best energy booster there is. While you are walking, you release "feel good endorphins" that are responsible for bringing pleasure. Consequently, you feel less stressed and anxious. So, forget about taking vitamins, that cup of java or an Energy drink. If you are feeling a little sluggish, chances are all you need is a bit of fresh air and a little walk.

d. Walking strengthens your heart

You might remember that phrase: "An apple a day keeps the doctor away!" but it could be twisted into "A walk every day keeps the doctor away".

When you are walking you heart rhythm accelerates, you pump more blood which increases your overall fitness including your heart and lungs. You also reduce the risk of getting heart disease or a stroke. It also helps you manage hypertension, high cholesterol and diabetes. So, go get your shoes and start walking!

e. Where do I start?

Although it's quite straightforward – you basically just have to get up and walk – there are a number of little things you can look into. To help you, I am listing a series of questions and answers below.

• Do I count minutes or steps?

It doesn't really matter just as long as you are out there walking. However, counting minutes or steps, is a great way to keep track of your progress. But it's also a number as in "30 minutes" or "5000 steps" every day, or a goal as in "walking 5 times a week" that you can reach. For this reason, it might be worth trying to choose one or the other.

• How do I reach 150 minutes a week?

The American Council on Exercise proposes to walk at a moderate intensity for 30 to 60 minutes, five times per week or to exercise vigorously for 20 to 60 minutes three days per week.

They also propose to do one continuous session and multiple shorter sessions of at least 10 minutes. You could, for instance, have two "30 minute" walks on the weekends and 5 shorter "10 minute" walks throughout the week.

These are ideal numbers however, and for many of you they may seem impossible to reach, either because they are too challenging on a fitness level or because you simply don't have the time. If you are not fit enough, just make a gradual progression of intensity, frequency and time. You can even start off with as little as 5 minutes a day. Your only goal, at first, should be to do it regularly.

If time is the issue, try to work around it. You could make sure you get a 15 minute walk every lunchtime. It may not seem like a lot but once you add it up it comes to 1 hour and 15 minutes a week. That's 65 hours a year! If you can manage to add one or two long walks during the weekend you are set to reach the AHA and ACSM standards!

• **How do I count steps? And How do I get all my steps in?**

A good idea might be to invest in a pedometer. A Pedometer is a little device that allows you to keep track of the number of steps you take during the day. A 2010 study done by the Journal of Medicine and Science in Sports and exercise says that the average American walks 5,117 steps a day. In 2014, Withings released an article in which they published the average number of steps they collected from their pedometer users around the world and the number of steps in the U.S.A. situated itself around 5815, while in countries such as France, Germany and the UK people were walking around 6300 steps a day. According to AHA, the recommended number of steps, if you want to achieve health benefits is 10,000 steps per day or more. And since research has shown that people using a pedometer tend to take 2491 extra steps each day, it might be a good idea to get one!

For those of you that have an Iphone, why not invest in an Apple watch: one of its cool attributes is an integrated pedometer. If you do not wish to invest in a pedometer but would still like to know roughly how many steps you are walking each day here are a few tips:

• 1 mile is approximately 2000 steps
• 12 average city blocks equals approximately 1 mile

If you do decide to invest in a pedometer, try the first few days not to set any goals such as reaching a certain amount of steps. Just set it on and see how many steps you achieve in a normal day. In this way, you will have a realistic starting point. After a few days, according to the number of steps you have achieved, you will have an average and will be ready to set a goal. Although 10,000 steps has been established as being the ideal amount per day, you might not be ready for such a big jump. You may even start at 2000, 3000 or 4000 steps. It doesn't matter. What's important is to just get started!

Note: Did you know that this "10000 steps landmark" was at first launched by a Japanese company in the 1960s to promote its pedometer and that it was based on the fact that "10000 steps sounded good" and wasn't backed by any research whatsoever? Since then, however, researchers have looked into these numbers and found that this number is actually quite accurate and have classified walking under 5000 steps as leading a sedentary lifestyle, 10000 as being active and over 12500 as being highly active.

We are all different however and have various levels of fitness. For this reason, it's important to establish *your* baseline: if at your initial starting point your daily steps are at approximately 2000, I would suggest that you walk around your block to see how many steps it amounts to: 200, 300, 500 steps and set a walk around the block once or twice each day as your first goal.

Then, once you get this goal anchored, try to find new and easy ways to add some more steps.

- You could for example decide to go up and down a flight of stairs that are in or nearby your home to add another 50, 100 or 200 steps, to tone your legs and butt and get your heart pumping.
- Next time you go to the supermarket, you could walk twice around the whole parking lot or… once you are inside, you could walk twice around the whole store before starting to shop.
- You could race your kids going up the stairs, while they take the elevator (let them give you a head start of about 30 seconds) and then switch roles.
- Make a phone call walk. We all have that phone call we dread to make, because we know it's going to take an hour. Take your phone outdoors, bring a pair of speakers and chat and stroll. This way you get two things done in one go. Tell the person you took 15-20 minutes (or more) time off especially to call them but that as soon as you get back home you will have to cut the conversation because you have got the kids homework to check, dinner to prepare etc.
- If you are lucky to have a treadmill at home, schedule a favorite TV program and walk your way through it. Many gyms have cardio equipment with a TV, so it's also an option there as well.

f. How to walk?
As I said before, no training is required, however, keep in mind the following:
- Keep your posture erect, stand tall. This means keeping shoulders back and reminding yourself regularly to pull them back. Keep your tummy in and your chin up, eyes looking forward.

- Swing your arms. I like to keep them bent and not dangling down otherwise my hands tend to swell from having the blood rushing to extremities after a while.
- Breathe and fill up your lungs. Remember that you should never be out of breath – Use the talk test to make sure you are at a correct speed: you shouldn't be able to sing beautifully but you should be able to have a conversation with someone.
- Smile as much as possible to the people you meet, or simply for yourself
- Check out my online P.E.T.s (Powerful Empowering tapes) and take one along with you.
- Or try out the "Reach your 5 senses Walk", see Change n° 57: *Empowering Walk*.

h. Equipment

You don't really need anything special to walk: what's important is to feel comfortable. You can even do it in your work clothes and walk to work. If you are worried about getting all sweaty, simply make sure you don't walk too fast. You can also plan on bringing a spare shirt and quickly change in the restrooms when you arrive.

You can also leave 5 minutes earlier and bring wipes and deodorant and have a quick perkup before you start working. My office has showers which is very convenient, especially in summer.

The one thing I would definitely invest in, is a good pair of walking shoes. Not all shoes are made for walking and you might end up with blisters or pain in different parts of your feet such as the heel or the Achilles tendon. Most major athletic brands offer shoes that are especially designed for walking.

No need to spend $100 but I do recommend buying them in a store as opposed to online. That way you can take the time to try them on and walk around. It's important that they feel comfortable and provide cushioning.

For the cold and windy days, a nice sweater might be all you need, or you may want to invest in a windbreaker, a scarf and a pair of gloves. I personally don't like to dress up too warmly. I know a lot of people layer up thinking that they will sweat more and lose weight. I don't know why but I have always felt that my body needs to breathe as well!

I prefer wearing a special long-sleeved running t-shirt. They often wick the sweat away, leave you feeling dry and protect you more from the wind than a normal t-shirt. I also believe in starting out feeling a little out of my comfort zone, that is, feeling like I could have worn an extra layer of clothes.

After a few minutes of walking my body starts to warm up. It may seem strange but under-dressing has the advantage of forcing your metabolism to work a little harder to keep your body warm, so you are actually burning more calories.

It's important however, that you never feel as though you are freezing, or cold and shivering. The goal here is to feel good and not to get sick or catch a cold.

This goal is probably one of the easiest ones to tackle: all you have to do is get up and walk. Call a friend and ask them to join you. Pull your shoulders back, breathe in deeply, look around and appreciate your surroundings and whenever possible, smile.

Try to create a practice that you look forward to by listening to your favorite music, watching your favorite TV show, calling someone up, spending a special bonding moment with you child or pet. If your goal is to add a daily walk, choose a realistic amount of time to do it. If this is totally new to you, choose a 10 or 15 minutes daily walk and stick with it. I would rather you do 15 minutes every day then 30 minutes twice a week. The goal here is to initiate a new habit.

If it is unrealistic and taking up too much of your time, there is a big chance you will get discouraged and soon quit. Make sure it's attainable. If you don't have much time but you want to do 30 minutes every day, I suggest you split the walks into 2 or 3 bouts of exercise, that way you are sure to get it done

For many of you, walking may seem too easy, but you would be astounded by its benefits. Just try it! Put a good pair of walking shoes on and walk at a fast pace. You will feel invigorated, energetic and totally revved up and probably come home with a refreshed mind!

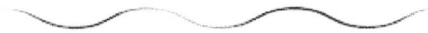

Change n°27
MINDFUL WORKOUT

27.

Nowadays, with our busy schedules, most people tend to race through their days and who knows how they manage to get everything done. This week why don't you decide to slow down and be more mindful. Take a look at what is going on around you, in a more detached way. Why not make a deliberate choice of becoming an "observer." The goal here is to take a step back and to look at yourself when you partake in any form of exercise: are you present or is your mind wandering somewhere else? Are you getting your exercise done because you have to or are you giving it your all? The way I see it: when you do something, give it your undivided attention. I would rather you do 20 minutes of exercise with intent, than one hour without it. Try it! Try being totally in the moment. Talk to yourself. Tell yourself what it is you are doing exactly: if you are going up the stairs, do it mindfully and feel your feet on the ground, your muscles contracting, your heart pumping and your body sweating.

If your body is your vehicle, are you the driver or a simple passenger?

A. Why be mindful or intentional when exercising?
a. Difference between absent minded and mindful exercising
The best way to understand why it's a good idea to train mindfully or with intent is to simply give it a try. When you DECIDE to do something, you bring INTENT. This intent puts you in a certain concentration mode and makes you FOCUS on what you are doing. You can either focus with your eyes closed, to grasp every sensation that is taking place within your body, or you can do it with your eyes open and really look at your muscles contracting and relaxing; whatever works best for you.

This focusing, you will come to see, creates ENERGY. And this energy brings CHANGE, in other words, RESULTS. Understand that it is one thing to simply exercise, and it's a whole other ball game to exercise with intent. So, it's your choice: you can either feel good or you can feel empowered and discover a new path: one of TRANSFORMATION.

Let's take the example of a bicep curl: the exercise consists of flexing and extending your arm. Make sure you start with proper posture: shoulders back, tummy tight, arms relaxed, legs slightly bent. Flex both arms while looking at your biceps. See them flexing. See the muscles contracting. Feel the contraction. Put intent into your exercise. When you reach the top, squeeze a few seconds and feel. Keep concentrating. You're not finished yet. While bringing those arms back down, keep everything under control. Don't just drop them. Mindfully bring your arms back into their initial position. Try doing this, 12 to 15 times. Then try to do the same exercise without any intent at all: by simply lifting your arms up and down, up and down again. Do you feel the difference?

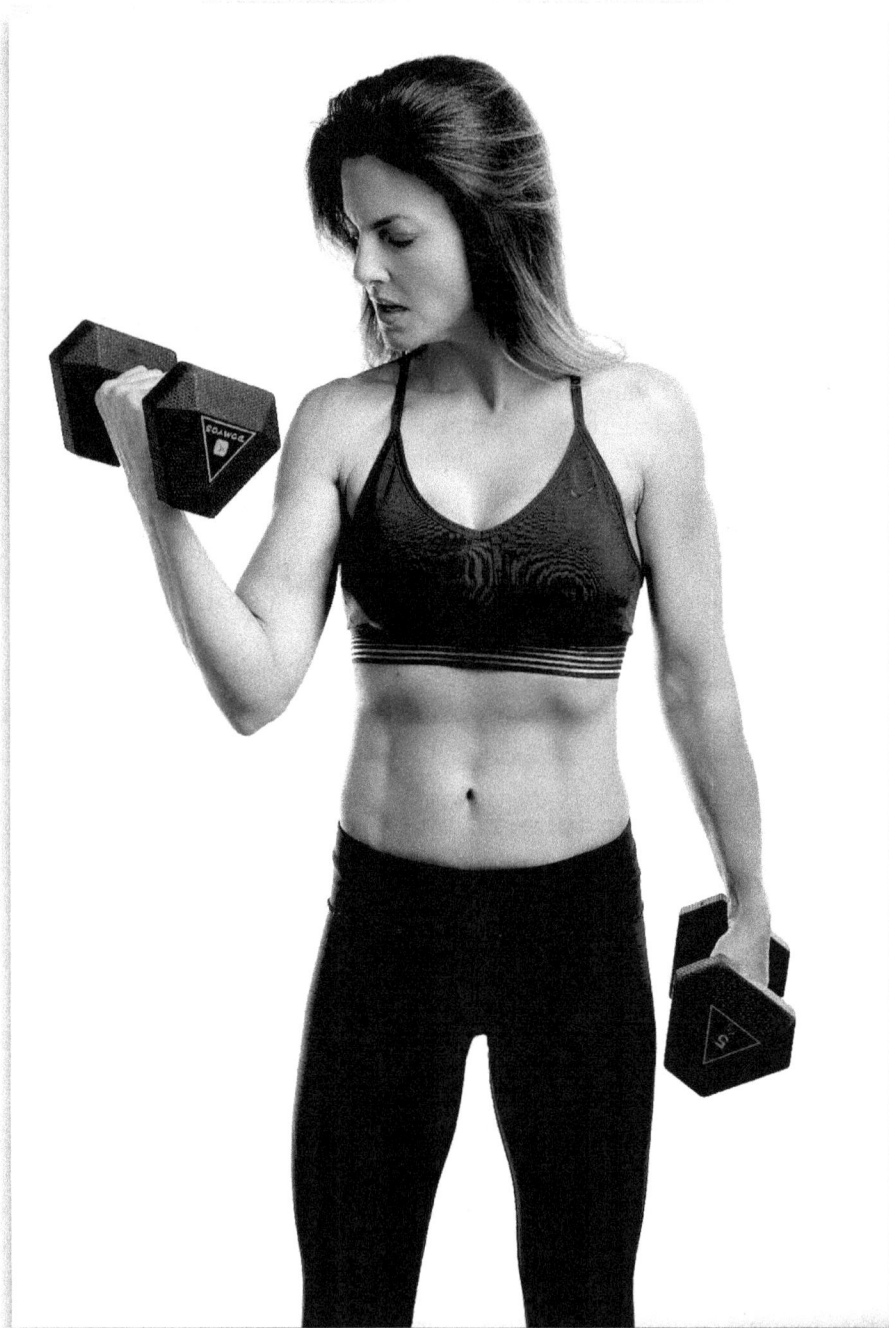

If you want results, "Intent" is the way to go.
Training with intent
will get you where you want to go, faster.

b. What if I am just a recreational exerciser?

Some of you might say: "But I am not a competitive athlete, why would I bother working out this way? My answer is: "Why not?" Yes, why not give it your undivided attention? Aren't you worth it? Even if you are just an occasional exerciser, why not give it your all and do the best you can while you are working out at the gym? Do it 200%.

Living mindfully means being totally present when you are doing something and not letting yourself get distracted with all that is happening around you, as well as inside your mind. Try, as much as possible to do things mindfully when working, talking to a friend, or studying. Also make sure you have moments when you can let your mind wander freely, such as in the car or when you take a break.

B. Benefits of training with intent

Working out with intent or mindfully also has other benefits:

a. It relieves stress

When you focus your attention on what you are doing, you don't allow yourself to be distracted by your surroundings such as noise or people talking. All this action that takes place around you is tiring your mind. I would even suggest that you turn your music off and learn to stay in tune with your body rather than a song!

b. A sense of accomplishment

When you give your undivided attention to something, you tend to be prouder of what you have accomplished. Once you have finished exercising, if you have given it your all, there is a big probability that you will feel a high sense of pride.

c. Helps to increase your self-acceptance

Focusing on yourself and on what you are doing can help you increase your self-acceptance. There is a certain power in determination that makes you stronger. As you progressively learn to focus on what you are doing, you will feel your inner strength grow and when leaving the gym, you will feel more confident and happier.

d. Learn to abstract the outside world

Training with intent and mindfully will progressively teach your mind to "zone out" and calm down. Think of it as a double workout: training your body to become healthy, but also training your mind to keep everything under control. Now how cool is that? Not only will you be beautifying externally, such as firming up your biceps or your booty, you will also beautify internally!

e. Focus. Intent. Presence.

Finally, by completely concentrating your attention on what you are doing, you are actually learning to increase your presence. Try as much as possible to expand this concentration to other aspects of your life, for instance by being more present when someone is talking to you or when you are with your children. People will feel it and believe me, will love the attention. So, learn to focus on one thing at a time: when you train, focus on the training, when you work, focus on the task at hand, and when you are with a friend, give them your undivided attention.

C. How can you integrate more intent and mindfulness when exercising?

a. Environment

The first important thing to consider is your environment. Does it suit you? Take a few minutes to look around and ask yourself: is going to the gym, jogging, or tennis really your thing? Do you find it more motivating to have people train beside you or, on the contrary, are you more of a solitary person? Maybe you feel too self-conscious about what others might be thinking. And how do you feel about training indoors or outdoors? Why not switch things around a bit? Sometimes, I jog to the gym ready for a great workout, but upon arrival I see that the place is packed and it's all hot and sweaty. I know, there is no way, that I will be able to focus on my training session. So, in such a case, what I normally do, is head back outdoors for a stress-free workout.

When you train, do you find that you tend to do the same thing repeatedly over and over again? Are you bored or do you often feel distracted? In this case, it might be time for a change in activity. The good thing about starting a new sport is that you have to give it your full attention and concentrate to learn the moves properly.

If, on the contrary, you love your activity, have a look at the way you train? Do you train with the same enthusiasm as your very first day? Probably not. Does it need a little bit of revving up? Why not take a coach for a while or sign up for a boot camp: if you are working out properly, normally there is no way you can have anything else on your mind!

If you run, walk or cycle, open up to your surrounding environment. Be curious and discover the names of the streets, the shops and the people. Be adventurous and follow some new paths. Become one with nature, observe the trees, smell the scents, recognize the sounds around you and see how they change from season to season. Sometimes the best way to forget what is going on in your mind is to try to focus on what is going on, on the outside. When things are buzzing inside your head, it's a good idea to open up, widen your perspective by focusing on something specific on the outside. This will help calm down the interior noise. I have tried it and know that it works. When I was diagnosed with cancer, my head was a constant chatter box and I just couldn't seem to quiet it down. I went out daily for some long walks and the fresh air was invigorating. One day, somehow, I decided to "forget" myself and to focus on everything that was going on around me: nature, the people, the sounds, the air going through my nostrils. It really helped me to disconnect from what was happening to me and it felt so good not to hear my mind blabbering away all the time.

b. Learn to be in tune with yourself

To bring more intent or mindfulness, the second thing you might want to look into is to be more in tune with yourself

For example, how do you feel before you exercise? Are you stressed, tired, mad or happy and enthusiastic? Write it down on a piece of paper and then head off for your workout. When you return check out how you feel and write it down. Chances are, all the tension has disappeared and you are feeling energized again. So, listen to yourself and take the time to see how exercise makes you feel.

I also really recommend finishing every workout with a few minutes of total relaxation: you cannot imagine how beneficial it can be for your inner-self to take the time to simply close your eyes, even if it's only for a minute or two. So, before you leave, treat yourself to a little bit of alone time, and listen to how you feel. Check out if you have any aches or pains, in which case in might be a good idea to switch activities or rest for a while. Do you feel jittery, as if you couldn't seem to relax? Many of us find it impossible to stop for two minutes: we are already creating a "to do" list in our minds, stressed about all the things that need to be done as soon as the workout is over. Try putting the list down, just two minutes, RELAX, BREATHE and let it all go.

Also check your rhythm and your breathing pattern. It's hard to focus when you are out of breath. If you are running, walking or swimming, try to synchronize your breaths with your steps or strokes. You can, for example, do 4 steps and breathe in, followed by 4 step and breathe out. This is all "trial and error" so you have to see what works for you.

Once you have found your rhythm, try to pay attention to technique. For example, if you are swimming free style, make sure you are stretching your arms out, keeping your fingers closed, pulling the water with your hands, bringing your arm all the way down to brush your thighs. This can basically be done with any other type of exercise: I can't stress enough the importance of focusing on proper technique and posture. It's just as important to center your thoughts on your training aspects, such as physical sensation and breathing, as it is to focus on proper technique.

Of course, I can only encourage you to learn, learn, learn: if you want to know more about becoming mindful, check out my website for more articles, take an online class and learn new tips on how to live in the moment.

Decide today, and from now on, that you are going to exercise with a purpose: the moment that you are out there, you will be giving it your all. Keep in mind that deep focus leads to increased energy flow to the muscles that are working, therefore better results in the long run. And remember:

Let go of what's troubling you and broaden your perspective.

This change of focus can be a good thing: We often tend to obsess over something, such as our weight for example. Why don't you "decide" to obsess over something else such as training with perfect form and technique, this way you will be getting your mind away from that number on the scale. Try it: change gears and forget about the weight. Move on to second gear and focus on technique and with the third gear steer your mind towards being more aware and feeling your muscles as they are working out. Once you change your pattern of thought and keep it away from the weight, redirect it towards thoughts to improve your skills, and get more results, that's when the magic starts to happen. This is what I mean by "broadening the perspective": leave what is troubling you aside and focus on something else.

Become passionate about it, have fun learning, start paying attention to how your body feels and you will see that those extra pounds will magically start disappearing.

And so, although at first it may seem contradictory to exercise and be more mindful at the same time, with one part implying movement and the other encouraging you to stop all movement, you will quickly realize that both are actually compatible. By learning to be more attentive to yourself as you exercise, you will surely learn a few things about yourself and will be growing on the inside and out.

c. Determined and Mindful Walking

When I walk, I don't just walk, I concentrate on the whole walking process. What this means, is that I totally invest myself into it and over time I have learned to be aware of my posture, my breathing and my thoughts. It requires a little getting used to and a little practice, but the outcome is really worth it.

The most important thing to do when you walk is to stand tall and believe in yourself. Pull your shoulders back, tuck your tummy in, lift your chin up and look ahead with determination. Avoid looking arrogant or superior. What we are looking for here is CONFIDENCE! At the beginning, when I started walking this way, I felt uncomfortable because it wasn't like me to boast my torso up and act assuredly. It felt as though by walking this way, I was looking down on others and that really isn't who I am. There is a solution to this problem however: Keep the shoulders back, walk with confidence but make sure you look at people with kindness in your eyes and smile whenever possible. When we think of confidence and determination, we tend to associate this with a hard and determined look but that really isn't necessary. You can totally stand tall and have a compassionate look in your eyes. Try it! From afar people will see you walking tall and looking confident and as you come closer they will see kindness in your eyes. What a surprising combination! And they will think "Now that's someone I want to meet!". It might be challenging at first to combine the two. Try thinking about something that brings compassion to mind such as seeing a fluffy puppy, or simply remembering something that you saw, that brought compassion into your heart or made you happy. Normally just the thought of these images will change your facial expression. And if you struggle with presenting compassionate eyes, then just try smiling nicely as much as possible. You don't have to smile at everyone. You can start by smiling when you see children or a dog, you can smile while you are talking over the phone, you can smile when you see a couple kissing or an old couple holding hands. Once you start looking around, you will see that there are thousands of good reasons to smile for!

So next time you go for a walk bring the two C's with you: Compassion and Confidence. Believe me, you'll feel the difference! When you get used to this during your walk, you will be surprised how you end up doing it every time you get up, whether to get a cup of coffee or just to go to the restroom. Remember one important thing: if you want people to believe in you, well you have to start by believing in yourself. Determined Mindful walking is a tool that can help you achieve just that!

Abdominal Training

But this is just the first part of my Determined Mindful Walking technique.

The second part concerns your abs. There is an exercise that you can include while you are walking, that tones your abdominals. It's a three-phase exercise.

The first phase is very easy to do, the second requires a little training and getting used to. The third phase requires practice and is more challenging. You don't have to do the 2nd or 3rd phase if you do not wish to. The most important aspect of this Determined Mindful walking is your overall posture and your attitude, so feel free to leave out phase 2 and 3 if you are not up to it.

How to proceed: You might want to practice doing these exercises while standing up and facing a mirror first. Once you have grasped the technique, you can move on to doing it as you walk.

Phase 1:

Stand nice and tall, feet shoulder-width apart. You must feel comfortable and stable. Keep your hands along your thighs or on hips. Keep your back straight, chest lifted and shoulders back. Start by inhaling slowly through the nose. Try to let the air go all the way filling up your lungs. Next, do a long exhale through the mouth while pulling your tummy inward. Try to imagine it touching your spine. Maintain this abdominal contraction through at least two entire breathing cycles of one inhalation + one exhalation. Make sure to keep your shoulders down throughout the exercise. Release and relax. Make sure to keep an upward posture the entire time. Repeat several times as well as regularly throughout the day.

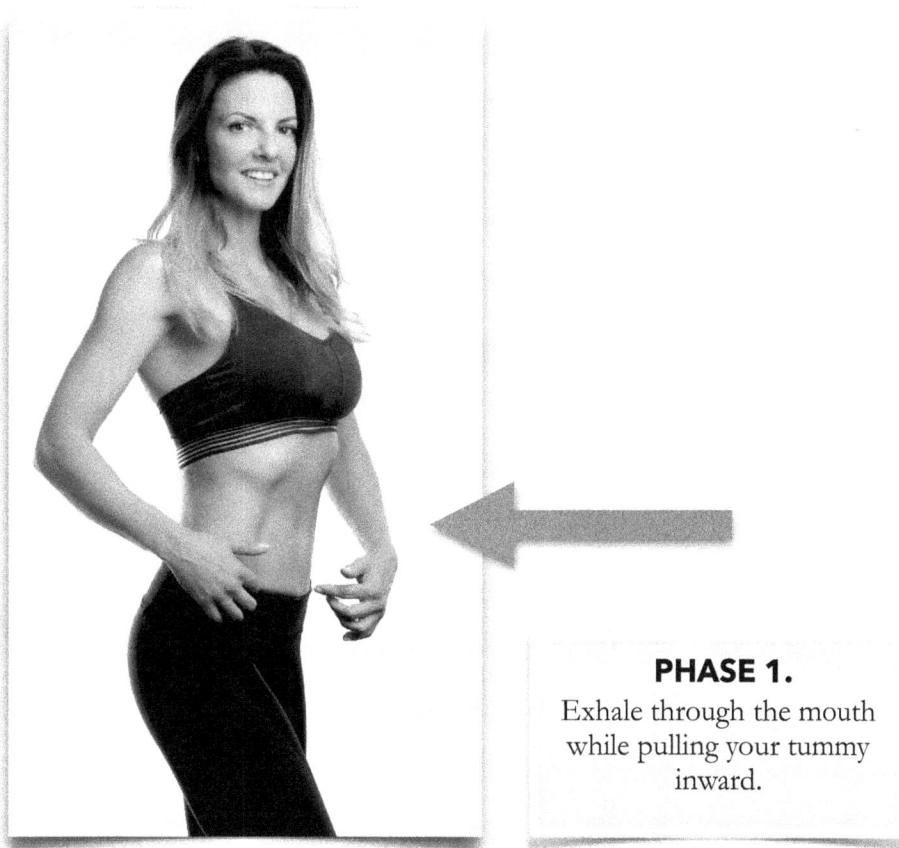

PHASE 1.
Exhale through the mouth while pulling your tummy inward.

Phase 2: Let's try to go in a little deeper now. This time, inhale through the nose, exhale through the mouth and, just as in phase 1, contract your abs by pulling your tummy inward. In addition, **you also want to try bringing both sides of your stomach together, like a compression wall.** You really want to feel both sides come together by squeezing them. This two-part stomach contraction engages all your muscles in that region and helps you consciously differentiate between the two phases. Make sure you keep your shoulders back and down.

Keep breathing normally through one more entire breathing cycle: inhale through the nose and exhale through the mouth while maintaining the contraction, tummy in, squeezed and compressed. You might release part of your abdominal contraction while inhaling. Just make sure to do the whole process again as you exhale. This second phase will require practice and some getting used to but keep trying and you will be amazed: you can actually work your abs just using your breath! Repeat several times and then relax.

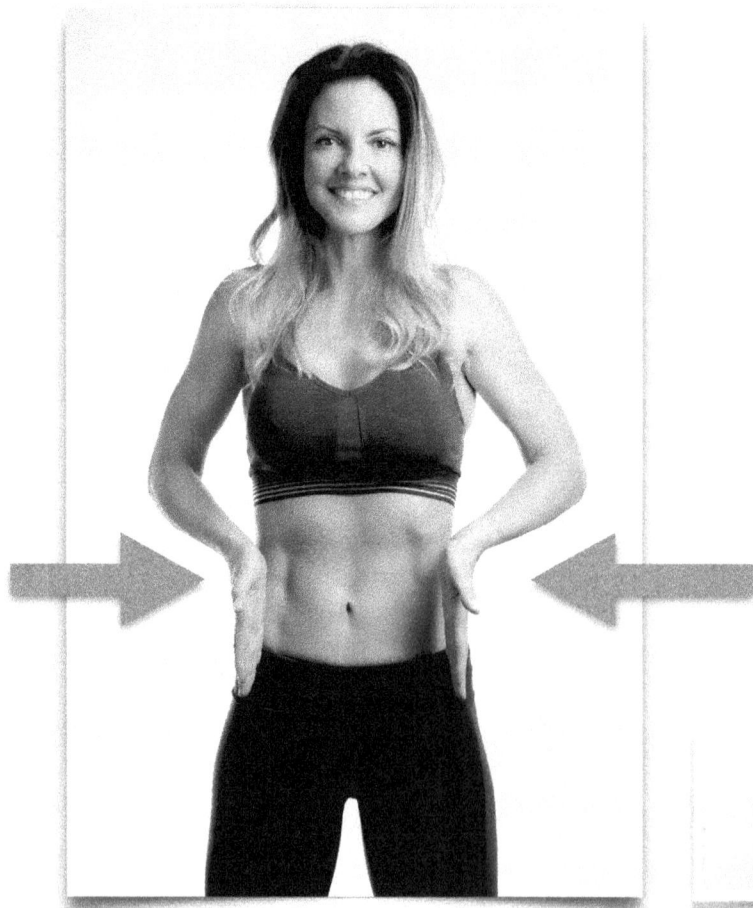

PHASE 2.

Squeeze your abs together like a compression wall

Phase 3: This part is more advanced and may seem too much for some of you. Feel free to leave this part out but, every once in a while, try to come back and begin working at an entire new level.

Once again, inhale through the nose, lift your chest up, shoulders down. Exhale and simultaneously **pull your abs upward** under your rib cage. Next repeat phase 1 and phase 2. This is how it goes: you pull upward, then contract, and compress. Maintain this abdominal contraction through two breathing cycles. Release and relax. Repeat several times. A tip: Place both hands on your stomach to properly feel your muscles exercising.

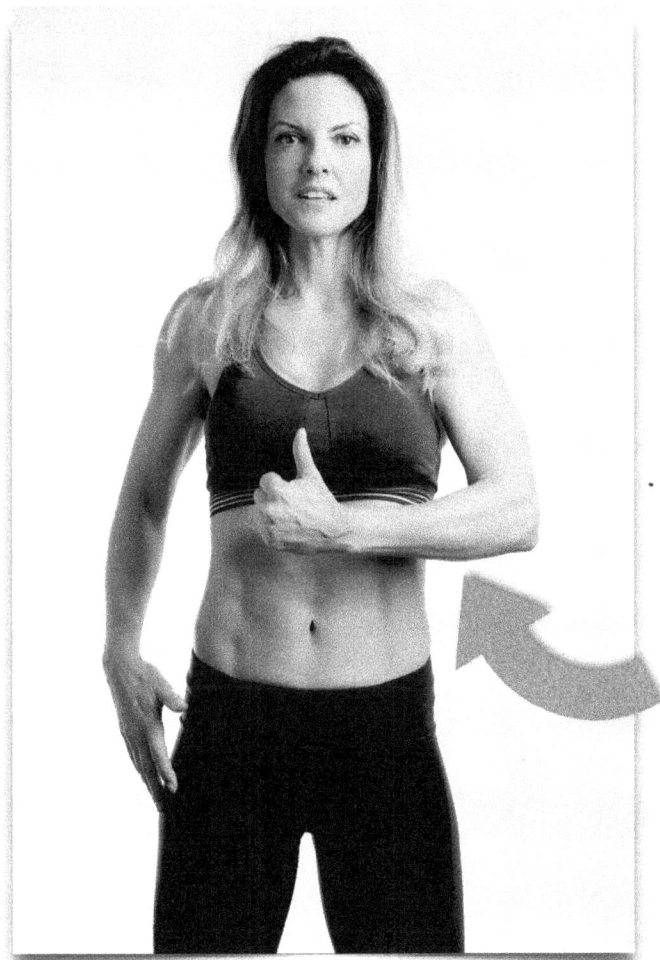

Phase 3:
Exhale and simultaneously
pull your abs upward
under your rib cage.
Next, repeat phase 1 and phase 2.

Forceful exhale option:
Each time you are exhaling you can either use a long slow deep breath, or three equal force exhales. With this exercise you will reach a deeper layer of abdominals.
All four of these exercises (3 phases + option) can be done lying down on your back, sitting down or kneeling. Have fun practicing them and remember, you can do them everywhere: while waiting in line, at the bus stop or doing the dishes.

Change n°28
HOT AND COLD

28.

EMBRACING HOT

Take a minute and see yourself soaking in a hot bubble bath or sipping on something hot like a nice cup of tea. It not only contributes to making your body feel good, it also has a way of making you feel more relaxed and calm. Read on and see what benefits you can get from bringing more "hotness" into your life.

A. Warm lemon water

a. Drink lemon water

The benefits of having a cup of warm lemon water first thing in the morning has been touted for centuries. One day, someone told me about her experience with this beverage and how she really felt the benefits. As I had been dwelling for a while on the idea of quitting coffee, I thought that this might just be the perfect substitute. When I got home, I decided that this was a change I wanted to tackle and I placed my coffee and beloved coffee machine in a box and stored it away in my cellar. Little did I know that quitting coffee cold turkey could have such challenging side effects. I had flu like symptoms and was literally falling asleep anytime, anywhere for almost a week. Clearly, I was no longer the one in charge: this brew had taken control over a part of me. This realization was just what I needed to strengthen my determination: I had to hang in there. Luckily, I had something to look forward to in the morning: my hot lemon water! The rest of the day I stuck with only water.

b. The benefits of drinking freshly squeezed lemon juice:

- Do you have bad breath, a dry mouth (coated tongue or no saliva), digestive problems, skin problems, headaches, or do you have unpleasant body odor? These are all physical signs of toxicity. Drinking lemon added to warm water first thing in the morning will kickstart the digestion process for the day and help cleanse the liver.
- Lemons have been known for centuries to be antibacterial and antiviral: they help fight against infections, colds and the flu thanks to their content in vitamin C, pectin, citric acid, calcium, magnesium.
- It will boost your immune system,
- It can help regulate your bowels if you are constipated and contributes to getting rid of intestinal parasites.
- It clears your skin and promotes energy and vitality.

c. The Lemon Juice Recipe:

- Add 10 to 13 ounces of warm water to half of a freshly squeezed organic lemon. Make sure it's fresh, firm and has a nice yellow color to it.
- Filter it so that there is no pulp in your drink. Eliminating the pulp will ensure that the lemon flows right through your body and doesn't stop to be digested in your stomach.

- The goal here is not to activate the digestive system but to cleanse it!
- Drink it immediately and be sure to wait 10 to 15 minutes before eating anything else.
- It is recommended to drink your cup of warm lemon juice with a straw: it has a high acidic content that can damage the enamel of your teeth.
- You can also try adding spices such as ginger or some cayenne and if you have a hard time with the bitter taste, you can, add a little drop of honey or maple syrup.

B. Drink warm water twice a day

Drinking warm water can be very beneficial. It might also be a good idea to alternate between warm lemon water and plain warm water. It is recommended that you drink a sufficient amount of water throughout the day. It doesn't really matter whether you drink your water warm or cold but, for many people, warm water is considered a holistic health remedy. The warmth can really help with digestion, so why not give it a try.

C. Hot! Hot! Hot! Enjoying a sauna or hammam!

a. Benefits of a sauna

Don't go for the wrong reasons: many believe that it makes you lose weight… A sauna is there to make you sweat and it allows you to relax, but those are not the only benefits. Here is a list to convince you to start using one:
- It will help you relieve muscle pain such as arthritis, muscle soreness after an intense workout and also migraines
- It will help you reduce tension and sleep better
- It stimulates circulation. Why not add an arm and leg massage to help with the process

Note: the temperature of a sauna is usually situated between 150 and 195° F (that's 66 to 91°C). Start off by doing 5 to 10 minute sessions and build your way up. You can do 10 minutes for example, get out to cool down for a few minutes and then go back in again for another 5 or 10 minutes.

> **Before using any product or making any drastic changes to your diet, consult your health care professional.**

b. Benefits of a hammam

Contrarily to the Sauna, where the air is dry, the hammam's humidity is around 99%. The temperature is usually situated between 75 and 120° F (25 – 50° C). You will want to build up the tolerance, which means that the length of your sessions should be reasonable and increased gradually. Normally people stay in hammams a little longer than in saunas. Read below to find out its benefits:
- Unclogs your pores and makes your skin look beautiful
- Helps you relax and feel calm
- Releases tension in your muscles
- Strengthens your immune system

c. How to use them safely and adequately
- While using a sauna or hammamDrink at regular intervals
- Build up tolerance to heat: be reasonable with the duration

- Be regular. Indeed, regularity will reap more benefits than doing it occasionally
- Take a cold shower after
- Use them for your general wellbeing and not for weight loss

d. Hot Yoga

Hot Yoga is definitely not for everyone but when I tried it, I was hooked immediately! You basically do a series of 26 hatha yoga poses in a room that is at 105°F (40°C) for 90 minutes.

Ask your doctor whether this is a discipline you can consider. Below are just a few of the benefits:
- You will improve your breathing capacity. Since you have to adapt to a strenuous situation of exercising in extreme heat, your breathing also has to adapt accordingly
- You will help your body rid itself of toxins
- You will increase your body's range of motion and flexibility
- It's hard. So, you are going to have to hang in there and accept being in discomfort for 90 minutes. This requires inner strength, the need to focus on the present moment, as well as determination. You will leave your session feeling proud of yourself for having done it!

D. Soaking up some sun

Sunlight stimulates the body's production of vitamin D, which plays a big role in bone health and soaking up a bit of sun can also really improve your mood. So, remember to step outside, go for a walk or have a coffee with a friend at a terrace café and let the sunshine in. You don't need much to reap the benefits: 5 to 10 minutes three times a week is enough but believe me, try lying in the grass and letting the rays of sun embrace you. Chances are you will want to stay there a little longer.

EMBRACING COLD

A. Ocean or lake swimming

a. My story

We have no idea to what extent our bodies and minds are capable of adapting until life really hits you in the face. Little did I know what was coming my way in 2016: cancer, divorce, putting my homeschooled kids back to school, job and apartment search,... basically having to start my whole life again from scratch.

That's when you realize that engaging in regular exercise, meditating daily, taking the time to be alone with yourself are essential: they are your life foundations. You can see your whole life going buck wild, but your feet will still stand on solid ground.

A few weeks after having been diagnosed with cancer, I decided to go for a walk and headed down to the beach. I am lucky to live on the lovely Mediterranean Sea. I stood there staring down into the water; it was beautiful and glittery and although we were approaching winter, the sun was nice and warm.

As I looked into the crystal-clear water, I felt this urge to jump in. I knew it was probably freezing, but it felt as if the water was calling me. I could have just striped my clothes off and jumped in cold turkey. All that life was putting on my plate at the moment, all those thoughts going around and around in my mind, all the fear that had started to grow within me… It was as if I was suffocating and desperately needed to breathe again. Then and there, I decided to do it and even though winter was well under way I ran in!

My very first feeling was that it wasn't as cold as I thought it would be. If I have to be totally honest, the hardest part was keeping my head underwater. But now, as a more experienced ocean swimmer, I must say that it's the most important part of the whole process: I literally would get a brain freeze. In a sense it was as if I was receiving electroshocks directly into my brain: I didn't have time to think or pay attention to what was worrying me, I had to focus my entire attention on my body and on the fact that I needed to adapt to the cold RIGHT NOW. I swam 4 to 6 laps and then took a cold shower to rinse all the salt off. I am not sure what it is about cold water exactly that makes me feel like I am on top of the world, but that's how I felt for the rest of the day. Did it come from the cold that literally reached my bones? Was it the fact that I felt proud for being able to throw myself into icy cold water? Was it the conviction that the ocean and its emanations were beneficial to me? Was it the brain freeze that helped me put things back into perspective? I really don't know, maybe it was all of them at once. But from day one I became addicted: this definitely was for me, and from then on, I went for my daily swim.

So, if your mind is going through hell right now, why not try something crazy as well: I really recommend ocean or swimming in a lake, but if it's not a possibility for you or just simply not your thing, why not try rock climbing, bungee or parachute jumping, going on a thrill ride at the fair, kart racing, or boxing? There are many options that require you to be totally focused on what you are doing. You could also, just take an icy cold shower!

b. How to tackle cold water walking and swimming

• With or without a wet suit
As the days got really colder, I opted for a shorty wet suit, a great shield against the cold, but you can also get yourself a full body wet suit and slowly work your way to not wearing one at all. That's what I did. Indeed, as I got used to it, I felt more and more capable of going in with just a swimsuit and I truly enjoyed the freedom of movement and the effect the cold water had on my body.

• Being properly equipped
The water is cold so it's important to come properly equipped: bring a towel maybe even a second one for your hair and warm clothes for when you get out. I make sure to always take a thick woolen sweater and a wind breaker. A bathing cap is also essential: I wear one and even sometimes layer two, one on top of the other. If you choose to use a wetsuit, ask for advice. I really feel that the shorty is a better choice as it allows you more freedom of movement.

• Go with a buddy

Although I went swimming on my own, I was never really all alone as there were always other swimmers there with me. Make sure, however, that you come accompanied. First of all, it will make the session more fun and you will both be more motivated to get in! Second of all, especially if you are a beginner, it's best to have someone with you for security reasons.

• Be mentally prepared

When you want to do something that puts you out of your comfort zone, it's important to mentally prepare yourself. You might find it helpful to make your very own P.E.T. (Personal Empowering Tape: see Chapter 1 – Change n° 05) and create a tape in which you show determination to go swimming and to getting into the cold water: "You can do this and you are going to feel fantastic!"

• Be consistent

As with anything new that you wish to tackle, consistency is key. Quit making excuses. Unless there is lightning, a storm or waves that make it impossible to swim, don't let anything stop you.

• Going in!

The hardest part is to actually get into the water. You may like running in but I don't really recommend it. Going in progressively is the safest way of doing it. The first few times, you might feel like only walking or wading in the water. Try to get in deep enough so as to have your legs submerged and then just walk. You might want to keep on a short sweat-shirt to keep the upper body warm. What I usually do is walk for about ten minutes and then I splash my upper body before diving in. These 10 minutes are usually sufficient to get half of my body acclimated to the cold water and ready to tackle the real deal.

B. Take Cold showers

I cannot emphasize enough the benefits of taking a cold shower. Today, I cannot live without them anymore!

a. The benefits are numerous:
- It improves your blood circulation
- You will burn more calories as your body has to adapt to the difference in body temperature
- It keeps your skin and hair healthy
- It makes your hair shinier
- It speeds up muscle recovery

I love doing it for only one reason: for the energy boost it gives me! I feel totally invigorated after having one, even an hour later!

b. How to tackle a cold shower?

Before starting, remember this: the goal here is to practice accepting discomfort. If you can manage to do it with little things, such as taking a cold shower, then it will get easier with the bigger challenges you set for yourself later on. The whole purpose of this book is to make you succeed at pulling through easy challenges and get used to being successful. After attaining a certain number of goals, you will feel more confident and believe it's possible to tackle some more difficult ones.

Doing it cold turkey! For some of you this option is open and worth trying: simply stand in your shower, put the tap on cold and let the water drizzle on you a bit to get your body used to the temperature and then go for it and enjoy this invigorating moment!

Doing it progressively If you are not brave enough to go cold turkey:
- You can decrease the temperature progressively
- You can start by showering only your lower body first: your feet, legs, thighs and buttocks and slowly, slowly, work your way up until you do your entire body
- You can alternate hot, warm and cold several times
- You can increase the duration: start with 10 to 20 seconds and work your way up to a nice long cold shower!

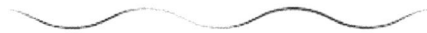

Change n°29
PHYSICAL ASSESSMENT CHECKLIST

29.

As we rush through our busy schedules, we tend to ignore all those little signals and alerts our body sends us, such as these:

"It was hard to get out of bed this morning" Hint - *You didn't get enough sleep.*

"I didn't poop today" Hint - *You're constipated, lacking water and fiber in your diet.*

"I feel pain in my stomach, I have gas and often feel bloated and uncomfortable" Hint - *You are not eating properly.*

"I have pain in my shoulders and neck region" Hint - *You have to work on your posture.*

"I feel drained and without energy" Hint - *Your life routine is out of balance.*

A. The Physical Assessment Checklist, meet Ms. P.A.C.

When we start thinking about it, the list of small aches and pains that we tend to ignore and tolerate, can be pretty long. One day, as I thought about this, I drew a human body on a piece of paper and placed arrows everywhere I had a physical problem, such as skin problems, pain or discomfort. I looked at my list and chose the one ailment that bothered me the most and decided to get rid of it once and for all. I would take care of the other ones the following weeks. I kept the drawing as a reminder of the different things I would have to look into the following weeks. That's how, one day, I came up with the idea of creating a Ms. P.A.C. that would allow my readers to make their own physical assessment by going over their various aches and pains.

All you have to do is scan your body from head to toe and fill out the empty boxes with your various aches and pains. To help you, you will find below the most common ailments.

Where are your challenges:
- Headaches and migraines
- Eye
- Ear
- Teeth
- Back and neck
- Aches and pains (such, shoulder pain etc.)
- Joint
- Skin
- Digestive problems
- Food Intolerance
- Constipation
- Mobility problems
- Weight problems
- Presence of a lump
- Sleep problems or insomnia
- Fatigue - Feeling tired – lack of energy
- Menopause

Once you have finished analyzing, select one and focus on it 200%. Give it your all. Decide to get rid of it once and for all. Some will need you to simply schedule a doctor appointment, such as seeing your dentist for that tooth that has been bothering you. Start off by getting rid of the easy ones. Then tackle the one that needs a little more effort on your behalf, for example, constipation. See your doctor, research it and find out what you can do at your level to improve the condition. Find out what foods/nutrients, vitamins and minerals can improve your condition. Remember that many problems are stress related, so find the time to slow down, relax more, meditate. It may be beneficial to visualize your problem disappearing.

Write a list of all the things you can do at your level and create a checklist to find all possible changes you can implement to improve and possibly eliminate your problem. Make sure to go over the list at regular intervals and each day make a conscious effort to overcome this ailment.

How to use Ms. P.A.C. and the Physical Assessment Checklist:
It would be an impossible task for me to write how to proceed for each and every physical problem. I am asking you to use your common sense, and read, consult, research and then apply what you have learned to make this ailment a thing of the past. There *are* things that you can do, at your level for most problems that you have, and with a little bit of consistency, you *can* most probably eliminate it.

Just to give you an idea, here is an example.

<u>Example:</u> Digestion: What can I do this month to get my digestive system back on track?

Do you feel bloated or sluggish? Are you constipated? Does it sometimes feel as though you have a knot inside your stomach? One has to admit that with the hectic lives that we lead, it isn't always easy to control what goes into your mouth. It is a fact however, that these poor eating habits create a buildup of waste and toxins in our intestines.

Most of our little aches and pains can much improve by simply switching a few things here and there. Why not take the time this week to clean up your act and set things straight! On the following pages, you will find a few different ways to improve your digestion. There is no need to follow all the advice: you can concentrate on several points or choose only one. Read on and find out what might work for you.

Ms. P.A.C.

1.

2.

3.

4.

5.

6.

7.

8.

9.

10.

11.

12.

13.

14.

15.

16.

17.

18.

19.

20.

21.

22.

23.

24.

25.

26.

27.

28.

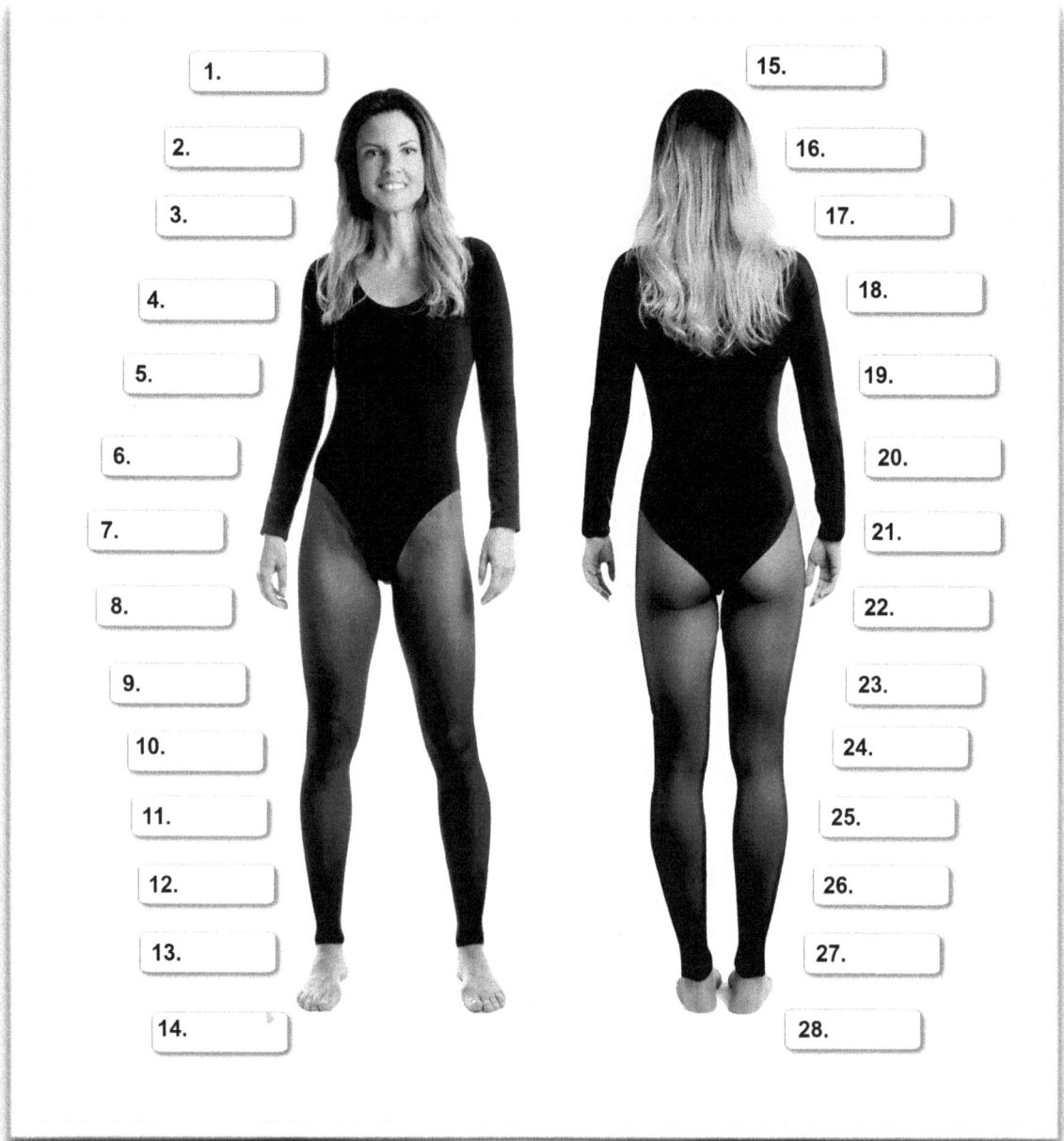

**Scan your body from head to toe and
fill out the empty boxes with your various aches and pains.**

B. Ideas To Get Your Digestive System Back On Track
a. Begin by consulting a specialist

The very first thing to do, of course, is to see your doctor and ask him what you can do to improve your digestion depending on what your problem is. Your goal this month could be to take his advice and to follow it. What's important is to get things straight and make your goal clear. Getting the help of a specialist who knows what is best for you, is by far the best thing to do. Becoming accountable to someone can give you that extra drive and incentive to do it seriously.

• Ask The Specialist About Supplements

Have you heard about Probiotics and Prebiotics? Ask your doctor or nutritionist about supplements they recommend for your condition.

If you want a regular bowel function, you need to have a healthy intestinal flora. A good way to help is to add probiotics and prebiotics to your diet. According to Webmd.com "Probiotics are good bacteria that help keep your digestive system healthy by controlling the growth of harmful bacteria. Prebiotics are carbohydrates that cannot be digested by the human body. They are food for the probiotics."

In numerous studies Probiotics have been found to ease digestive stress, help absorb nutrients from your food more efficiently, balance hormones, and boost your energy and immunity.

If you choose a simple solution, you can find probiotics and prebiotics naturally in certain foods before attempting to take them in the form of supplements.

What foods contain probiotics?

Yogurt, Kephir (fermented milk), miso (fermented soja), sauerkraut, fermented soft cheeses.

What foods contain prebiotics?

Artichokes, bananas, garlic, leek, onions, endive, asparagus, oatmeal…

• Ask The Specialist About Natural Colon Cleansing

You have quite a few to choose from: from herbal teas, laxatives, or enemas but also magnesium. You also have the choice to undergo colon cleansing with colon irrigation, high colonics. In this case you should consult a colonic hygienist or a colon hydro-therapist. Via a small tube, the hygienist flushes water (warm, hot or cold) several times into your colon at different intervals. After a few minutes, there will be a reverse effect whereby you let all the water come back out. This allows for great internal cleansing that eliminates a lot of accumulated waste. It may seem a bit daunting, something you feel you absolutely could not do, not even in a thousand years… I was very hesitant the first time a friend talked to me about this technique. But being curious, I chose to do it anyway. The specialist really puts you at ease and there are no odors as everything comes in and out via a tube. I used to do have a colon-cleanse in the spring and in autumn. It was like decluttering my home: a great way to start the change of season this way!

Today my eating habits are so healthy that I no longer have any problems with my digestive system and am regular. For this reason, I no longer feel the need to get colon cleanses.

b. Slow things Down

Digestion starts in the mouth: saliva is the magic potion that helps the whole digestion process. How do you produce saliva? By chewing. So, the more you chew, the more saliva you produce. It's really important that your food reaches your stomach completely chewed and loaded with saliva. The more, the better for your digestive system: it really takes a load off your digestive system's work. This is an important point that only needs a little getting used to. So, TAKE THE TIME TO CHEW YOUR FOOD!

c. Getting To Know The Different Parts of Digestion

For your digestion to work properly, this means that:
• your liver must be uncluttered,
• your intestines must be unclogged,
• your kidneys must eliminate properly the toxins your body needs to get rid of.
So why not try to find a natural way to clean up your act. Below you will find a list of the foods that can help you in this process.

1. Foods to help detox the liver
• Artichokes: eat one every day for 10 days
• Horseradish: cut into slices and eat with a dab of salted butter or grate it over your salad.
• Strawberries, when in season, have a bowl each day for 10 days.
• Lemons: squeeze half of an organic lemon and add warm water. It's great to do this first thing in the morning and to wait a bit before having anything else.
• Ginger and turmeric: add some to your freshly squeezed juices!
• Dandelion: get an organic herbal tea and drink a cup every day.

2. Foods to help detox your intestines:
• Leek: eat them steamed, boiled or cooked in a pressure cooker.
• Prunes: eat some for breakfast every day for 10 days. Simply place 4 or 5 of them in water and let them soak overnight. In the morning, warm them up. Start by drinking the juice and then eat the fruit.
• Fiber: try adding more to your diet by eating more whole wheat bread or by making sure you are having enough fruit and vegetables.
• Figs can also help to detox your intestines. Just eating one can bring 2 grams of fiber!
• Avocados: the healthy fats keep our digestion moving and lubricated.
• Eat a light and early dinner to allow your whole digestive system time to rest. Make a vegetable soup. Drink the broth and eat the vegetables separately with a little olive oil. If you wish to finish with something sweet, have some cooked fruit, such as apricots, apples, peaches or a Greek yogurt.

3. Foods to help detox your kidneys:
• Asparagus
• Celery
• Cucumber
• Raisin
• Grapefruit

• Drink lots of water
• Green tea: make a big jug and drink it throughout the day
• Reduce coffee, alcohol and chocolate for 10 days

d. Check Your Eating Habits

To clear up your digestive system there are certain bad habits that you can try avoiding, such as:

• Eating and munching outside your meals: try as much as possible to give your body a break by eating at regular intervals.
• Eating on the go or "unaware eating": many of us tend to eat because we have to and often end up doing several other things at the same time. It's important to take a break and eat consciously.
• Make sure you drink a sufficient amount of water every day and 1 or two cups more, if you exercise. Drinking helps to filter out the accumulated toxins. Check to see whether your urine is clear: it's the best indicator that you are getting enough. Don't forget that we are talking about water here and not fluids in general. Soft drinks, coffee, alcohol can in no way substitute for natural water.
• Not getting enough fiber? Eat more fruit and vegetables to make sure you get enough in your diet. This is truly what made a difference for me. When I really focused on eating fruit and vegetables at every meal, I never had a problem with constipation again. And ever since I have gotten into the habit of eating most of my vegetables raw, things have really changed and I really saw a big difference.
• Eating fried and processed foods: make them an occasional treat and once in a while avoid them completely for one week or ten days. As a rule, try as much as possible to make your meals from scratch.
• Listen to yourself. Are there any foods you have a hard time digesting? Avoid them for a while or if you really can't, try eating them separately/alone. I love candy, the gummy bear type, however I know that when I eat a few, that "jelly-ish" substance gets stuck somewhere along the way and stays put for days. Although I'll have a few occasionally, I really make a point to avoid eating them altogether.

e. Try different techniques to help your digestive system:

1. Have you ever tried self-massage?

It's an effective way to help your digestive system eliminate excess wastes and toxin buildup and thus cut down the stress you are putting it through.
The massage is quite basic.

- If you only have under 5 minutes:

Start by drinking a glass of water: it will help with the process.
You can do the massage with bare hands or you can use some body lotion or essential oils, such as tarragon, clove, peppermint, oil of oregano or marjoram as they are recommended to help with digestion.

• Decide whether you want to do it standing up, lying down, with bent knees or sitting on a chair.
• Place your hands on your stomach and take the time to inhale deeply while letting your stomach expand

- Contract your abs as you exhale. Repeat, several times.
- Create a slow circular motion with your hands but apply some pressure with your fingers. You can make your fingers go clockwise in an area that is a little painful or hard, stay there and gently massage these spots.

- **If you only have 15 minutes:**
- Continue doing the massage for a little longer
- Try to vary the hand movement:
  - Go left and right.
  - Make your fingers walk all over your stomach
  - Do large circular movements circling towards the left, pressing down when hands are at the left-hand side of your navel and pressing up when coming up on the right-hand side.
- Finish with another glass of water to help eliminate the toxins that have built up inside.

A preferred time of day to do it is first thing in the morning and before going to bed but do it when it's convenient and you are sure to have the time to massage yourself thoroughly. Do it daily to reap incredible results!

2. Have You Ever Tried Digestive Breathing?
This exercise may seem a bit long, but don't let it discourage you, it is quite simple and straightforward.

Step 1: To begin, lie down, preferably on a mat and place your hands on your stomach. As you inhale, expand your tummy letting your hands gently press down into your belly. Breathe out and relax. Repeat 5 times.

Step 2: Place your hands on the floor beside you for support and bring your knees up to your chest. Slowly let your knees drop to your left side, while keeping them comfortably folded high up on your chest. While breathing in this position you are actually doing an internal massage inside the abdomen and producing heat for your digestion. Stay in this position for a count of 5 breaths.

Step 3: Slowly bring your knees back up towards the center and keep your back flat on the ground. Place your hands on the floor beside you for support and let your legs stretch out in front of you, bringing your legs down. As in step one, place hands on your stomach and as you inhale, press your hands gently down into your belly. In this position, you are energizing the spine. Continue for 5 breaths.

Step 4: Next, place your hands on the floor beside you for support and again bring your knees up to your chest. Slowly let your knees drop to your right-hand side. Keep your knees folded comfortably high up on your chest. While breathing in this position you are actually focusing more on your mental energy, coolness and relaxation. Stay in this position for a count of 5 breaths.

Step 5: Bring your legs back to the center. Stretch them out in front of you, back down onto the floor and breathe 5 more times. Slowly get out of the position.

We are not really aware but breathing is part of the digestive process. Taking the time to breathe consciously can help alleviate many common disorders like indigestion or heartburn. So, it's well worth trying!

3. Are You Exercising Enough?

Not exercising? No need to sign up at a gym. Just get up and go for a walk, go have fun with the kids, go for a bike ride, shoot a few hoops…

4. Your body knows how to express itself: Are you attentive to what it is telling you?

When a baby is hungry, in pain, tired, they only have one way of letting you know: they cry! Your body is quite similar to a baby's since it has no other way of letting you know that something isn't right aside from sending out pain signals. Learn to stay alert and attentive to the information your body is delivering. Just like you would with a baby. If your body is crying, stop, assess what is happening and address it quickly.

<u>Being attentive: Example n° 01</u>

Taking the time to observe what you eat and how you feel afterwards will really help you determine which foods work and which ones don't.

A friend of mine suffered for several months from extreme fatigue. She was in her twenties and said that everything, at one point, felt overwhelming. She would come home feeling exhausted and would break down crying and just couldn't seem to understand why she was feeling that way. She consulted several doctors, had blood tests done and for a while, her doctor focused on iron deficiency. But weeks went by, and despite the treatment, she saw no improvement whatsoever. Finally, they tested her for gluten intolerance and the results were clear: she suffered from coeliac disease, which meant she was allergic to gluten. Although it was a little tough and sometimes frustrating to have to switch to a gluten free diet, her energy levels quickly came back to normal and she was back to her old happy self again. She was surprised that she became allergic as an adult in such a sudden way but it does happen. After a few months on her new diet, her energy came back and she was finally able to move forward with her life: I was so happy to learn that she was pregnant and able to lead a happy, healthy pregnancy!

<u>Being attentive: Example n° 02</u>

I exercise a lot and, every once in a while, I feel a little pain in my knee, or my shoulder, neck or back. Usually, for me, that's a signal to back off for a while. What I normally do is switch my training around: I completely cut out the running and replace it with walking and swimming, or I do absolutely nothing for a few days and simply allow my body to rest.

Swimming or taking a break really helps me and it allows parts of my body that are often overextended to get the rest they deserve. I enjoy moving and sports so much, that the idea of getting injured and having to stop for an extended period of time, seems like hell. I always think in terms of the "long run." And so, with this goal in mind, I must address my minor aches and pains regularly to make sure they don't grow and progress into an injury that will, most probably, take months to heal.

<u>Being attentive: Example n° 3</u>

At one point in my life, I experienced difficult nights. I would wake up and find it challenging to fall asleep again and then even more difficult to get up in the morning and tackle a day at work. I was going through problematic times and figured that my sleepless nights had something to do with my situation.

But in fact, it had nothing to do with my sleeping problems.
I decided to quit coffee and wine to clear my body of its toxins and had withdrawal issues because of the caffeine. It took my body almost a week to accept living without the java. As for the wine, it had become a pleasurable moment that allowed me to unwind after work. No withdrawal issues here, although I will admit that I missed that "wine moment" at the end of the day.

Always in self-observation, I had noticed something in the past: when I had a glass of wine, I felt drowsy an hour after the drink: I would have no difficulty falling asleep quickly, but I would usually end up waking up two hours later feeling fully alert. After quitting the glass of wine, I was no longer waking up in the middle of the night. I continued to observe my sleeping pattern and it was clear to me that the wine had something to do with my waking up at night. Believe me, that really helped me stick to living without it and it became clear to me how certain types of foods can directly affect my life and my overall wellbeing.

So, step back and take the time to observe yourself and your habits. Could it be that one of them has a bad effect on another part of your life?

Fatigue can come from a number of different reasons and it's important to address it. Maybe it simply comes from a lack of sleep, but it could also be something more serious. Don't ignore the situation. Take your life into your hands and find out what the problem is. When you wake up in the morning feeling energized and enthusiastic, it makes life so much more enjoyable for yourself and the people around you. If you are getting enough sleep, eating reasonably, as in right amounts and sensibly with a variety of different foods, getting some form of exercise, of at least 30 minutes every day whether walking, running, riding your bike… and undergoing a normal amount of stress, then there is no reason why you should lack energy.
If you are following these guidelines but still feel tired, you really should consult a doctor to help find the source of your problem. However, from my experience, most of the time, simply going to bed earlier, slowing down, meditating and eating properly is all that it takes to get you energized and up and running again.

As I have said before, use a little common sense and be honest with yourself. If your problem needs medical attention, then your doctor will have the proper answers. But you will come to notice that many of your little ailments have something to do with your lifestyle and can be treated by simply twitching a few things here and there or allowing your body to rest and recover.

Change n°30
7 DAYS TO MOVE
IN 7 DIFFERENT WAYS

30.

Exercise, for me, is a passion: I just couldn't live without it. How about you? Do you love working out or do you dread it? I know that for many people exercising is uncomfortable, painful, challenging and the mere fact of thinking about starting an activity can seem like an insurmountable task.

Or, maybe you do workout regularly. If so, what do your workouts look like? Are you like just conveniently repeating the same training session over and over again? Sticking to the same routine is easy: no need to think. You enter a certain comfort zone in which you do your usual workout, shower and go. How's that been working for you, in terms of results? Although routine is comfortable and can actually make you feel good, when it comes to getting results there is an important factor to take into consideration: your body needs to be challenged regularly. I know what you are thinking: it's already hard to get your workout done, if you have to become creative and bring variety, it makes things a lot more complicated. No need to panic. Where fitness is concerned there are thousands of opportunities and ways to bring variety.

And so, as I thought about this, I wondered: what if you changed the way you viewed things and instead of looking at it as only exercise, decide that you are simply going to have more fun? For those of you that exercise regularly, why not, every time you get your workout done, do one thing to make it more fun and challenging?

Read on and discover how, by adding the "fun factor" you will completely change the way you view exercise!

A. Ideas To Make Your Workouts More Challenging And More Fun

Change the reason *why* you exercise. An important step here would be to see exercise and the reason why you exercise with a new set of eyes. Have you always exercised to lose weight? Why not change your viewpoint: train because you want to be a role model for your children, family and friends. Are you training to add muscle mass? Why not focus on specific goals such as succeeding in doing 10 chin ups and 20 double-unders? Probably the most important thing when it comes to staying motivated is to understand that our thirst for variety is in fact a desire to fight boredom and still find the enthusiasm to keep coming back for more. Why not train to be able to share more sporty moments with your kids? Why not train for a contest, to lower your cholesterol level and reach a certain number, to become more flexible and knowledgeable, to improve your posture and self-esteem? Why not change your mindset and see yourself as the sporty type, a healthy parent, a fitness competitor? Be the role model you aspire to become. Become that today.

Sign up for a fitness event and start training for it. Very often, setting a goal for a certain date can be highly motivating.

Try a new activity or vary the activities you partake in. When was the last time you went for a bike ride, jump roped, played frisbee, went to the countryside or nearby woods for a walk, went to the pool to do a few laps, went roller skating or ice skating, horseback riding, snowshoeing, played ping-pong, did a relay or a race, accrobranching, hiking, paddling, scuba diving, played tennis…? The list of activities is endless. Check out my list and decide to do as many new activities as possible and to just have fun.

If you are training at home, turn up the music, it can be a great source of motivation. Create several playlists with all of your favorite motivational songs to ensure you have great music for your next workout.

Watch inspiring movies about sports or that encourage you to develop your potential:
• Spirit of the Marathon
• The Hoosiers
• Rudy
• Step up
• Karate kid
• Rocky
• The way of the peaceful warrior
• Why not watch Ray Mears' Extreme Survival series?

Make your workout shorter, but more intense. Set your mind to doing a 20, 30, 40 or 50 minute workouts and give it your all. Try even doing only twenty minutes, but give it your undivided attention. Learn to be efficient and make good use of your time!

Create your very own training journal - check out Change n°25: *Your Transformational Journal,* for more details about creating one.

Hire a personal trainer - *Change n° 31: "Train Right".* You don't have to find one in fitness. Why not try boxing or outdoor training?

Compete. Sign up for a competition or an event. Were you competitive in high school? Why not sign up at a local club where you could play your favorite sport and rediscover the joys and thrills of competing? Are you into fitness? Why not sign for a fitness contest or masterclass? The goal here is not so much to win but to get your adrenaline going again. Do you think you are too old? Too fat? Too whatever? It's never too late. Do you like tennis? Sign up for a tournament and start practicing and training again. Do you enjoy running? Sign up for a race and challenge yourself to beat a certain time. Do you enjoy yoga? Sign up for a yoga retreat.

You could also check out what event or race is coming up near you and register. Where I live, there is an annual 8 km Christmas race and also a Christmas bath in the sea. You can partake in a half marathon that enables you to cross three different countries, France, Monaco and Italy. We also have a "couple bi-athlon" where you have to do the whole race with a friend.

Monaco is just a bus-ride away from beautiful canyon spots and there are numerous long mountain hikes just minutes away. There is an amazing hike I have always dreamed of doing called the GR20, that crosses the island of Corsica allowing you to cross the island from North to South, offering breathtaking views.

Look around your area to see what your region has to offer. I am sure there are lots of fun activities to do.

Reward yourself. Yes! The day you can jump rope for X number of minutes non-stop, go buy yourself those nice running shoes you've always wanted. The day you can do X number of laps in a row at the pool, you will go and buy yourself some really cool goggles! The day you manage to do 10 perfect pull-ups, get a shot of yourself and frame it. For a big achievement, you could also reward yourself by hiring a photographer for a photo shoot.

Train with a friend. Each session, take turns deciding what activity you are going to do. Make sure you have fun and choose a partner that is a friend and not someone who is overly competitive and will put you down or make you feel like a failure. You are team mates in this and are both there to support each other, laugh and crush it.

If you are not into exercise, find some fun activities that will get you moving and go have a great time!

- I suggest that you speed walk around a mapped-out area where you live and then take your time to walk through it at a leisurely pace
- Clean up the house: turn up the music and dance and sing your way while cleaning
- Garden
- Go for a walk or make your dog happy by taking him out for a walk: chase him, play with him, throw a ball and pretend to race him to retrieve it. Believe me your dog will love it!
- Go roller-skating or ice-skating
- Try orienteering and explore finding your way in the woods
- Go have fun at the beach while swimming, walking in the water or on the beach, playing volleyball
- Play Wii-sport
- Play frisbee
- Play with the kids: hopscotch, jump rope, hula-hoop, racing
- Why not practice doing handstands or somersaults
- Try rope climbing
- Challenge yourself with monkey bars
- Beach volleyball
- Walking on the beach: walk one way on the beach and the way back in the water
- Put on your favorite movie or TV series, one that makes you laugh and exercise at the same time. This way you can get a 20, 30, 60 minute workout done depending on the length of your program. You can easily do this on a treadmill, bike or elliptical trainer. Let the commercials set your intervals: pedal or walk at a steady pace while watching and then increase the intensity and focus during the commercials. Or you could decide to exercise every time there is a commercial: watch your favorite show and every time there is an intermission, go up and down the stairs or walk twice around the house.

- Book a sports holiday where you can engage in multiple of sports activities
- Get a fitness app and start a program. There are many fitness coaches out there, that propose great workouts.
- Get a fitness watch or a pedometer and set daily achievable goals
- Set ahead of time one tiny goal a day for the week to come, such as a certain number of push-ups or sit-ups, to go for a walk, to take only the stairs and so on.

If your goal is to lose weight, research different ways to get your cardio in and your heart pumping: go for a walk, take a flight of stairs, hop scotch twice, run to the next tree, stop at a bench and go up and down 10 times. It's easy and will get your heart pumping. Start by doing short sequences and add more active moments throughout the day. Remember that it all adds up.

At one point, I would train in the morning and then sit down to work with my children all day since they were homeschooled. I realized, however, that my days were intense early in the morning but then mostly inactive the rest of the day. I knew something had to change and I made the extra effort to move more throughout the day. I took the stairs every time since I lived on the 9th floor and added a nice long walk in the evenings. Our bodies are meant to move and not sit all day. Find little things that you can add to your every day to get yourself moving more often.

Try to add a new component to your fitness regimen: balance, core, stretch, strength, power, endurance… If you only do cardio or weights, why not decide to challenge your body differently: You could integrate all 5 elements of fitness: aerobic, strength, stretching, core and balance. Just like you need to balance your plate with different food groups, your exercise regimen needs to be balanced as well. Develop the benefits of each component. For example, for flexibility: over the years our range of motion reduces. Making sure you add elements of flexibility that will enable your body to maintain its natural range of motion. Have a break in your normal routine in which you do your regular training for 3 weeks and the 4th week you do one or several totally different activities. For example, if you go to the gym, why not go swimming or biking for one week out of the month? Or simply walk or do some recreational activities in order to let your body rest.

Change components such as pace, distance, type of exercise, equipment and intensity. Do you always do the same thing when you workout? Change. Add new drills, use your bodyweight to exercise such as doing push-ups/pull-ups/lunges. Use weights, machines, elastics, bands, ropes, balance balls, BOSU, weighted balls and kettle bells.

If you usually do a 30 minute jog in the park, find a hill and run up and down 10 times and then do a 10 minute light jog. Or you could try sprinting 10 times. Spice up your workouts and see how you can make them more fun and put an end to routine. Train according to temperament. Do you like to be in the company of others or do you prefer flying solo? Think about it and find activities that match your personality. If you are a social type of person then why not do activities that get you out of your home, that allow you to be around other people with whom you can talk and share an experience. Why not try Zumba or dance based classes, for example, or team/group-based sports, like volleyball or basketball? Are you more of a solitary type? Then why not look into cardio machines, yoga, walk/jog, tai-chi, one on one training, circuit weight training or hot yoga? Do you need to be pushed and challenged? Try H.I.I.T. training, spinning classes, boot camps, or parkour.

Take some time to see what really suits you. Maybe you are part of those who always say: "Exercise is not for me." But what if you simply hadn't found the kind that suits *YOU*?

Have a sports buddy. Trying to engage in new activities will enable you to build relationships. Fitness or sport relationships are fulfilling but in a different way compared to normal friends. When you train together, compete with others or form a team, there is a special connection that is created. A whole lot of emotions are experienced such as joy, frustration, anger, or empowerment to name a few. When you share them with others, it creates a special bond between you.

Try High-intensity interval training (H.I.I.T.): it's a workout that alternates between intense bursts of activity and fixed periods of less-intense activity or even complete rest. For example, a good starter workout is running as fast as you can for 1 minute and then walking for 2 minutes. **Tabata Training** is one of the most popular forms of high-intensity interval training (HIIT). It consists of eight rounds of ultra-high-intensity exercises in a specific 20-seconds-on, 10-seconds-off interval.

B. Take Up The 7 Day Activity Challenge: 7 Different Ways to Move in 7 Days

The goal here is to select and engage in a different activity each day. Below you will find a whole list of great options. Each day tick a box and write the date next to it.

You might ask: shouldn't I be taking a day off? Now that's a pertinent remark. I agree that you do need to take a break, but only from intense training. You don't want to be exercising full on, 7 days in a row. For this reason, you will also find a whole list of recreational and fun activities that you can safely enjoy, even if it is your rest day.

Please note that although bringing more variety into your exercise regimen is most definitely associated with having more fun, I must warn you that there is such a thing as too much variety. If you are trying to master a certain discipline, your body needs time to adapt. Bringing too much change won't give your muscles enough time to adapt and this would defeat the purpose. Indeed, how do we progress? Through repetition. If we always do something different or new, we cannot progress and improve. So, variety is good but only to a certain extent. In this change, my aim is to accentuate the importance of enjoying the activities in which you engage in: to bring more fun, laughter and joy. Many people tend to think that the only way to exercise is to get on that treadmill and walk/run for 40 minutes, or workout vigorously at the gym. I wish to pinpoint the importance of enjoying what we do. We also tend to think that certain activities, such as playing frisbee or walking the dog, don't count as exercise. But anything that gets you off that couch is exercise and the mere fact of adding a bit of fun and laughter to your exercise regimen can go a long way. It will help you stick to being more active. So, get up, grab that racket, your roller skates, flippers and goggles and go have some fun!

7 Different Ways to MOVE in 7 DAYS

Today, I...

1

2

Today, I...

Today, I...

3

4

Today, I...

Today, I...

5

6

Today, I ...

Today, I...

7

Alphabetical LIST of ACTIVITIES

WORK SPACE

- ☐ Acro branching
- ☐ Archery
- ☐ Aqua aerobics
- ☐ Aqua biking
- ☐ Aikido
- ☐ All-terrain vehicle racing
- ☐ Baseball
- ☐ Boxing
- ☐ Badminton
- ☐ Beach volleyball
- ☐ Baton twirling
- ☐ Biathlon
- ☐ BMX
- ☐ Bodybuilding
- ☐ Basque pelote
- ☐ Catch
- ☐ Cheerleading
- ☐ Cricket
- ☐ Climbing
- ☐ Canyoning
- ☐ Cross country skiing
- ☐ Cycling
- ☐ Capoeira
- ☐ Curling
- ☐ Canoeing
- ☐ Crossfit
- ☐ Diving
- ☐ Dog walking
- ☐ Dancing
- ☐ Elliptical
- ☐ Fishing
- ☐ Frisbee
- ☐ Fencing
- ☐ Figure skating
- ☐ 5 K
- ☐ Football
- ☐ Gymnastics
- ☐ Gliding
- ☐ Golf
- ☐ Hiking
- ☐ HIIT training
- ☐ Hockey
- ☐ Horseback riding
- ☐ Hula hoop
- ☐ Handball
- ☐ Half marathon
- ☐ Hurdles
- ☐ Hurling
- ☐ Hopscotch
- ☐ Ice skating

- ☐ Interval training
- ☐ Jumping jacks
- ☐ Jogging
- ☐ Juggling
- ☐ Judo
- ☐ Jump roping
- ☐ Kayaking
- ☐ Kite surf
- ☐ Karate
- ☐ Kickboxing
- ☐ Kart racing
- ☐ Longboarding
- ☐ Laser tag
- ☐ Lacrosse
- ☐ Lumberjack
- ☐ Logrolling
- ☐ Meditating
- ☐ Mini-golf
- ☐ Mountaineering
- ☐ Mud race
- ☐ Marathon
- ☐ Motocross
- ☐ Netball
- ☐ Orientation walks
- ☐ Orienteering
- ☐ Olympic weightlifting
- ☐ Pilates
- ☐ Parachuting
- ☐ Paragliding
- ☐ Ping-pong
- ☐ Padel
- ☐ Polo
- ☐ Pole climbing
- ☐ Pole dancing
- ☐ Paintball
- ☐ Pool (snooker)
- ☐ Parkour
- ☐ Pétanque
- ☐ Powerlifting
- ☐ Rafting
- ☐ Roller skating
- ☐ Running
- ☐ Rock climbing
- ☐ Rope climbing
- ☐ Rope jumping
- ☐ Racketball Rodeo
- ☐ Rugby
- ☐ Rhythmic gymnastics
- ☐ Relay race
- ☐ Surfing

- ☐ Skiing
- ☐ Swimming
- ☐ Skydiving
- ☐ Wingsuit flying
- ☐ Softball
- ☐ Skateboard
- ☐ Snowboard
- ☐ Spinning
- ☐ Sambo
- ☐ Snooker
- ☐ Sprinting
- ☐ Squash
- ☐ Sailing
- ☐ Sled
- ☐ Shooting
- ☐ Stairs
- ☐ Street workout
- ☐ Synchronized swimming
- ☐ Scuba diving
- ☐ Snorkeling
- ☐ Sports car racing
- ☐ Snowmobile racing
- ☐ Sex
- ☐ Trampoline
- ☐ Table tennis
- ☐ Triathlon
- ☐ Tag
- ☐ Tennis
- ☐ Tennis against a wall
- ☐ 10 k
- ☐ Toboggan
- ☐ Trapeze
- ☐ Trail running
- ☐ Trial
- ☐ Tree felling
- ☐ Unicycling
- ☐ Underwater target shooting
- ☐ Windsurfing
- ☐ Wakesurfing
- ☐ Wrestling
- ☐ Water polo
- ☐ Walking
- ☐ Walking in water
- ☐ Weightlifting
- ☐ Woodsman
- ☐ Yoga
- ☐ Yoga Mudra
- ☐ Zumba
- ☐ Other_____

Change n°31
TRAIN RIGHT

31.

So, this is it! You have decided that this week you are going to start leading a healthy and fit lifestyle. But where do you start? What do you do? The problem is that these two simple questions are often a source of discouragement, and the reason why so many of you have abandoned this project in the past. So, why not put all chances on your side and decide to hire a trainer: let them handle the "how", "how much", "where" and "what". The only two questions you will first need to tackle are "when do we schedule" and "why we are doing this?". It's so much easier to start things off when you have a shoulder to rely on and someone to lead the way.

I would like to take the opportunity to make one thing clear: Your trainer cannot do the work *for* you. They can be supportive and encouraging, but most of the work has to come from you. Your trainer will indeed give you a great workout but once you push past those gym doors, you must leave your excuses outside and be committed to participating 100% physically and mentally. While you are working out with your trainer make a point of learning everything there is to learn. Ask questions, do your best to train correctly, get all the feedback you can get, buy books about fitness and healthy eating and discuss what you learned with your trainer. All the while, keep in mind one important thing: Your ultimate goal is to be able to work out on your own without the assistance of a trainer. So, make sure to make the most of every single session!

Of course, money is an issue here because trainers can put a big hole in your budget. But isn't it time you started taking care of yourself? Aren't you worth the investment? We are talking about your health here, your self-worth and well-being. The way I see it, nothing else is more important. So, grab your running shoes now and like 8 other million Americans, book a session with a trainer and let today be the first day on your path to a healthier and fitter YOU!

A. Why Hire A Personal Trainer?
If you are still not convinced about the difference a trainer can make in your life, then read on and see why it's worth investing in one.

a. Learn proper form and technique. Probably the most important reason to hire a trainer is that they are knowledgeable and will teach you proper form and technique. Good personal trainers know their stuff. How many times do I see people not exercising properly at the gym: lifting too heavy, not executing the movement correctly, not doing the exercise with proper form or posture, not focusing enough on what they are doing or not breathing properly. Hiring a trainer is the surest way of getting things right. This is especially true at the beginning. Make sure you get off to a good start and after a while it will become second nature. Not only will you learn how to do it right, but you will also train to see results.

b. A clear plan of action: not sure exactly where to start or what to do? Your PT will have things written down for you on paper and will give you a clear plan of action: they will get your started with an assessment to have a baseline, and will give you a detailed workout.

c. Tailored training. This is one of the reasons why you really need to hire a trainer. Your PT will tailor an exercise program according to your specific needs. We are all built differently and want different things. Your trainer will take you along the right path to reach these specific goals.

d. They'll push you a little harder. This component is more important than you think. Most of the time when people workout they tend to quit as soon as it gets a little uncomfortable. Your trainer knows when you can do more or will encourage you to push past your comfort zone. By training this way you will reap greater results. If you are looking for muscle definition and visible results, this is the way you want to go. Some of you want to lose or gain weight while others want to add some muscle mass, or maybe succeed in doing 10 chin ups. A good trainer will lead your way to success.

e. Lower your risk of getting in jured. This is a good point. Your PT will help lower your risk of getting injured. We often throw ourselves into a fitness program without considering several important components such as how many reps, how long should you train, how many times a week? Let your trainer break it down for you and guide you when it's time to rest and avoid chances of getting injured.

f. A source of motivation. If you find a good trainer, they will find the words to get you going and coming back for more. With time, you will get to know each other, and they will know how to push and encourage you.

g. YOU will be the center of attention: when was the last time you had someone's entire attention, taking care of only you? You deserve it!

h. Workout variety and creativity. Your trainer will bring variety and creativity into your workouts. Often when we are on our own, we tend to always do the same thing over and over again. If you want to improve/grow, you need to stimulate your muscles in a number of different ways. It's important to get your body wondering what you are going to do next. Variety and creativity are also important for you mentally: doing something different can be challenging, but also fun. What better way to keep you motivated and coming back for more when you are enjoying yourself.

i. No results? Are you in a rut? Have you been training for years but are not really getting the results you are looking for? A trainer might be just what you need: They will know how to boost your motivation, how to challenge you to push past your comfort zone and show you the path to reach visible results.

j. Hire a trainer to learn a new sport or form of exercise. Have you always wanted to try boxing, biking, swimming but didn't know how? Find a coach that will teach you how.

k. Keep track of your progression: often enough, we train randomly but without a clear plan of action or tracking any progress whatsoever. Your trainer will note your progression and keep you informed regularly about your success. This alone is a great source of motivation.

l. Your trainer will challenge you. While some of you are in for more strenuous training, others may not be. Nevertheless, it is important that you feel challenged. Your trainer will do just that for you. You will be trying new exercises, climbing and jumping. Slowly, slowly you will see yourself succeeding in doing things you never thought possible.

m. Your medical concerns. Do you have an injury or a specific medical problem? You might want to have a trainer by your side to make sure you are training according to your condition. A good trainer will know what exercise can help lower your cholesterol, lower your body fat or what to do when injured, so you can still workout while allowing that specific body part to recover.

n. Prepare for an event. If you are planning a race, a sport or a personal event, such as a high school reunion, your PT can help you get ready and in top form for D Day. Take the stress out of the preparation and let your PT shoulder you and lead the way.

o. It will be educational. Yes, I love learning and I know I keep encouraging you to learn and study. Many people believe that exercise, such as lifting weights, is something superficial and that trainers know only how to flex their muscles. But exercise is a science and a good trainer should go through each exercise, analyze it and explain what muscles are involved and how to use them properly. You will learn the vocabulary linked to training such as eccentric/concentric, pushing past muscle failure, plyometric as well as how to increase or decrease the difficulty of an exercise, and a lot more.

p. They'll help you set realistic goals. Sometimes we have this image in mind that we wish to achieve. A good trainer should be able to help you choose a realistic goal, so you won't be disappointed or frustrated in the future. Maybe they will help you break down your goal into smaller more achievable ones. For this reason, it is important to choose a good trainer and not one that will sell you a bunch of unrealistic dreams.

q. You will be accountable. Once the appointment is set, you are accountable. Your trainer will require that you do certain things like eat less of a certain type of food, walk more and so on. Every time you see them, an update on what you have done since your last session will be expected. It can be an additional source of motivation to stick to your goal.

r. Take a break from your problems. A session will be a full-on session. Your 30 minutes or one hour session will be a 200% session where you will have to give your all. If you train this way regularly, you learn to exercise with an empty mind and it's nice to focus on something else than your problems.

s. You will work all important components of fitness. Stretch, muscles, cardio, balance, relax and rest.

t. A trainer can be a good listener. Many times, when someone has weight issues it is often linked to an emotional problem that has been bottled up inside. Training and having a friendly ear can help you free these emotions and work past them.

u. You will have a good spotter. Depending on what type of training you are doing, you might need a spotter. Whether you realize it or not, there are good and bad spotters. A good one has to assist you just the right amount. Too much will take out the benefits of the exercise and too little could make the exercise too challenging. Normally a good trainer will know exactly how much assistance you need. Have you always wanted to succeed in doing chin ups? Well hiring a PT who will spot you, might just be the solution you were looking for.

v. You will feel inspired. Normally a good PT should be a role model when it comes to exercise and diet. Working out alongside someone who is fit and healthy can be a real source of inspiration: you would like to become more like them. You could see that it is possible to be fit, eat healthy and be happy. Many people tend to be convinced that leading a healthy lifestyle is boring. Working out alongside someone who leads a healthy lifestyle can really change the idea you have about cutting out junk food, going to bed earlier, instead of partying, and exercising instead of watching TV. Your trainer can truly become a role model of healthy lifestyle.

w. Help with finding solutions: what's your excuse for not exercising? Family, work, obligations, no social support? Already tried in the past, but was unsuccessful? Too tired or lack of energy and motivation? Health issues that leave you uncertain about where to start or make you feel uncomfortable working out with others? Too self-conscious? Your trainer will know what to do, put all the excuses aside, and keep you busy.

B. How to choose a good Personal Trainer: my 10 prerequisites!

N° 01: Credentials. The very first thing to take into consideration is the trainer's credentials: ask for fitness certifications. Look out for trainers with accreditations in the US or in the country you live in. In the US, look for C.S.C.S., ACSM, NASM, ACE. Look online on their website as most are registered based on area code. In France, trainers are required to have passed the "Brevet d'Etat".

N° 02: Price. Prices can range between 20 and 70 dollars an hour but can reach up to 120 to 150 USD/Hour. How much can you afford? How much are you willing to invest? How many sessions do you wish to take? Consider the following: maybe one session a week with an excellent trainer is more worthwhile than two with another. Or on the contrary, two or three cheaper sessions are what you need to make sure your workouts are done.

Note: some trainers have online videos for off days that offer the possibility to add in extra workouts for free. It might be something to look into. If one on one training is too expensive, maybe you can cut the cost by bringing a friend along or proposing a shared session with one of the trainer's clients.

N° 03: Word of mouth. If friends or others are "hooked", getting noticeable results, enthusiastic about training with them and keep on asking for more, chances are the trainer is a good one. Always keep in mind, the aspect of personality compatibility. Indeed, not every trainer is a perfect fit for you. Ask for a trial session to see if you click. Another good idea is to look out for trainers at your gym. Keep your eyes open to see how they train, and their attitude. An idea might be to ask your doctor, physiotherapist or other medical professional if they can recommend a good trainer for your needs.

N°04: They are close by. You absolutely need to take travel time into consideration. If the trainer you have hired comes to your own home, this is not an issue. However, if you are required to drive to a certain location, you must take into consideration the conveniences: is it close by? You don't want to add costs for gas, parking, and highway, or stress while searching for a parking spot, or battling traffic.

N° 05: They are available. Will it be challenging to book a session? You already have a busy schedule and can't accommodate others. Ask straight out about their availability, the cancellation policies and how many days in advance you have to book your session.

N°06: Your Trainer's specialty. What does your trainer specialize in? Many trainers have a specialty, such as boxing, yoga, relaxation, posture, weight loss, diet and nutrition. Find one that offers what you are looking for. Before signing up, keep in mind the activities you enjoy and those you don't.
Note: Also keep in mind... some of you just don't like training. Maybe what you are really looking for is a dietitian, a weight loss clinic or a specialist that can create you a personalized weight loss plan. With time, once you have lost a little bit of weight, you will feel like adding a bit of exercise.

N° 07: Mentality and Compatibility. Unfortunately, you will most likely know about this after the first session. You don't want your trainer repeating what you have said or hear them badmouthing another customer, nor do you want to hear condescending or racist comments. You are not paying them to know what they think, you are there to train. Remember, you have a right to speak up if something is wrong or bothering you. You are the one paying so in right to demand optimal service.
There are many different types of trainers out there: some are tough and that might be exactly what you are looking for, or maybe not. Are you looking for a Seals type of training? Get that type of coach. Do you want to reduce your cholesterol? Find a trainer that knows the problem and has already helped numerous patients through exercise and sound diet advice.
A special note: please respect your trainer! Although you have hired them and are paying, they deserve your respect. A friend of mine, who is a coach in Monte-Carlo, told me that one of his customers whistled him to come to him like a dog, in front of other people. My friend was offended and felt humiliated. But he addressed it intelligently. Throughout the session he processed how to go about it in his mind and before leaving, he politely told the customer that the gesture had offended him. The customer, who had done it a little bit jokingly, was quick with sincere apology and never did it again.

N° 08: Your Communication. Before going to meet a trainer, set a short list of issues you wish to address. As a rule, never sign up for multiple sessions straight out, even if the cost is worthwhile. I recommend trying out at least three sessions before signing any long-term commitment offers.

Once you signed up, take the time to ask questions. What is their attitude like? Are they interested in what you have to say? Do they answer your questions? Are they attentive, listening? Or are they distracted and constantly interrupting you, acting like a know it all? This is something to take into consideration. You want someone who is interested in YOU. You are the one paying for the session. Do you have health issues? Talk about them now and see whether they can and know how to address them. One trainer might be more suited for a certain type of training. If they are a good trainer, they will be honest and maybe give you the contact details of another trainer that can really help you.

Also make sure that your PT clearly understands your goal or that you have both decided upon a clearly measurable one to achieve it. Leaving your first encounter with a goal clearly set, demonstrates that your PT has listened and you know where you are going and what steps are required to get there.

Note: If you have been training for a while with a specific coach and things are not going well, show some respect and face the situation. Many customers stop calling or stop coming. Even though it is uncomfortable, set things straight. Tell the trainer you are:

- *Sorry*
- *Things are not working out*
- *You are less motivated*
- *You are not getting results*

Be polite and graceful. It will be unpleasant for a few minutes, but your mind will be relieved in knowing you did the right thing.

N° 09: Is he insured and C.P.R Certified? No exceptions here. Just make sure your trainer is covered and insured. As for C.P.R., most Personal Training diplomas require that you take a C.P.R. course which prepares PTs in case their clients get injured. He can then assist you and give proper advice if such a situation arises.

N°10: Do they practice what they preach? I am not saying that you have to look like a top model athlete to be a good trainer, but it does make sense that your coach should look fit and healthy. I have been through ups and downs with moments of deviation in my life but have constantly made fitness and healthy eating a priority and have always come back on the right path. Just like the suggestions and guidance I am sharing with you in this book: I don't just write or jot ideas down on paper, I have tried them and learned to apply them in my daily life before proposing them to you here on these pages. There has to be consistency in what the person is proposing and what they actually do or it will make outsiders skeptical.

C. Meeting a Personal Trainer the first time

Make sure you discuss the following with your PT before hiring them:
- How much: is the cost per session. Are there packages, can you bring a friend to cut costs?
- What is the number of sessions the PT thinks are necessary to achieve your goal?
- Availability. Does the trainer have readily available time slots? How many days prior must you book your session?
- Cancellation and refund policies: what happens if you have to cancel? Under what circumstances can you get a refund?
- Length of each session: how long is a session? Can you schedule for 30 minutes? Remember in 30 minutes you can get a good workout so it might be worth looking into. If your budget is limited, it might be a good solution to come early and do some cardio, proceed with the 30 minutes trainer session and finish off with some stretching. It's a good way to cut the costs and still get an awesome session. You could also do some switching around. For example, take 3 half hour sessions per week: first half hour, have your trainer work with you on the cardio, while getting tips, advice, recommendations and motivation, continue to do the weights and stretch alone. Next half hour session, first do the cardio alone, then weights with the PT, and end by stretching on your own. And finally, for your last session, begin with the cardio, continue with the weights and conclude with a good stretching session with your PT.
- Discuss with the PT what is required from you outside your training sessions Do they expect you to train sometimes on your own and if so, what should you practice?
- What is your PT's experience or special area of expertise?

D. Training at the gym or at home?

a. At home:
- If you are a little self-conscious, training at your home can eliminate the one issue that's keeping you away from exercise.
- When training at home, your trainer gets to see your environment. It might be a good idea to program a kitchen session where you both go through the kitchen cabinets to see what needs to be chucked away or maybe replaced with another ingredient.
- You can divide your workout into half the time indoors and the other half outdoors.
- You will have the equipment and knowledge to exercise on your own at home on days when your trainer doesn't come.
- You can save money, travel and preparation time plus the cost of the club.
- You don't have a good gym close by? No more excuses: anytime is a good time to train. Remember, your home is open at all hours. Although it may need some getting used to, eventually it will become really convenient to train in your own home.
- You will be able to concentrate totally on what you are doing, be more focused. No one is there to judge you and there is nothing to distract you either.
- You can put the music you like as loud as you wish.
- You can adjust the room temperature to your liking.
- If you want to do circuit training, you won't find someone else on the piece of equipment you need.

- You can wear whatever you want, to see your muscles work or to be comfortable. No need to wear long hot leggings. Wear shorts and let your legs breathe. You could even, if you are up to it, train in your bathing suit and get to really know your body.
- If you wish to buy some equipment, all you really need are a mat, a ball, a few dumbbells and elastics and you're all set. There are a lot of natural pieces of "equipment" out there ready to be used such as stairs to climb or do push-ups on, a bench for step-ups, or a chair for dips.
- You lack motivation to get off the couch? The PT will come to your doorstep. No more excuses.
- You and a friend of yours have toddlers or babies? Book a one-hour session at nap time and cut the costs of having a baby sitter. Pay only half the session since your friend is training as well or else why not take 30 minutes each.

b. At the gym:
If working out at home is impossible, then let's have a look at the advantage of training at the gym:
- It offers the possibility for added variety and this is an important factor.
- Men lift heavier weights and might do exercises that require specific equipment, such as using a variety of different heavy dumbbells or a chin-up bar. Although it is possible to buy these, it will inevitably require higher costs as well as more storage space at home.
- Sometimes it is important to leave your home environment when training. This is especially the case for stay at home moms.
- You don't want your kids or spouse there to interrupt your session.
- You can book a session during lunch hour and be free in the evenings. Make sure you bring a little snack along at work to eat around 11 am so you are not famished during your session.
- Working out while surrounded with others can be a real source of motivation. You might even end up finding a training partner which could give you the added boost you need.

No excuses. Years ago, I had a job that only had one-hour lunch breaks. That didn't stop me from going to the gym. I was lucky enough to have a gym very close by and would walk over, do an intense 40-minute workout, shower, and walk back with lunch in hand. As I said, no excuses. 40 minutes is better than nothing. The way I see it, even 20 or 30 minutes are better than nothing. Go work out!

E. If you really can't afford a Personal Trainer, what are your options?
What if, even with your best efforts, you really you can't afford to hire a trainer? You didn't think I would let you down, did you?
If you have read the part where I explain why it's important to hire a trainer, I will show you below ways to override these reasons and still get the needed boost to train and reach the goals you wish to attain.

WHY HIRE A TRAINER?	SOLUTIONS IF YOU CAN'T HIRE ONE
They will motivate you	Train with a reliable friend
You will be accountable	If you train with a friend, learn to be both accountable to one another. Each of you should send messages to one another other every day including photos of weight progress, meals and detailed training. Photos are great because they show portion sizes and are proof of how much you weigh. It's important that both of you be honest and say when you are not doing ok, are eating too much or skipping training sessions. It's ok to deviate but your friend will help you get back on track.
Tailored training	You don't know what to do exactly? Don't let that stop you. Just get out and do something. **See the world as your gym**: take the stairs, shoot hoops, go for a walk, go for a swim, play hula hoop or jump rope with your child You see a bench, step up and down 10 times. There is an elevator, race your kids by taking the stairs. You have 5 minutes: do 10 jumping jacks, 10 easy pushups, 10 Squats, 10 abdominal reps. Repeat 2 or three times depending on level of fitness.
Learn proper form and technique	First of all, keep things simple. The simpler the better. My advice is often to use movements that you would in ordinary life. If something feels awkward, don't do it. A good idea is to choose 3 or 4 exercises:1 for the upper body, 2 for the lower body, 1 for the abs and core region for your next session. Repeat the whole sequence 2, 3 or 4 times. To make sure you are doing them properly, look online and watch videos to see how to do them with proper form and technique, read a book or magazine that goes through the different steps. Check the reference section of the book for ideas.

They will challenge you	Why not challenge yourself. Sign up for a race, a photoshoot with a friend, a sports event.
Medical concerns	Ask your doctor what is best for you or what to avoid and follow their instructions.
Educational	With internet, the opportunities you have today, are endless. Check out the reference section of the book for ideas.
Set Realistic Goals	Sit down with a true friend and try to set goals together. If you are trying to lose weight, try to remember the weight you were able to maintain in the past for over a year: this probably is your ideal weight. I am not saying you cannot go below this point, but it's already a landmark giving you a realistic weight you can set as a goal. If, on the contrary, you are trying to bulk up, remember to check your diet as it is an important component. There is no limit to bulking up.
Take a break from your problems	Program a getaway session every week that allows you to breathe. Go for a long walk at the beach, a hike in the mountains or go dancing. Do more things that make you happy.
A good listener	Program a one hour walk with a friend where you each get a ½ hour to blabber about your problems.
A good spotter	Use props, elastics Learn to ask for help at the gym Train with a friend. A piece of advice for your friend: she should help you just enough so that you feel challenged but still manage to do at least 6 to 8 repetitions.
Get inspired	Why not become a source of inspiration for others: a friend, your spouse, your children, your colleagues? Decide to become a role model and start setting an example.

You also have other options that might cost a lot less. Have you ever considered:

Online training programs? It's very reasonably priced. You can do it when it suits you. There is a big variety of different workouts and trainers out there and there are over 65 million videos online.

Workout Apps? Most fitness stars offer programs and apps to download. It can be very motivating to workout with someone you admire. There are also apps that offer a lot of different workouts according to your tastes and goals. Many offer how-to videos and the possibility to track your progression.

Swapping trades? I had always wanted to get boxing lessons. I knew this personal trainer that proposed boxing training sessions and was really tempted, but really couldn't afford it. To my surprise one day, he came up to me and asked me if I could give him some English lessons. I immediately proposed to swap trades: 1hour of English in exchange for one hour of boxing. It was a win-win situation. See if there is a way you can swap trades: tennis lesson for a computer course, or a swimming lesson for a dance lesson.

On-Demand Class Streaming? Today you literally have the possibility to find any class you want and do it in your own home. What do you feel like doing: Zumba? Core training? An abdominal session? You name it and you can surely find it. No more wasting time in traffic. No need to be at the gym at a certain time. You can have your very own personal instructor in your own home at any time of day or night for an affordable rate.

Get the proper training to become a trainer? Nothing can beat self-service!
If you are passionate about fitness or leading a healthy lifestyle, why not study to become a personal trainer, or a health and lifestyle coach? Learn your way into fitness. You don't have to be super fit to study fitness. Start reading books about health and nutrition and why not search around for a high-quality course and exam you can attend. It will be cheaper than hiring a coach and that way you can train anytime anywhere: you'll know exactly what to do!

Conclusion
There is no doubt that hiring a trainer is an investment but remember it's only temporary. Very soon you will be flying on your own. You can ease off progressively by taking one session every two weeks and then move on to once a month. That way you are still accountable and if you get a little demotivated, that training session might be just what you need to get back on track. Start things off right and learn to train correctly to build a good foundation. Progressively you will feel capable to move forward on your own. This is your life and health we are talking about, remember… you are worth it!

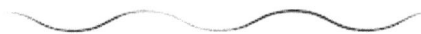

Change n°32
SELF~SUPPORT

32.

One of the biggest lessons in my life has been the importance of learning to love myself. It's probably, when I think of it, the most important lesson of all. Most of our problems come down to these two points: first, we don't accept ourselves the way we are, and second, we would like others to be more like us or do things the way we like them done. Kind of nonsense when you really think of it. Why on Earth would we want people to be like us, if we don't like the way we are in the first place? Well that reflection gave me a good laugh!

As I already mentioned previously, as a child I was often on my own for long hours at a time. I got used to being alone and learned to appreciate these moments and actually longed for them. I truly believe, however, that Mankind was meant to live in the company of others. Indeed, while interacting we learn, we dialog and exchange ideas which allows us to grow. Other people do things differently, which makes us question ourselves whether what we do or think is right or wrong. We observe others - how they react in different situations - but then, we also observe ourselves - how *we* react. Indeed, we have an intrinsic need to exchange, and for this reason, being often alone, I got in the habit of dialoguing with myself. I would take the time to ask myself many questions, I would observe my attitudes in life and sometimes I would even get mad at myself, feel ashamed or on the contrary, feel quite proud. I also learned to be there for myself: to pat my shoulder when I was feeling down and to tell myself reassuring words when I felt like crying.

In fact, I had learnt to become friends with myself, and one of the best things about having a friend is that you are allowed to be yourself. Indeed, there was no need to pretend being someone else. I could pinpoint my flaws: I knew when I was wrong and when I had over-reacted. This honesty I developed within myself helped me grow and become more humble.

There was a problem however and it lay in the fact that all the feedback came from myself as I only rarely got the opportunity to interact with other people. And so, when the day came for me to get back into the ring of life and confront others for real, I found it very difficult to get past Round 1: believe me, I got knocked out many times. I am using a boxing metaphor, because that's what it really felt like for me: a battle. Every time I stepped out my front door it was as though I had two worlds to confront: the outside one with all the people and its situations, but also my inner one, with the thousands of questions that dwelled in my mind. "What should I say?" "What was the best way to react?" "What would I have to do?" For many years I struggled: it was really hard and at times felt like utter torture.

With time, however, I learnt to accept the awkwardness of being with others. I also learnt to be really grateful for being there for my own self. When life was tough, I knew I had somewhere to go to and that there would always be someone there for me. When I was going through divorce and cancer, that little voice inside me was always there to tell me to hang in there. I truly realized as I traversed this difficult period of my life, how lucky I was to have lived my childhood years the way I had: it had enabled me to spend a lot of time connecting with myself and getting to know who I really was. Because let's face it, when times get rough, even if you have family and friends, if you are struggling with a situation, all in all, you are on your own. And that's when you realize that, that person inside of you, is truly your best friend.

Did you ever sit down and wonder why you enjoy the company of your best friend? What are your friend's qualities? What is it that they do that makes you feel like seeing them again? Below, you will find the main qualities of a true friend. I will further explore the importance of each and every one of them, and how you can be more this way yourself to become your very best friend.

A true friend is:
- honest
- a good listener
- not too judgmental
- expresses empathy
- kind
- encouraging
- protective
- respectful
- knows how to keep a secret
- fun to be around and you enjoy simply sitting around with

So how can you become your very best friend?
To become your best friend, you simply need to make sure you have these qualities and act towards yourself more as a friend would.

A. Honesty
A person who is honest will speak without pretense and be frank enough to tell you things the way they are. It's a person who is trustworthy.

For some, a relationship is based on good looks and pretty lies, namely being told what they want to hear. But a strong relationship is based on honesty and sincerity. It's so important to know that you have a special someone who cares enough to speak the truth because they sincerely want what's best for you.

a. Your friend is honest
You love your friend because they love you enough to set you on the right track. It might sometimes get you upset, but deep down inside you know they mean well and tell you certain things because they care.

b. Being honest with yourself

To become your very own best friend will require you stop lying to yourself and start being totally honest about your feelings, your actions and your thoughts. I mean, nobody is going to hear you, so what have you got to lose anyway? So, go right on ahead and admit you were jealous, angry, hurt, envious and then try to understand why. Take the time to talk to yourself just like a friend would and learn to put things back into perspective.

Example:

You have a colleague who really annoys you at work. You keep telling yourself it's because they are the problem, but let's be honest here. Could it be that this colleague has a great personality or is better than you at work or is physically more appealing? Why not take a minute to think about that. Try to admit it to yourself: I am jealous because they have a great personality, are more efficient than me at work or have a better physique than I do. Hey! Let's face it: there will always be someone better than you, but that's no reason to spend your whole life feeling miserable about it or making this person pay for it. Take a minute to accept the fact that someone is better in certain ways. I would even suggest, at one point, to be totally honest and to compliment them for this quality to "get it off your chest". Chances are, they might even open doors and you could learn to enjoy their company after all. It might be worthwhile to observe them to see what makes them "better," according to your standards. Are they more professional, a better listener, more positive and outgoing? Learn from your "opponents" and start asking yourself what you can do to improve yourself as well. You could also make a list of your talents and strengths and take a bit of time to sit down with yourself for a visualization session in which you see yourself feeling more confident.

You could do all this, or…. you could go back to work and not change a thing: continue feeling jealous, go on criticizing your colleague, totally denying the truth while still feeling miserable. It's up to you to decide.

Over time, honesty about how you feel will help you open doors, not only towards others but also the inner doors that you carry within.

My son, Diego, has books to read for school and since reading is not his "thing" we often enjoy reading them together. The last one was *The Giver* by Lois Lowry. In this story, the main character, when confronted with an emotion, was obliged to express it and would spend a certain amount of time to figure out the "right word" that expressed exactly how he felt. Is it lust, is it fear, is it jealousy…? Take a step back and find *the* word that fits exactly what you are experiencing right now and acknowledge it totally. Open doors to honesty and you will be one step closer to becoming your best friend ever.

B. A Good Listener

A good listener, according to the Cambridge dictionary, is "someone who gives you a lot of attention when you are talking about your problems or things that worry you and tries to understand and support you."

a. Your best friend is a good listener

Let's face it, it's nice to have someone on a daily basis to talk to about our ups and downs, things that happened to us, whether funny or sad. It's someone we enjoy and may even need to share things with.

You know when something happens to you and you get that urge: "I just have to call up or text "so and so" to tell them." Both of you share a good laugh or you feel some kind of relief from the fact that you were able to get a load off your chest and it feels nice to have a reassuring voice that confirms you were right to react that way, or to the contrary, that you are all wrong and should put things back into perspective.

b. Take some time to listen to yourself

In our busy world, we seldom have time to be alone with ourselves. However, aloneness is essential. You make time for your family, your work, getting the groceries, but you also need to find some time to be with yourself, in order to get to know who you are, what is troubling you and what you really want. To succeed, it is essential to slow down, observe your reactions, your thoughts and attitudes and learn to be objective in your analysis.

Take the time to see what is troubling you, then find a solution in order to give some sound advice. This is the second step to become your best friend ever.

C. Non-judgment and expressing empathy

Being non-judgmental is to find yourself in or observe a certain situation without judging others. It goes a bit with empathy since you need the capacity to put yourself in other people's shoes and be understanding. Every single situation could evoke a thousand different reactions. Think about it. Why should others react the way you do? The same holds true the other way around. Other people don't know what you have been through, they haven't lived your life. What you are doing now and the way you are handling it, belongs to you and holds to a million different factors that others have no clue about whatsoever. If you have a friend she has probably been around for a while and she probably knows your ups and downs and just how much you can handle.

Your child is having a tantrum at the supermarket. People around you see the tantrum and you can just feel the weight of their judgment. But do they know that you spent the day at your mother's place because she was ill? Do they know that on your way back home you realized there was no more milk for the kids and that you urgently had to stop to pick some up? Do they know that your child wasn't able to get a good nap because you woke her up when you reached the grocery store? People often are quick at judging and forget that life isn't always linear and easy.

I remember one time I was on the plane and sitting next to me was a young mother with her 1½ year old child. There isn't much room on these planes and when children are this young they usually stay on the mother's lap. The baby was obviously in pain, maybe the ears, maybe just uncomfortable and the mother struggled for a long time to put her child to sleep. I am never able to sleep on a plane and so I just sat there doing my best to catch at least a 10 to 15 minute snooze. At one point, an old lady walked past us, and I saw her looking at the child next to me with disapproval. Being judgmental and thinking that she knew best, she bent over me to grab the pacifier that was in the baby's mouth. The baby of course woke up startled and started crying. The poor mother, who was sleeping as well, woke up with the fear that something had happened to her child. The old lady just stood there with the pacifier in her hand saying: "He's too old to have one!"

I, as well as all the other passengers on board, finished the flight with a crying baby and a poor mother doing her best to quieten him up.

I find people to be very judgmental when it comes to raising children, but they are the same for everything else we do in life: how we dress, what we do and how we do it. It seems as though "what others do" is their favorite topic of conversation. Just goes to say: whatever you do, people will judge you. So, do what you think is best for yourself.

a. A good friend is not judgmental and shows empathy

A good friend loves you the way you are. They know you put on a few pounds and don't feel good about it, they know you are heartbroken and are not inclined to smiling just yet, they know you're tired because you have been handling a lot lately and understand why you are a little aggressive, they know you have money problems and are having a tough time making ends meet. True friends don't judge, they put themselves in your shoes and understand.

b. Practice being less judgmental towards yourself. Take a step back and put yourself in your shoes!

What about you? Don't you think that there are enough people criticizing and judging you on a day to day basis? Do you really need more criticism from yourself?

If you want to be your best friend, you are going to have to accept this third step and stop judging everything you do so harshly and putting yourself down all the time. Hey! You know what? You are doing the best you can with what you have, with what life has given you. Stop criticizing yourself and give yourself some slack. You might want to start with being less judgmental with others and practice expressing empathy towards them: learn to stop in your tracks and notice when you are being judgmental towards other people. Next time you feel like criticizing, put yourself in the other person's shoes and make a conscious effort to understand. Gradually, with this realization, start seeing how you behave the same way with yourself. Talk to yourself the way a friend would: "Everything is going to be all right. Maybe you should cut out a few things from your busy schedule and slow down. Maybe you should not watch TV tonight and get an early sleep…"

Learn to pat yourself on the shoulder and be less hard on yourself. If anyone, *YOU ALONE* know what you have been through, so give yourself a break.

D. Being kind and encouraging

A person who expresses kindness is a person who shows tenderness and consideration and has a helpful nature.

A person who is encouraging is someone who gives you courage, confidence or hope.

a. A friend is kind and encouraging

When you are going through tough times or are feeling down, your friend is there offering you kind words to make sure you know that you ARE special and that someone really cares about you.

When I found out I had cancer, after the initial shock of the news, I was in a sort of daze. My true friend Rachel asked me to go out for lunch so we could talk about it. When I arrived, she handed me a special healing bracelet, which I am still wearing today, and told me that she was totally freaked out about my cancer. She was so scared about not doing the right thing or saying the wrong words that she actually bought a book about the do's and don'ts when you find out a friend has cancer.

It was so kind of her and in a way so funny that she actually read a book to make sure she did the right thing, that we both broke out laughing. But it helped me realize that my cancer was difficult for those that were around me as well: How does one react? What does one say? What can one do? Both the bracelet and the fact that she was concerned about doing and saying the right thing to help me, were beautiful gestures of kindness. I will never forget. Thank you Rachel!

b. Be kind and encouraging to yourself

You put on a few pounds. Don't hate yourself for it. You made a mistake at work, don't be too hard on yourself. You lost your temper with the kids again, go hug them and patch things up. When you get off track from your diet or your exercise routine, don't beat yourself down. Things don't just happen overnight.

> *Change takes time, understanding, questioning, trial and error.*

We all search for a quick fix, but forget we have a whole life to learn, to practice, to get to know ourselves.

The way I see it: my whole life is a learning process. Sometimes, I will be good, sometimes great, and sometimes downright dreadful. What's important is to understand that when you make these mistakes, it's not over. You were just trying. So, get up and try again.

Take weight-loss as an example, food, for many, is a struggle. I know that today I am at peace with my plate, but I have had my ups and downs and have learned to get to know myself.

I am 53 now and when I look back I am glad I didn't give up. Just remember: getting off track once in a while, a week without training, eating a bit of junk food… it's all ok. Just get back up and keep believing it's possible. You're simply on the road to learning. I wish you continuous success. Take some alone time and write down a few kind words of encouragement to yourself. You can also *Create Your Very Own Personal Empowering Tape*, a P.E.T., that's Change n° 5, in which you go over your past achievements, encourage yourself to move on, keep believing, and express faith and confidence that you will succeed.

E. Protective

A person who is protective is someone who shows they care.

a. A friend is there to protect you

When things are going wrong, a friend is there to protect you. They are concerned about your health, your welfare, and your wellbeing.

b. Learn to be protective of yourself

To become your best friend, you have to learn to be attentive to your own wellbeing. Learn to listen to your inner voice and try to catch telling signals when something is not ok. Learn to open up a dialog between:

- You and your body: are you feeling pain anywhere? Are you feeling tired? Have you lost all patience? Are you not sleeping well or maybe not enough?

- You and your mind: do you hold anger deep inside that you keep harping on? Are your thoughts more on the negative side? Do you feel lousy or down?

Stop. Breathe. And take some time off to spend it with yourself. Sometimes, simply closing your eyes and resting for 20 minutes can be enough to get yourself back together. Or simply take the time to do something you love, like singing, exercising, gardening, fixing or spending some time on the car, going for a motorcycle ride - you name it. That's all it takes to feel centered and at peace again. We all have ways of reconnecting with ourselves to feel better. Some of us will feel comfort in food: cooking and eating, indeed, can be great ways to relieve pain or bottled up emotions. However, I highly recommend finding other ways to reconnect. Maybe a book, a movie, a walk, being creative, writing down how you feel and what you can do about it.
If you want to be your best friend, you have to be there to make sure your body and mind, including your emotions, are addressed. Don't ignore your inner signals. Be there for yourself.

F. Respect
When we talk about respect we imagine someone who is courteous towards you and who shows regard towards your feelings.

a. A friend shows respect
A friend won't intentionally hurt you. They will be careful and attentive to how you might be feeling and will think of you and not only of themselves. They will want you to be happy and will wish you the best.

b. Be respectful towards yourself
The day you decide to respect yourself is the day you stop depreciating yourself. It's the day you put your foot down and express how you feel and what it is that you really want or will no longer tolerate.

Don't you think it's time now to start focusing on your qualities instead of your flaws? List your good qualities down on paper. Then, try to find ways to become even better at them: read a book, take a lesson, do some research, instead of wasting your time dwelling relentlessly on your flaws, start focusing on improving your gifts, strengths and positive qualities. Concentrate on doing and improving what you love and are good at. Everybody needs to know that they are useful. Everybody needs to feel proud of themselves. Once you have boosted your self-esteem by doing things that you love, notice how compliments start flowing towards you. Then, and only then, can you start tackling a flaw, something that is pulling you down, such as your weight or your laziness. So, every time you overeat or are lazy again, you have something to turn to that makes you happy again. It will help you focus on something else and get you back on track.
Respecting yourself means that you never put yourself down, never depreciate yourself.
So, stand in front of your mirror and look into your eyes and smile. Know that you are there for yourself.

G. Know how to keep a secret
a. A friend knows how to keep a secret
What are friends for? They offer a shoulder to cry on or share a good laugh with you about the silly things you have said and done. They are also there to share your deepest secrets. At times, it feels good to get things off your chest, to have an attentive ear and get some advice. You will often admit to your friends things you would not like everyone to know. If it's a true friend, you know they won't be judgmental and will want to sincerely help. You also know they are trustworthy and will not reveal your trusted secrets.

b. Learn to be quiet and keep some secrets to yourself
Inside each and every one of us there are a many, many different emotions. Learn to name and be aware of them. Learn, whenever possible, not to blabber about everything and to keep these emotions to yourself. Not everything needs to revealed or expressed. If you want to become your very best friend, it's important that your "you and I" have a chat every once in a while and share their little secrets.

Example: I was at the gym the other day and I saw two women looking at me and laughing. At first, I wasn't really sure that I was the source of their amusement. After a few moments, however, it became clear that they were indeed making fun of me. It was obvious they were trying to make me feel uncomfortable. I stopped a few moments to consider this situation. I had a friend of mine at the gym and I could have gone up to speak to her for reassurance, but I chose not to. I had no wish to make this situation worse or to play the same game. Instead, I thought about it and it hit me that if they were wasting their time laughing at me, if they were trying to destabilize me, it was probably because I made them feel uncomfortable. I stopped in my footsteps and looked at them: they were obviously struggling with their weight and it made me further realize that they were jealous and trying to make me lose my self-confidence. I acknowledged this and kept it to myself. On future occasions, I encountered them and had the opportunity to talk them separately. I did my best to encourage and flatter them about true things they had improved and the laughing never occurred again.

Had I chosen to go talk to my friend about it, they would have known and it would have only made the situation worse. Many times, when I am angry or hurt, I intentionally choose to keep things to myself and not share anything with my friends. Indeed, I have found that dwelling on a situation often made me feel worse inside. Although it's not always the case, I do feel that, quite often, a friend even with the best intentions, will end up worsening the situation by telling you that you were right to be offended, mad or hurt and they will actually find other arguments to prove that you are right. By dwelling over certain situations, things can actually feel worse inside and leave you feeling angrier, more frustrated and even more resentful than you were in the first place.

When I was struggling through cancer and divorce, I intentionally chose to stay alone because I knew that if I saw a friend we were bound to talk about what I was going through, and although I know my friends only had the best of intentions, I would inevitably find myself with my anger and resentment reemerging. For this reason, I find that sometimes things are better left to rest. Stirring it all up adds up to nothing.

If you want to be your best friend, it will be nice to know that there is strength in letting your inner friend hold on to some of your secrets. One thing is certain, this one will never betray you.

H. Fun

a. A friend is someone you have fun with and whose company you enjoy

When you are with a really good friend, it's so nice to know that you can simply be "you". You can speak your heart out, you can cry or laugh your head off, you can be grumpy or silent and you know they will love you just the same. These moments create a unique bond between both of you. As the years go by, looking back upon them will make you realize how much they contribute to making this special person, a friend.

b. Learn to have fun on your own and enjoy your own company

Make a point of spending some time alone where you can be yourself. Put on some loud music and sing and dance or make yourself a little picnic, grab a good book and let yourself laugh and cry freely. When you are alone, allow to feel your emotions. Nobody is there to judge you, so let that inner you be its real self. We spend our days being in control and on top of things, but when you learn to become your best friend you are free to laugh about the goofy stuff and cry about irrelevant issues. Who cares! Set your "inner-you" free for a bit. Let it all come out. Becoming your best friend goes hand in hand with spending some time to let all those inner emotions run lose.

To conclude…many times, I hear people say that "the day they have lost all the weight", "the day they meet that special someone", "the day they own a house or some other object" they will be happy. But they have got the equation all wrong. Happiness starts within. Learn to be happy in aloneness. Get into the habit of nourishing your inner soul by expressing honestly how you feel and by being attentive to your specific needs. If you find happiness on your own, it will no longer be essential to meet someone, lose the weight or own something. The day you find happiness after having spent some time alone, you will no longer live in fear. You will be at peace with your plate and lose the weight, you will no longer fear being on your own or losing someone, you will no longer feel the need to own things and will find joy in the simple things in life. Indeed, the moment you come to understand that nothing is more important than that special friend inside of you, you are sure to be on the path to true happiness.

When it comes to training for results and reaping the benefits, most professionals agree that we must integrate the 5 following fitness components: endurance, strength training, flexibility, core and balance. All of these are essential and increasingly so, as we age. However, I find that there are two other important components when it comes to working out, that have been left out: being present, totally focused on our workout and training with proper technique.

B²: **B**rain and **B**ody invested in a 200% workout
E²: **E**ndurance and **E**quilibrium for a stronger heart and improved balance
S²: **S**tretch and **S**trengthen for toned muscles and reformed posture
T²:Technique and **T**ranquility: train with perfect form and unwind

Below I will go through the importance and benefits of each one of these components with an added emphasis on being present and using proper Technique.

A. " B² " stands for investing both your Brain and Body for a 200% workout

You have to BE THERE 200%: People tend to think that training simply involves getting their body past those gym doors, but they totally forget the necessity of bringing their mind and intent into the equation.

Many times, when I am working out, I see people chatting around and texting, sometimes even reading a book or a magazine. On a scale of 0 to 100%, what percentile would you rate the quality of their training? Talking, texting, reading, I would say, although your body is getting somewhat of a workout, we can affirm that if your mind and intent do not enter the equation than you lose as much as 80% of your workout's quality turning it into an almost useless session. One could argue the necessity of making their workout pleasurable and I won't deny that it's better than nothing: at least these people are at the gym doing something and not on their couch at home. But let's be honest here: why did they come and workout in the first place? Was it just for the distraction? Didn't they come to get results? To get rid of those saggy arms? To tone up their abs? To get more muscle definition? And so, I feel like saying: let's stop lying to ourselves here and face the facts: if you want results, if you want to change, you need to invest both your Body and Brain: B².

Give it your All and do your Best.

When I was younger I would stay at the gym for 1½ hour, usually do 40 minutes of cardio, 30 minutes of weights and balance training and 20 minutes of stretch and relaxation at the end of the session. But the day I gave birth to my first son, it was a struggle to get even one hour in. Most of the time I had 40 to 50 minutes maximum. I still wanted to get all of the parameters in and so I jam-packed my sessions to make the most of every minute I had. Usually I would do 20 minutes of cardio, 15 or 20 minutes of weight and balance training and end with 5 to 10 minutes of stretching and relaxation. And you know what? To my surprise, I started seeing more visible results than I ever experienced before. People started coming up to me to ask me how I got my arms and abs so defined. Although I had indeed shortened the amount of time I invested in cardio, I made sure that it was more intense by running faster or doing interval training. And when I hit the weights I made the most of my 20 minutes: instead of resting in between sets, I would work an antagonistic muscle, perform a set of abs or do some balancing exercises. And I always made sure to stretch and relax at the end of my session. If I really didn't have the time, I would try to make up for it later when I was at home.

And I pondered about this. Why was I getting more results? I had ALWAYS done my workouts conscientiously. I was never the talking type. The difference lay in the fact that I made the most of my workout: I knew that I only had 45/50 minutes and I gave each minute my all. I was determined and focused 200% on what I was doing, giving every movement my undivided attention, literally staring at my muscles while working them out. Not only was my body working out, my mind was there completely invested in the training session. And that made the crucial difference.

And so now I tend to say that I would rather you work-out full-on for 20 minutes instead of a whole hour without intent.

Try it! Walk past those gym doors determined to do your best workout ever! Stay fully alert and focus on every single movement you do: feel your body working out. Feel your muscles contracting or stretching. Keep your eyes focused on what you are doing and not on what is going on around you. Stay centered. Put your brain into the equation by directing it to question and analyze everything you are doing and why you are doing it. Use your full potential and be there 200%. I have already explained this notion in Chapter 3 Change n°27: *Mindful Workout*, in which I explain the difference between exercising and exercising with intent but it's so important to understand that your mind has to be lit up 100%. Part of my B.E.S.T.[2] workout is an equation in which your body and mind work out hand in hand, both giving it their all.

Use your mind 100% + invest your body 100%
= 200% chance of success
intent/focus   + implication   =   success

I will not go into too much detail concerning "Endurance and Equilibrium" "Strength and Stretch" as you can find information everywhere. As with everything you do, be smart and sensible: think first, be informed or go ask a trainer or physical therapist how to perform an exercise and what they recommend according to your personal goals.

B. " E² " stands for Endurance and Equilibrium training

1/ Endurance training

a. What is endurance or cardiovascular training?

According to the Cambridge English Dictionary endurance is "the ability to keep doing something difficult, unpleasant, or painful for a long time."

If you search further, "endurance", in regards to physical fitness is "the ability of an organism to exert itself and remain active for a long period of time, as well as its ability to resist, withstand, recover from, and have immunity to trauma, wounds, or fatigue."

b. Why engage in cardiovascular training?

- Your heart will be healthier
- To reduce your stress level
- To have some alone time to think things through or on the contrary to clear your mind. Some people can even reach a meditative state
- To improve your sleep
- To feel more energized
- To improve your mood
- To increase your ability to do certain tasks like lifting boxes, sprinting to catch the bus, climbing up stairs
- To reduce your risk of getting injured
- To develop body awareness and get to know yourself better
- To help control your weight
- To develop your capacity to accept discomfort and strengthen your determination
- To have healthier, stronger muscles and improved bone density
- To enjoy higher self-esteem and improved confidence
- To gain a sense of accomplishment
- To add new and different activities to your exercise program

c. How to develop your endurance?

Answering this question depends on where you are at, right now. If you are sedentary, then start off with 5 to 10 minute bouts of exercise such as walking, running, walking and running, biking, doing the elliptical machine. If you can, try to do a second round later on during the day. Slowly focus on increasing duration, before tackling intensity. Your long-term goal is to build the duration of your cardiorespiratory activity exercise to 30 minutes on most days of the week.

Once you have reached that goal, you can start looking into increasing intensity, alternating longer distances, adding walking up the hills or stairs, using variable terrain, such as running on the beach, in the woods and accelerating or doing intervals.

d. How many times to reap benefits?

If you are a beginner, start working out one day and resting the next. This way, you will either get 3 or 4 workouts throughout the week. If you already engage in some form of physical activity, then you can train on most days of the week. Make sure you get one day off during the week to let your body recover.

2/ Equilibrium training
a.What is equilibrium or balance training?

Balance/equilibrium is the ability to maintain your center of gravity over your base of support. This type of training involves a series of exercises designed to enhance muscular control and improve interpretation of information from the senses by creating controlled instability. According to the N.A.S.M., the idea behind balance training is to stress or challenge a person's individual limit of stability. So, during an equilibrium session, your goal is to aim for your balance threshold, which is the limit you can perform an exercise without losing control of your center of gravity.

b. Why engage in equilibrium training?

The benefits of balance training are numerous:
- Develops and improves coordination
- Helps in joint stabilization
- Promotes body awareness
- Improves posture: for perfect balance you need to hold yourself properly
- Brings variety to your workout
- Gratifies with quick results and improvements
- Engages your core muscles, also the muscles of the hips, thighs, glutes and lower back in a different way than a normal weight training session would
- Decreases your chances of getting injured especially as you age: loss of equilibrium is one of the leading causes of injury as we get older
- Improves your reflex system: When you first attempt this form of exercise you have to be fully focused and think about the movement you are executing. The more you practice, the more your body and mind integrate it and movements becomes automatic
- You can use balance exercises between sets of high-intensity interval training or just simply add them to your weight training workout
- Allows you to exercise when injured, so you still get some form of training done
- Teaches your body and mind to adapt to new situations
- Enhances performance in all sports; especially recommended for improving your running technique
- Allows you to recover faster if you are injured

c. How to develop equilibrium?

There is a huge variety of exercises to challenge your equilibrium. Some can be done on the ground with no equipment at all. Or you can find in most gyms, an array of equipment such as balance disks, wobble boards, BOSUs, foam rolls and so on. If you wish to workout at home you can easily find all you need at your local store or online. Just make sure you start off easy. The goal being to improve your balance and avoid getting injured.

d. Working on my equilibrium

Your balance workout can be done at any time throughout your workout as long as you warm-up beforehand. I like to integrate it into the weight training part of my session. Instead of resting after a set of biceps curls or a back exercise, I will integrate either an abdominal or a balance exercise. Remember that you should try to improve your balance in all planes of motion and not just the frontal plane.

Note: *The first few times, you might want to start off by keeping a chair nearby, just in case.*

If you are just starting, select two or three easy exercises. Once they become easier, you can always make balance exercises harder simply by not relying on any support, increasing the duration, closing your eyes, trying a new piece of equipment, or adding a bit of movement. Here are a few exercises to choose from:
- Practice regularly standing on one leg. Remember to switch and do on both sides.
- Practice standing on leg with your eyes closed
- Get yourself a wobble board and every once in a while, take a break and stand on it. It will put many of your senses in alert mode
- Try standing up and then sitting down without using your hands
- Practice walking on the balls of your feet when doing chores at home
- Try doing a few yoga poses such as the tree pose, the balancing stick or the eagle pose
- Here is a multi planer exercise: Stand tall with your hands on your hips and lift your right leg in front of you. Do the exercise slowly. Without touching the ground, bring your leg down back to the center and then lift the same leg out to the side in a controlled manner. Once again bring your leg back down to the center and then extend your leg behind you and finish by bringing your leg back down to the center. Repeat the same exercise with the left leg.
- Do your abs on a stability ball or a BOSU

C. " S² " stands for Stretching and Strengthening:
1/ Stretching
a. What is stretching?
A good stretching program would be one that causes permanent (plastic) elongation of soft tissues without causing or contributing to injury. Your goal is to increase R.O.M. - range of motion - available at the joint or joints being stretched.

b. Why stretch? What are the benefits of stretching and lengthening the muscles?
- To increase your R.O.M. and flexibility
- To stretch and lengthen your tight muscles
- To improve your posture
- To help prevent injury
- To promote blood circulation
- To ease, get rid of or prevent back pain
- To reduce soreness. I find that when I stretch I have less or no muscle soreness the next day
- To calm down after your workout: use stretching to de-stress
- Because you will feel so good afterwards!

c. How to stretch? What techniques can be used to develop flexibility? How much and how long, to get best results?
The most important thing to remember about stretching:
• Always stretch a muscle once it has been warmed up and never before. Try to engage in a mild aerobic exercise for at least 5 minutes to get your temperature up and your blood pumping to the tissues, before attempting to stretch. Walking, a slow jog, doing some knee

lifts or butt kicks for the lower body and some arm rotations for the upper body are great ways to get your "engine" ready to stretch. Stretching is not the best way to get your body ready and is, in fact, not recommended: indeed, if your body is "cold" the stretching could lead to injury.

- Never stretch to the point of pain. You can get slight discomfort when you stretch, but it should never be painful.
- Being flexible or not, greatly influences posture, so try to stretch all of your body's major muscle groups to create overall balance.
- How much? You can stretch daily, but if you are short on time, try to stretch at least 3 times a week.
- How long? To reap most benefits it's best to perform 2 to 3 sets of each exercise and hold the position without bouncing or forcing for up to 30- 60 seconds. Do each exercise in a controlled manner and make sure you release slowly when coming out of each position.
- There are many different types of stretching techniques. As usual, I am here to encourage you to research and inquire. Read, watch videos, consult a specialist and see what's best and what works for you. Stretching is essential. Even regular exercisers tend to forget its benefits.

All types of stretching should be performed only after an adequate cardiovascular warm-up.

• So, when should you stretch? At the beginning, during the session or at the end? There is no optimal time to stretch just as long as you are sufficiently warmed up beforehand. If you are not that much into stretching, or if you are often short on time or tend to skip it when done at the end of your workout, then try to fit a few active stretches in throughout the session.

I, personally, really look forward to this moment: I find it pleasant to take the time to relax and wind down when I am done. If you do it at the end, make the point to close your eyes, breathe calmly and come into communion with your body.

2/ Strength training
a. What is strength training?
Resistance training is the name given to an exercise that causes your muscles to contract against some form of external resistance, such as dumbbells, barbells, resistance bands or even water bottles. This resistance can also be provided by using your own body weight, as when performing push-ups or chin ups or when partaking in partner-assisted manual resistance training in which the resistance is provided by a training partner. People tend to directly head to the weight stack but there are many other different options to get your muscles contracting.

b. What are the benefits of strength training?

As we age, we lose 5 pounds of our muscle mass every decade after the age of 30. Therefore, it's important to increase or at least try to maintain our muscle mass. Here are the numerous possible benefits:

- Slows down or even reverses the aging process by building muscle mass and strength
- Raises metabolic rate which can help you burn more calories throughout the day
- Helps you burn more fat
- Increases your metabolism
- Adds to your strength
- Improves your appearance. Wouldn't you like to have jiggly free arms, nice guns or a toned butt?
- Creates a toned appearance
- Changes the way others relate to you or see you
- Brings added self-confidence
- Many people when they reach a certain age have difficulty lifting themselves up off their chair due to lack of muscles in their lower body. It's good to know that it is never too late to start lifting weights. You can increase your muscle mass even if you are over 70 years of age.

c. Tips for effective strength training?

Make sure you choose the appropriate amount of weight. I often see people lifting weights that are way too heavy for them. They perform poorly and have the added risk of getting injured. Make sure you can execute your movement with proper form for at least 12 to 15 reps before increasing the amount of weight. Keep in mind to work all your major muscle groups – the chest, back, shoulders, arms, abdominals, and legs. You must think harmony and balance. Many people tend to train only what they see or what is "in fashion" like pecs, abs, or buttocks, completely omitting the importance of building a harmonious body.

If you want to bring variety into your workout, always keep in mind to perform your exercises with:
- proper form, good technique and excellent posture
- proper resistance, while not too heavy
- proper speed, especially not exercising too fast

If you keep these factors in mind at all times, you won't go wrong and will keep injuries at bay. Make sure to keep your head in neutral position: avoid looking up or down. Think "My head stays in alignment".

Always stand nice and tall with your shoulders back and down. I can't stress enough the importance of reminding yourself incessantly throughout your workout to make sure that your shoulders are:
- relaxed, by avoiding tension
- pulled back while maintaining a nice straight posture
- and down

Correct posture also means keeping your back's natural curvature when performing an exercise. To find your optimal posture, simply stand tall up against a wall while making sure that your head, upper back and buttocks are in contact with it. Again, make sure your shoulders are pulled back and down and several times throughout the day, check how you are holding yourself by doing this simple exercise: it's a good reminder of what your posture should feel like.

When performing an exercise, keep your elbows and knees slightly flexed: you do not want to lock your elbows or your knees. Also avoid hyperextending. You want to perform your exercises with full range of motion while making sure to stop just before you feel that your elbows or knees are about to lock. You don't want to over stretch your ligaments or impede proper blood flow.

d. How many times should you strength train?
The number of times required for resistance training varies according to the individual's needs and desires. "When health-related benefits are the desired outcome for the program, ACSM has proposed that 2-3 days per week using a full-body resistance training program is sufficient. Additional days may be necessary for intermediate and advanced trained individuals for continued strength related gains." Seek professional advice if your goal is hypertrophy, power, or endurance.
Try to work all major muscles of the body – your chest, back, shoulders, arms, abdominals, and legs – while doing 8 to 12 repetitions and 1 to 3 sets per exercise. Repeating 2 to 3 three times a week is the best way to see results. If you just started resistance training and are aged 50-60 years and above your aim should be to reach 10 to15 repetitions.

D. " T² " stands for Technique and Tranquility
1/ Technique
Technique is the foundation of any sport
When it comes to training, it is of utmost importance to build your foundation. What's the point of working out if you are not performing the exercise properly? You want to reap benefits from your workouts, right? Who wants to make matters worse? Although this might seem obvious to many of you, it's not the case for most people working out at the gym. Just like in anything you do: there is a technique and it requires proper training. Do it the right way: seek professional advice and start building yourself a better body using proper technique.

Starting simple
If you want to build a proper foundation, then go back to the basics. The simpler, the better. Variety, adding more weight, going faster or doing complex exercises can be added gradually, once you have mastered the basic techniques.

Training also involves your brain and becoming more knowledgeable.

If you are doing recreational activities the goal is to have fun and to feel good. But if you are working out at the gym or engaged in a regular sport or activity, it is essential that you do it with proper form. Start getting into the habit of questioning what you do: how do you execute this exercise correctly? Which muscles are involved? Why and what are the benefits? What parts of your body need to be improved or corrected? Do you have round shoulders? Do you carry excess fat around your hips and abdominal region? Are you too thin? Are you often out of breath and need to improve your cardiovascular health? Learn to adapt your training accordingly. Start working out intelligently.

Far too many people workout without having a clue or with only a slight notion of what they are doing and why. Learn to question yourself and understand what you are doing. Are you executing the movement properly? What part of the body are you supposed to be challenging? Do you feel those muscles being challenged? There are certain exercises, such as the lateral pull down, that work your back and the cable triceps exercises that are seldom executed the right way. One glance is all I need to know if the person has a clue to what they are doing or what the purpose of the exercise is.

Don't copy someone else or assume that some random person at the gym is exercising properly. Do your research, apply what you have learned, listen to your body's feedback, be in tune with the muscles that are supposed to be challenged. Aim for a perfect technique. The best and easiest way this can be done is by learning from a qualified professional such as a trainer or physiotherapist. If you are looking to get benefits and results, it is absolutely essential to get your information from the best source.

Let's look at this differently. Let's say you want your children to learn how to play basketball or do gymnastics. What if I told you to just drop them off at a local park or gym club and have them imitate what others are doing? Would you do it? No, of course not. You would want them to learn it the right way while avoid getting injured. If it's not good enough for your kids, then it's not good enough for you. I can't insist enough on the fact that you either do it right or better off not do it at all. I hope I have convinced you that this is the only way you will get a better body and enjoy true, long lasting results.

Quality vs. quantity: More is not better
Many times, I hear people tell me that they have worked out for one, two or even three hours! But how did they train for that length of time? Were they able to sustain the whole time a proper form and perfect technique?

More is not better.

Focusing on the quality of your training is far more important than how long you actually stayed in the gym. Are you just repeating the same old routine every day or week? Do you work out regularly, but without knowing exactly what you are doing? Keep in mind that repetition and practice are not the only factors that will help you improve. You want to achieve perfect technique. Your goal is "quality training". Developing your skills and abilities and making sure that you are performing them perfectly: this is your top priority.

Remember what your Mamma used to say: *"If at first you don't succeed, try and try again."*? Well I feel like changing this quote:

> ## If at first you don't succeed then question, research and then try again.

And when you reach the point where you feel like you have trained properly, continue to question, keep on researching and strive to reach excellency. Data and scientific results are constantly changing. Learning is an ongoing process, so once you learn something don't ever assume that it will remain forever true.

Look, Listen and feel

When you are working out it's important to look at what you are doing. Are you executing the movement properly? How is your posture? Get those eagle eyes out and scrutinize everything. If you can't see for yourself, why not ask a friend to film you. This is great with any sport. My fiancé regularly films my workouts and I only need to view them once to see whether something needs to be corrected.

Looking also involves eyeing at what *others* are doing. Start by checking *their* posture: if their back or shoulders are rounded or if they are locking their knees, then they are not training with proper form. While lifting weights how is their body "behaving" itself? The core should always be stabilized and under control. What about the way they handle their weights: is there any swinging or swaying involved and are they focused throughout the *entire* movement, which means during the contraction but also as they are releasing and returning to the starting position. Indeed, you will notice that many times people put intent during the contraction phase of the exercise but then simply let their arms or legs "drop" as they release.

Learn to listen to what your body is saying. Does the exercise feel awkward? Is it causing you physical pain? Chances are you are doing something incorrectly. Sometimes a little practice is all it takes to help you get it right, but many times we omit to listen. And if you feel any pain after or during the workout you must immediately stop and let that body part rest for a few days. Your goal is to be able to train until your old age, so it's important to manage yourself properly. The listening part can go a long way.

Lastly, it's important to really feel what you are doing. Feel your abs or your muscles contract, feel air coming through your nostrils and your heart pumping, feel the sensation you get from stretching and elongating your muscles. Looking, listening and feeling are important components that can really help you improve your technique: get them involved in the process!

I really enjoy working out regularly and I am lucky to be able to train at different gyms on a regular basis. It is an unfortunate fact however, as I push past the front door, to notice that most clients are there for the wrong reasons:
• They feel that they have to
• In order to get another workout done
• If they don't exercise, they will feel guilty

And so, as I observe them, I can tell that they are not into their workout at all. Some chat a lot, others are on their phones, many are there to pass the time, to "kill" another work out..., to ease their conscience. But why is it that these people, who come to the gym regularly, without ever getting any visible results, never seem to question themselves about why they don't change?

Isn't it just so convenient to blame the outside world or genetics!

I would like you to stop here for a moment: if you are exercising and not getting results, then *you* are the only one to blame. Be honest for once and for all and start taking responsibility. You *can* change things. Yes, even if your entire family struggles with weight issues. What is your mindset like when you are working out? Are you really, *really*, giving it your all? What are your beliefs regarding your capacity to succeed? Do you work-out with the inner conviction that no matter what you do, you can't change your genetics? What is your attitude throughout the day concerning your diet and exercise? Do you constantly lie to yourself and others about the amount of calories you really ingest and how you really work out? I could go on and on and ask you to answer a great number of questions.

But what I suggest from my heart is to be completely honest with yourself, take responsibility for your current state, and then decide to do something about it and *change*.

E. Tranquility

Once you have completed your session, I can't insist enough on the importance of lying down and relaxing, even if just for a few minutes. Take a moment to breathe, feel your bodily sensations and just let go completely. Remember that it is necessary to instill a dialog between you and your body. Learn to listen to what your body has to say and how it is feeling. So whenever possible, simply lie down on a mat, close your eyes, let everything go and feel. Be grateful for your training and proud that you have given it your all during your workout. A few minutes is enough, but if you can add more time for a meditation or visualization session, it would be even better.

You will find suggestions to develop this point in various parts of the book. Feel free to check out Change n°18: *Visualize* and Change n°50 *Meditation, Mindfulness and Prayer* if you would like to find out more. I also invite you to check out my website and chose a P.E.T. to listen to while you are relaxing to focus on improving a particular aspect of your life.

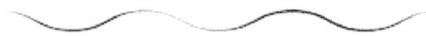

Change n°34
YOU CAN CHANGE!

It's 4 a.m. and little Mary is making her way onto Earth. She has been in her mother's womb for the last 9 months and is now ready to come into this world. But she is not alone. As she feels the urge to push, a little angel is close by. The angel is there to offer her guidance and encouragement and so, as Mary feels the force of her mother's womb contract, she also hears the angel whispering wise words to her in a soothing tone of voice: "Hello Mary! My name is Happy. Have no fear; I am here to accompany you on this short journey. In a few moments you will be starting a new life on Earth. But, before entering this new world, I would like you to take a few minutes to listen.

You have a mission on Earth. Of course, you are free to accept or ignore it. The choice is yours.

You can either live each day without giving it much thought, brandish a sword and shield and get through life in survival mode, incessantly fighting, ducking life's obstacles and shielding yourself for protection. Or you can decide to become a Knightess with a mission to find yourself, to find and create *your* truth. It won't be easy as you will have to do it amidst this world's turmoil and challenges, but it will be a great source of satisfaction and pride and will enable you to tackle your life in an entirely different way, turning it into something exciting as you search for what I like to call your "pot of gold" or "your holy grail". The ultimate goal is to leave this world so much stronger, so much wiser, with pride in your heart for what you have accomplished.

Before coming on Earth, you are given a set of tools: your Body, Heart and Mind. Try to keep your weapons, that sword and shield, at your feet and make use of these tools instead. See them for what they are: amazing gifts. You must learn to use and treat them wisely and with tender loving care. Understand that these tools have other worldly powers and you alone hold their reigns.

In a few moments you will be on your own and from now on it will be up to you to decide how you choose to make use of them. Constantly observe yourself and learn to master your Body, Heart and Mind. Beware however, as these tools can either help or hurt you. Think of a knife, it can either stab or carve, it can either kill or save someone's life. The situation can easily turn the other way around with your body, heart and mind controlling you, in which case you will inevitably end up being at their mercy.

Should you choose, however, to become their master then you will be able to attain high levels of mastery and wisdom. You see, your Body, Heart and Mind will be constantly tempted by greed, various desires, and the urge to react in certain ways. You must let them know that "you" are the one in charge here. Just like children: you must be firm and raise them in a "tough love" kind of way. Should you choose to become a Knightess with a mission then you will see that every single thing that happens becomes an experience. And every encounter is an opportunity to grow and get you one step closer to becoming a Great wise Knightess. You will be on *The Path*, the one that leads to true happiness.

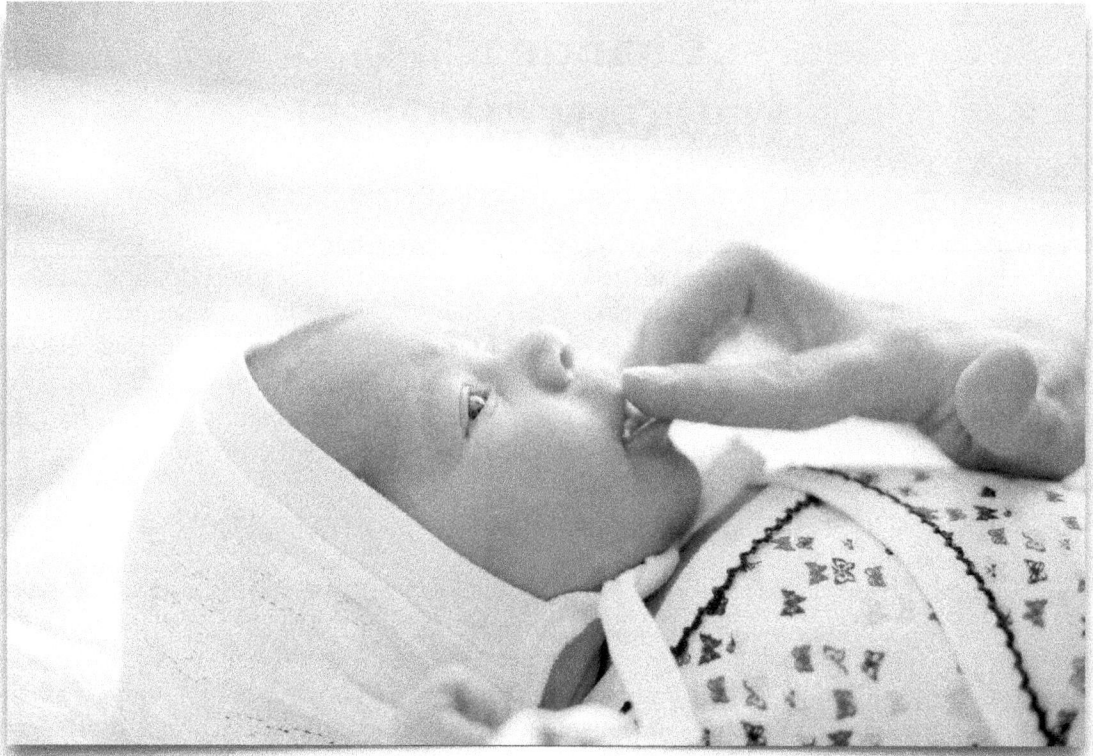

Every child receives the visit of an angel just before birth. What we reveal to each and every one of you however must remain a secret. For this reason, you will not remember a single word. It is your job now, your mission on Earth to dig down deep, and uncover this buried treasure.

To help you, however I have placed my words, somewhere inside you, in your "soul", and they will reveal themselves to you in the form of intuitions, feelings and yearnings. You must learn to listen to these sensations. Your Body, Heart and Mind each have a language of their own and you must learn to be in tune with them, be able to decipher their messages, be more attentive to their wise words and their warning signals. If you do so, you will become your very own guide; no need to find another Knight or Knightess, no need to have a King or Queen.

There will be sure signs that you are not on the right path. Indeed, when you are not listening to who you really are, when you lose yourself in routine and Earthly matters, life will be leading you down a certain path and you will be receiving specific signals such as feeling depressed, sad or having bottled up anger. When you find yourself in such a state, press the pause button, look and listen for answers within you.

Your life has to be thrilling, little girl. It's up to you to make it that way. The secret is to learn to listen to your inner voice and be in tune with what you really want deep down inside. You won't always be on the path. You will fall off track once in a while. It's normal and to be expected. We all succumb to temptation, greed, jealousy and anger at times. Just don't stay stuck inside these emotions for too long. Always remember your mission and get back on "The Path."

The angel knew that in a matter of seconds little Mary would be entering this new world to begin her very own Path. And so, as she gazed down at Mary with loving eyes, she also leaned forward to place her index finger over the baby's mouth leaving her mark just below the baby's nose, the *Angel's Mark*, most commonly known as the "Philtrium."

"Shhhhhh! now little Mary. This secret can never be revealed. It is henceforth your mission on Earth to search for it, to find your truth and live accordingly. Don't lose yourself. On the contrary, your mission is, to find yourself. Off you go my beautiful little Knightess. Good luck. Make the right decisions and remember: You *can* make a difference. You *can* change the world."

38 years have gone by and Mary has become a woman. She is married to Bob and has 3 children. She is currently working as a secretary: not a very gratifying job, but occasionally she feels needed and appreciated for her work. She still loves her husband, but somehow their relationship feels more like they are housemates than husband and wife. Their children have always been a source of great satisfaction, but lately her adolescent daughter has been getting at her about the extra weight she gained and spending more and more time out of the house, slowly slipping away.

Mary is sitting on her bed alone, and staring at her reflection in the mirror. She can't help but notice that she has put on more weight. Probably another 10 pounds she figures. She doesn't know exactly. She stopped going up on the scale when she reached 175 pounds. "What's the point of starting her day off with bad news…" seemed to be the sensible way of ignoring the problem. She keeps on staring at herself and finally breaks into tears. This has been happening quite regularly lately, her crying. She doesn't know exactly why. Her life isn't all that bad. She has a roof over her head, three beautiful children, food on the table. It's true that with her husband things have been a little tense between them recently. She has a feeling that everything she does has a tendency to annoy him. Come to think of it, the same holds true for her: she has been acting more and more impatient and exasperated towards her husband. The thing is, she just knows that he is going to do something that will upset her again. She remembers how in love they used to be and how, she couldn't wait to be with him each day. How things have changed… Mary sobs even deeper…

What happened to Mary? On the outside most people would regard her as being a rather fortunate person: she has it all, right? But behind closed doors, Mary feels sad and although she does her best to hide it, she knows she is sinking into depression.

The angel has kept her promise however and has sent quite a few messages, signs and signals. Mary never really paid attention to any of them, preferring to ignore them, by keeping busy with all the hustle and bustle that occur each day and watching TV and munching on junk food in the evenings. She really enjoys these moments. They keep her mind off of things.

Mary has never taken the time to question herself about the meaning of her life. Those amazing super powers she was given, her Body, Heart and Mind well she has simply taken them for granted. Her body gets her around, her mind allows her to solve minor problems, and her heart… well her heart yearns to be loved.

It's been a while since she felt loved by her husband, but she finds satisfaction in the love she receives from her children and her sister, Bianca, with whom she is fortunate to share a very close relationship.

What about you? How have you chosen to use your tools? Are you listening to your inner voice? Are you searching for that buried treasure? What is your mission here on Earth? Are you going to keep getting up every day to repeat the same day or are you going to find ways to turn on that inner spark of yours and bring some passion into your life? A tip: if you are getting up in the morning and feeling excited, then you are on the right path. If you are not, then start digging inside of you, search for *your* pot of gold, the only sure way of finding your happiness. It's time to understand that you are here for a higher purpose.

Mary's mission on Earth is most certainly not to meet her husband, Bob or to have, three children. Her husband and children are there as lessons to teach her patience, unconditional love, resilience and so on. The problem comes from the fact that we are raised in believing that happiness comes the day we meet our prince charming or our princess and have children. The stories always end with "and they lived happily ever after" don't they? But does it really happen that way? I often wonder why we keep filling our children's heads with these fairytales? We have come to Earth as spiritual beings with a mission to find, call it whatever you want, our truth, inner wisdom, self-love, inner peace. We are on a Path, on a quest in which every single thing that happens, every person we meet... is a lesson, an opportunity to learn something about ourselves, to test our super powers and fine tune our capacity to handle them.

But let's get back to Mary. She is 42 now...
Bob has moved out. Things were just not working out between them: their numerous arguments had kept him away from the house more and more until he finally gathered the courage to tell her that he met someone else and was leaving her. After the initial shock, Mary had to admit that it was for the best. She was tired of all the arguing and sick of having the children witness the scenes...
Mary decided that she wasn't going to waste any more time feeling sorry for herself. That part of her life was over. On the contrary, she tried to have an honest look at her situation: no more arguments, now she was free to live her life according to how *she* chose to live it.
Although her husband was out looking for a new youth by dating many different women and chasing worldly things, Mary aspired to find a deeper meaning to her life by savoring moments of peace and quiet and enjoying quality time alone, with her children, friends and sister.

She decided not to play the victim anymore. What was the point of wasting the rest of her life in that role? She wanted to make the most of the time she had and complaining was not part of the plan.
She began focusing on important things and taking special care of her needs. She embarked on daily walks and occasionally, she would do a few lunges, push-ups and a good stretch. She also decided to observe and change a few of her eating habits. Nothing too drastic: she simply made sure that she was eating fruit and vegetables at every meal and

adding this little ritual whereby she would sit down once or twice daily to enjoy eating something simple, like an apple or a carrot in total awareness. She liked the idea of making an offering to her body.

Surprisingly, the weight went down and she really felt as though the walks were invigorating and breathing life into her. Now when she looked at herself in the mirror, she no longer saw her body as "ugly" or "undesirable". Indeed, she became aware that her body was in fact a beautiful gift that accomplished miracles each day and that she not only neglected it, but also let it deteriorate. Actually, it was worse than that, in the past *she* ate excessively and made bad foods choices which led to high levels of cholesterol. Her doctor put her on medication, but she refused to go down that path and had managed to convince him to put the treatment on hold for a few months: she was going to prove to him that she could get the counts down. It turned out to be fun and exciting to see the levels actually declining. It became clear to her that she had a hand in her health: the cholesterol was clearly a consequence of her poor eating choices. But another thing became clear: if she was capable of worsening her health, she also had the power to reverse things. She had the possibility to improve her overall health and wellbeing.

It's strange when she thought of it, how all these years she was so passive and always came up with excuses - excuses which she actually believed - to justify why she couldn't lose the weight and exercise.

But things seemed to have gradually shifted in her mind and she was slowly becoming the Master of her own body.
She started to see her body as a temple. She understood that she had to make peace with it and start to treat it with respect and gratefulness. Her body was no longer something she was ashamed of, it became a beautiful gift that had the power to heal, to create life, to bear children. It was also a body that procured her great pleasures such as the pleasures of eating, receiving a massage and making love. Mary had a revelation the day she realized that if she wanted to live according to her life purpose, she had to start purifying her body and mind and respect certain rules. And the best and easiest way was to eat healthier foods, take care of her body and exercise regularly.

What about you? How do you see *Your* body? Do you see and treat it as a gift? Do you make good use of your tools, your Body, Heart and Mind, or have you let them take control over you? Have you strayed? If so, you need to get back on The Path. You need to become that Knight and Knightess with a mission. The good news is that it's never too late. So, instead of trying yet another new miracle diet or a new piece of gym equipment or protocol, try to face the problem head on. Understand that if you are eating too much, it is most probably because you are trying to fill a void.
Remember what the Angel said: "Your Truth will reveal itself in the form of intuitions, feelings and yearnings. You must learn to listen to these sensations."
Do you feel sad, angry, depressed? Many times, you may get the feeling that you are lost, alone and unloved. That's how you know that you have strayed. But you are simply off track.
So, grab my hand. You are not completely alone. I would like to give you a little push here.

Start questioning yourself: what makes you happy? What are you passionate about? And then, set out to do it more often. Become good at it. Excel and start seeing sunshine filling up your life. The idea is to get your mind off the food. You have much better things to do on this Earth… you have a mission. Time is ticking. Start turning your routine into an adventure! Come on, all of you Knights and Knightesses hop on The Path! Start tuning in with who you really are, become that person you aspire to be.

Redirecting your attention to finding your life's purpose is the best way to start. Even if you are not passionate about anything yet, focus on doing things that make you smile, happy and proud. The more you live this way, the more you will see yourself rising in the morning, hopping out of bed, excited about the day to come. Then you will know that you found Your Path.

After years of living in a lost state, Mary was starting to change. She couldn't explain exactly why, but now there lied a certain form of hope within her that gave her the drive she needed to move forward. When she thought about it, it felt kind of like "faith." It wasn't faith in a God or something religious, it was faith that she was onto something. It felt as though this new path she was on, made sense. It felt right and she was feeling happier and more serene.

Mary was also very supportive of her sister, Bianca, who had been diagnosed with breast cancer. They both had taken the time to talk it through and became aware of the responsibility they each had in regards to their own health and illness. Her sister lived in the shadow of a controlling husband for years, living according to his desires and beliefs, never daring to speak her truth. At first, she blamed the outside world, including her husband for her cancer. For a while, she even convinced herself that *they* provoked her tumor. But she quickly realized that it wasn't so. She had been living an unbalanced life – between who she was, what she aspired to be, and how she was actually living. In fact, the real culprit was herself for accepting a situation in which she denied herself the right to be the person she really was. She ended up seeing the tumor as a sign, a message that things had to change. It was a real wake-up call.

Just like Mary, Bianca had also come to realize that her body was in fact an amazing vehicle, an extraordinary tool that was constantly receiving and reacting to messages from the outside world. This inter-reaction became extremely clear: exterior events provoked emotions that in turn created either visible or invisible reactions. They then manifested themselves in various ways such as headaches, stomach pains, skin problems or excessive eating and so on. Her Body, Heart and Mind processed every piece of information it received according to her inner truth and values. How she truly felt deep down on the inside somehow found a way of expressing itself and often left stigmas. In a sense these stigmas were like a message in a bottle.

Both Mary and Bianca understood this. Being happy and healthy not only meant nourishing their body with good, wholesome foods, they also had to harbor beautiful loving thoughts within their minds and live in accordance with their hearts. Living in anger or in peace, having negative or positive thoughts about themselves and the people around them, but also ignoring or deciding to listen to their heart all contribute to each and every one's overall well-being. The Mind, Heart and Body work hand in hand. For the body to function well, the Mind and Heart have to be happy and serene, thus the importance of laughing more often and doing things that make one smile.

Bianca had always loved horses and decided to renew her childhood passion. She really looked forward to these moments and had actually seriously started considering quitting her job as a dental assistant and live her passion fully. This would mean a 360° turn in her life, but the idea was slowly becoming an exciting new reality. As for Mary, she became very passionate about how the body manifests itself, the signals and messages behind different ailments, as well as the negative effects of stress on her general wellbeing. Consequently, she grew aware of the importance of slowing down and decided to turn to meditation and visualization.

She had tried to visualize in the past, but to no avail. Now she understood that she could not be in a state of sadness, resentment or anger all day long, and then expect to get results from visualization by simply sitting down and imagining the life of her dreams. It just didn't make any sense. She had to be in a state to receive. Visualizing is kind of like "asking" for a desire to come true. But how could she expect to receive a gift without the feeling of deserving it. She needed to get down to business, get the work done first, and then, and only then, could she be in a state to ask for a reward. And so, just as she had managed to maintain her body under control, she also needed to become the master of her own thoughts. They both went hand in hand. She decided to really focus on harboring higher thoughts by fixing her attention on positive subjects and clearing her mind of all the negative ones… she tried her best to stop criticizing and made sure she focused on kindness and compassion. It was hard work, but it didn't take her as long as she thought it would. She soon realized that she was feeling happy on the inside and once in a while she would even catch herself smiling for no particular reason. That's when it hit her: the necessity of being in the right state of mind to receive. She was proud of all the work she accomplished and it felt right: she was now entitled to reap the benefits. Moreover, her mind felt a lot freer to meditate and visualize. She was also able to focus on her desires throughout the day. Her life was starting to be exciting!

In this story there are no beautiful princess and no prince charming riding on a white horse, but it still has a happy ending. Both Mary and her sister, Bianca, have become Knightesses and blossomed into two amazing women. They still have many years ahead of and so much more to learn. Indeed, *The Path* is limitless. The minute you start thinking that you have reached a certain level of mastery, it means it's time to start thinking, questioning and searching again, as it is a never-ending process. You can learn until your very last day.

And inevitably D-Day will come. You know when it's time to leave this Earth. That Day, your angel will be there, waiting for you. She will have one question to ask: "So, how did it go?" I hope, from the bottom of my heart, that in that moment, you will be able to look straight into her eyes and say: "My life? It was amazing! When do I get to start again?"

A special note: This story talks about Mary and Bianca, but it very well could have been anyone else's or your story. Each and every one of us comes to Earth as a potential Knight or Knightess and with our very own special mission.

Change n°35
THE CELLULITE CHALLENGE *35.*

I am not a cellulite specialist or a doctor, but I firmly believe that whatever it is you wish to change, there is always something you can do about it at your level: so, step back, question your habits, look at the whole picture, write everything down, reflect, add a little common sense...and then...

Start Your Revolution!

Although I highly recommend seeing a specialist in whatever you attempt to do, I simply want you to understand that there are ALWAYS things that you can do to achieve your goals. So, if you have cellulite, get off that chair and start doing something about it! Remember to take a before and after picture using same lighting, same position, same place!

Just like everything else I do, when I decide on a goal, I like to research it and try a number of different little things while adding them progressively in order to get results. And please, stay away from promising adverts that say their special cream or product will get rid of your cellulite in no time. If miracle products existed, believe me, we would know about them.

As I have mentioned before, I do not believe in depriving myself of anything: so, no drastic measures either, such as no longer eating certain types of foods or doing 4 hours of exercise in a sweat suit. The smart way to do it is to start drinking more water, eliminating and walking regularly. Just as it makes sense to me that sitting all day cannot possibly be good for me and my hips, butt and legs, it also makes sense that if I eliminate properly, if I have more overall muscle and less fat, if I am more active and get more blood circulating, that my body will look and feel a lot better.

A. What is cellulite anyway?

Cellulite are lumpy deposits of body fat especially on thighs, hips and buttocks, also found on the arms and stomach region that give a puckered and dimpled appearance to the skin surface. Some people compare it to an orange peel. It usually affects women more than men. According to Medical News Today it is estimated that between 85 and 90 percent of women over the age of 20 have some cellulite so the good news is that you are not alone on this ride!

There are several grades of cellulite ranging from mild, moderate to severe and each grade is according to the number of visible depressions you have.

I do not pretend to have a special remedy against cellulite, but I do believe that if you put all your energy into it for the next few months, if while using some common sense, you are consistent and persistent in this endeavor, well then you will surely see improvements in the overall aspect area of your legs, hips and buttocks.

Please stop lying to yourself that you have tried it all and nothing works. It's time to be honest and to put all your cards on the table and have a good look at what you are doing wrong and what could be done to improve the overall aspect of your body.

B. What can I do about it at my level?

You will find below a helpful list of things that I have progressively integrated into my lifestyle and are now second nature to me

• Drink more water check out Change n°13: Hydrate and make sure you drink more every day.

• Juice more. Check out Change n°14: Daily Dose of Goodness.

• Get outdoors more and fill your lungs up and breathe. You will feel energized and revved up.

• Stretch more and get your blood circulating. If you are sitting down at your office all day, get up regularly and stretch.

• Sit and stand tall. Your body can accomplish all it has to do in a much better way, if it is properly aligned. I can't let go of the idea that if our body is in alignment, it will have less pain and it will function a lot better anatomically and physiologically.

• Let your skin breathe: Don't wear tight fitting clothes all the time. Allow your body to breathe. Aside from the fact that wearing tight fitting clothes prohibits return blood flow to the heart which forces it to work harder, it also has an effect on your blood circulation which is one of the causes of the appearance of varicose veins, and on your digestive system. Wearing tight clothes around the waist line, like tight jeans or skirt doesn't allow your stomach to expand as much as it needs to in order to digest properly. By wearing tight clothes, although it is not the cause of cellulite, bad blood circulation can provoke the development of fat nodules in the thighs.

• Massage your legs and get the blood circulating. Although I do not believe in magic creams, it definitely is a lot easier and so much more agreeable to use one when massaging yourself. But basically, any cream will do, so no need to spend a huge amount of money for a special caffeine or a specific cellulite cream. I like to use unscented 100% Shea butter cream. It smells a bit like petrol and for that reason many people have a problem with it, but I absolutely love what it does to my skin.
Note: according to the American Journal of Clinical Dermatology who reviewed 17 studies, with over 600 patients "there is little evidence that topical treatments (in other words, creams) have a potential positive effect on the appearance of cellulite."

• Get a massage done professionally or try the professional endermologie LPG Cellu M6 technique, which is basically a massage done with a machine.

- Lie down on the ground and give your legs a break by placing them up against a wall for a few minutes. Your legs will thank you for it! Why not try an inversion table!

- Take a cold shower. If you can't handle "head to toe" cold showers, you might be able to handle letting cold water run over yours hips, thighs and buttocks. Shock these parts into thinking: "what on earth is she doing now?" You will see that your skin will instantly feel firm and once you get used to the cold, it will be invigorating.

- Walk in the ocean, sea, lake or pool where it is shallow enough to walk. Your hips, thighs and buttocks will feel the resistance and when you walk out of the water your legs will feel light and you will feel invigorated.

- Try pool biking: when you are pedaling you are pedaling against the water which adds 12 times more resistance, than if you were cycling outdoors. The water resistance is much better for your muscles, bones and joints and it will get your blood circulating, your lymphatic system activated and can really help you get rid of that cellulite. Also, one hour of aqua biking will get you burning between 600 and 800 calories. This is a must, if you want to bust that cellulite.

- Add more fruit and veggies: see Change n° 15: The Big 5 Challenge.

- Sleep better. Make sure you get enough shut eye. Not that this will directly affect the aspect of your legs, but after a good night sleep you will be more positive and able to tackle your day with a positive attitude. You will also be less likely to crave junk food and feel energized enough to hit the gym or head out for a walk, jog or swim… you name it. It's just common sense that after a good night sleep your day will be so much easier to tackle compared to a day after a restless or short night.

- Eat a healthy and balanced diet. This is obvious.

- Go swimming. If you want to reduce the orange peel aspect of your skin, well then you have to burn all that fat, since fat is what turns into cellulite. Swimming is a great way to help you get rid of it as are other cardio exercises such as running, jump-roping, cycling and many more. The good thing about swimming is that it offers resistance, so it tones and strengthens your entire body. Compare it to other cardiovascular exercises and you will see that you get a full body workout: indeed, swimming engages your arms as well as your legs. You also tone your abs and back by soliciting your core muscles. If you choose to swim in the ocean, the saltwater also has a great effect on the quality of your skin as it clears the pores and makes your skin look healthier and tighter.

- Try Pilates to increase the tonicity of your body.

- Try Hot Yoga. The good thing about this yoga practice is that it engages endurance, flexibility, coordination, balance and strength. With the temperature at 105 degrees, you will be sweating a lot which will help cleanse your body. Indeed, when you sweat you don't only eliminate water, you also rid your body of its toxins and can burn up to 1000 calories in a "90 minute" session. Furthermore, the poses stimulate your organs by compression and relaxation which helps them work more efficiently.

- Do the "Stand Tall Walk" more often. Try walking nice and tall, chest up, shoulders back and shoulder blades down. Maintain this posture and walk on variable terrain to get your heart pumping: go uphill, upstairs, or create variety by alternating your speed while walking, light jogging, running, sprinting or by using a jump rope or a hula hoop… get both your heart and your behind pumping!

- Air out your house and apartment every day, even when it's cold. Bring healthiness into your life. Although you might be wondering what this has got to do with cellulite, it's important to realize that your home and body are the same: they both need to be cleansed of their pollutants. Air out your home and keep it clean! Get outdoors, breathe some fresh air! Keep your insides clean, as well, by eating lots of fruit and vegetables, drinking water and eliminating properly.

- Do body scrubs: I like the loofah exfoliating sponge, but you can also use a loofah sponge strap body scrubber, a loofah soap, an exfoliating body scrub glove, a body shower sponge towel, a loofah scrubber…you name it!!

- I have read different studies on the subject and this is how we could summarize its action: body scrubs are good for you and can really improve blood circulation, but let's get things straight: no matter how much you rub the surface of your skin, it's impossible to change the structure of the skin's lower layers.

• Try coffee scrubs. I really enjoy this and make my own:
-½ cup of coconut oil
-½ cup of raw sugar
-1 cup of fresh organic coffee grounds.
Mix all ingredients together. There will be enough for two months if you do it three times a week. Take a scoop of the mixture and spread all over your legs, thighs and buttocks. Massage firmly for 5 to 7 minutes. You can use a timer. You might want to be in the shower to do this because it can get quite messy. Then wrap your legs, hips and buttocks with celowrap and wait 15 minutes. I usually like to take the advantage of doing a face and hair mask at the same time and I also have a natural teeth-whitening product that I like to use. This way I get the most of my time and really feel great. After 15 minutes, take off the celowrap and rinse, preferably with cold water. Your legs will be as soft as silk!

- Boost your metabolism: Low metabolism is linked to increased cellulite. The higher your metabolism, the more calories you burn. You can boost it by eating more protein and making sure you eat enough throughout the day. Drink cold water: your body uses more energy to heat the water up to body temperature. Drinking water also curbs your appetite and helps you eliminate. Try H.I.I.T. training: doing quick and very intense bursts of activity can really boost your metabolism and also helps burn more fat. Take cold showers or train in the cold your body will have to work harder to maintain its temperature. Finally, lift weights/do some weight training. Indeed, the more muscle you have, the higher the metabolism.

- Do squats, lunges, step ups, kick-backs, all great butt exercises. Do specific exercises that target your hips, legs and butt. Remember to completely focus on the exercise you are doing and to contract, squeeze, while really feeling the muscles that you are soliciting.

- Commit to Walking 2000, 5000, 10000 steps a day. Decide on walking a certain number of daily steps and stick to it.

- Keep a diary of your progress. Write down everything you do every day to improve these aspect of your physique: butt, legs, thighs, hips, arms. Check out Change n° 01: Your "Daily Positive Checklist". Find photos of what you would like to achieve, but also take some shots of your personal progression.

- Eliminate more. It goes without saying that if you want to rid your body of cellulite, you need to make sure that your digestive system is functioning properly and that you are going to the bathroom on a regular basis. Drink lots of water and make sure you have fruit and vegetables at every meal. Sometimes it's enough to do the trick.
- How much coffee or alcohol do you drink? Although coffee and a glass of wine can taste really good, they are both toxic to your body. Focus on doing everything to cleanse and clear your body of all its toxins. If you are up to quitting completely, that's fantastic but if you are not really ready to jump to such extremes, try cutting down. I know that alcohol makes me drowsy and I saw a huge difference in the quality of my sleep when I quit coffee altogether.

- Hit the weights and don't hesitate to train heavy. The more muscle mass you have the firmer your skin will be. Many women hesitate to lift weights fearing that they will appear too muscular or bulky. I have been lifting weights for over 30 years and I can assure you that I am far from looking muscular. If you want results, nothing beats the combination of being more active, lifting weights, eating a healthy diet, drinking more water and eliminating on a regular basis. To help you and make the process more fun, I have created a cellulite challenge. Read below to get more details.

3. Why not try the Cellulite Challenge?

Fill out your daily Cellulite Challenge checklist. It's like a game: Each day, simply try to fulfill as many points as possible. Consult your checklist many times throughout the day and see what immediate positive action can be taken that will get you one step closer to getting a great looking physique!

My Daily Positive "Cellulite" Checklist

Here are 35 different ways to help you get rid of your cellulite.
Set a goal to tick at least 5 boxes every day. Your ultimate goal: ticking at least 15!

- I Went to bed earlier. Don't minimize the importance of sleep!

- I Juiced

- I Walked. Try variable terrain: stairs, hills, sandy beaches, mountain hiking

- I Did specific exercises for my hips, butt, legs and arms_____

- I Drank more water 1 2 3 4 5 6 7 8 9 10 11 12

- I Massaged my hips, legs, buttocks

- I Took a cold shower or a Hot/cold shower

- I Walked in the ocean, lake, sea, pool or, eventually biked in pool

- I Ate more fruit and veggies 1 2 3 4 5 6 7 8 9 10 11 12

- I Did the coffee or a body scrub

- I Exfoliated my skin with an exfoliating glove, loofah or brush

- I Took a Pilates or a stretch class

- I Oxygenated my home. I oxygenated myself by reconnecting with nature

- I Did the inversion table or lied down with legs up against the wall

- I Wore lose fitting clothes

- I Worked on my posture

- I Eliminated 1 2 3 times

- I Cleansed myself (enemas) or had it done professionally

- I Got a massage: lymphatic drainage, cellulite specific massage

- I Created my P.E.T. "I am getting rid of this cellulite" tape and listened to it

- I Read a book or an article about getting rid of cellulite

- I Watched a video or program about getting rid of cellulite

- I Ate a healthy breakfast/snack/Lunch/snack/dinner

- I Walked 10000 steps or the amount set as a goal _____

- I Wrote in my "Special Diary", glued photos, focused on my goal…

- I Took the time to look at myself in the mirror, to learn to love myself

- I Didn't do_____. For example, today I didn't smoke, drink, eat junk

- I Visualized myself looking amazing

- I Had a Yoga session

- I Sat nice and tall with legs uncrossed to allow a good blood circulation

- I Did a H.I.I.T. workout (High Intensity Interval Training)

- I Fasted and let my body have a break and cleanse toxins

- I Saw a professional to help me rid myself of my cellulite

- I did Aquagym, swimming laps, flutter kicking

- Other _____

The idea is to tick as many boxes from the checklist you possibly can, throughout the day. Remember that this is a gradual process. At first you will only tick in a few boxes, but quickly you will see how fun it becomes and you will be trying to tick as many as possible. So, stick it in your notebook, on your fridge, in your agenda…and see how motivating it can be to increase your number of check marks!

Remember that your goal is not to force or punish yourself into doing things but to focus on bringing positive elements into your life, such as bouts of exercise, learning about cellulite, taking care of yourself. Focus on learning, having fun and on embracing change.

Change n°36
AN EXERCISE CHALLENGE 36.

If your problem comes from a lack of motivation to start exercising, then a fitness challenge just might be what you need, to kick start your willpower. Most fitness challenges are not time investing and yet, surprisingly, give results. What have you got to lose anyway?

Below you will find a whole array of different fitness challenges to choose from. Take the time to read each one and see which one suits you best.

A. 15 Different Fitness Challenges to Choose From
1. Upper body challenge
Many times, a fitness challenge implies doing one exercise, a certain number of times for a predetermined number of days. As an example, you could tackle a push-up challenge. Below, I will develop programs for both the upper and lower body, but keep in mind that you could very well decide to take up 3 different exercises and alternate them every day. For example, if your goal is to increase upper body stamina and strength, you could: Day 1, do push-ups, Day 2, dips and Day 3, some Burpees or pull-ups. It's really all up to you. But once you've decided upon a certain challenge, stick with it. Don't start adding or changing components. What is essential here is to learn to do something to completion, to get into the habit of accomplishing an entire challenge from beginning to end. The goal being to cumulate more and more successes in your life, make yourself proud and sky rocket your self-esteem.

Let's say you have decided to do a certain number of pushups every day, the number you will choose to do, depends on your initial level of fitness. If you are an advanced athlete, you could decide to either do 100 repetitions every single day for an entire week or you could very well start off by doing 20, 30 or 40 repetitions and progressively increase the number of reps each day. Let's say, this would help you reach 25, 35, 45 and why not 50 repetitions by the end of the week. In order to establish your challenge, first warm-up by doing a 5 minute brisk walk and then by doing big circles with your arms, 15 times forward and then backwards. Repeat several times. Once your warm up is complete, count how many push-ups you can do in one go, either against the wall, on your knees or real push-ups. The number of repetitions that you can do becomes your baseline. So how many did you manage to do? 20? 10? One? Even if your baseline is one, don't panic! Believe me, you are not alone. A push-up is a challenging exercise but with practice, you will start increasing the number of repetitions in no time.

Remember that you can choose to do the set number of repetitions all in one go, or you can spread them out throughout the day, whatever is easier for you, just as long as you get the predetermined amount of reps done every day.

A little note for the ladies here: Many women tend to work their lower body and totally overlook the fact that it is so important to work their arms, shoulders, chest and back as well. As we get older, upper body strength is essential to accomplish a number of daily activities such as pushing ourselves off a chair and carrying our groceries. Doing the push-up challenge will help you increase your upper body strength, arms - namely the triceps - chest and shoulders. Are your arms flabby when you wave goodbye? Indeed, push-ups are a great way to strengthen this part of your anatomy.

If done correctly, it can help improve your posture. Before tackling the challenge, make sure to get professional advice so you are sure you execute the exercise properly. Keep in mind that you are seeking to strengthen your upper body and avoid getting injured or worsen your posture. If you are too weak to do a normal push-up, as I said before, start off easy by doing them on your knees or off a wall. See how many you can do and build up from there by adding 1 push-up at a time every day or every other day. You can also start by doing 10 normal push-ups, then move on to doing them on your knees and do an extra 5 or 10, until you can no longer push yourself up off the floor. This is called reaching muscle failure. To build upper body strength and stamina, you could also choose the pull-up or dips challenge. Same principle.

Here is a 30-day push-up challenge if you are starting off with one push-up. Up to you to decide the length of your challenge: 7, 10, 14, 30 days according to the number you wish to achieve. At the beginning, you might want to practice doing one, two or three push-ups several times throughout the day to get your body accustomed to the exercise and allow for faster progression. Let's get started!

AN EXERCISE CHALLENGE WITH PUSH-UPS

Day 1	1	Day 11	6	Day 21	9
Day 2	2	Day 12	Rest	Day 22	9
Day 3	3	Day 13	7	Day 23	9
Day 4	4	Day 14	7	Day 24	Rest
Day 5	5	Day 15	7	Day 25	10
Day 6	5	Day 16	Rest	Day 26	10
Day 7	5	Day 17	8	Day 27	10
Day 8	Rest	Day 18	8	Day 28	Rest
Day 9	6	Day 19	8	Day 29	11
Day 10	6	Day 20	Rest	Day 30	11

Remember: If it's too hard, ease things up by doing knee push-ups or doing them off a wall. If, on the contrary, it's too easy, you can harden the challenge by varying your push-ups: for example, by placing your hands wider or right under your chest or by placing your feet up on a step or bench. You can make things more challenging by executing your push-ups slowly or by doing a one second pause when your chest reaches the ground. You could also do a spider push-up: you start standing up and bend down forward placing your hands on the ground. Slowly crawl forward until you are in a push-up position. You do your push-up and then crawl backwards and come back into a standing position.

2. Lower body challenge

For the lower body challenge, you can basically do the same thing as for the upper-body, but you choose one exercise that targets your lower limbs, such as squats, lunges, or step ups and just make sure you get the predetermined number of reps done each day or on the scheduled days. As above, adapt according to what you wish to achieve.

A LOWER BODY CHALLENGE
Example of a Beginner/Intermediate squat challenge

Day 1	30 squats 3 x 10/day	Day 11	40 squats 20 2x/day	Day 21	48 squats 24 2x/day
Day 2	30 squats 3 x 10/day	Day 12	40 squats 20 2x/ day	Day 22	48 squats 24 2x/day
Day 3	30 squats 3 x 10/day	Day 13	40 squats 20 2x/ day	Day 23	48 squats 24 2x/ day
Day 4	Rest	Day 14	Rest	Day 24	Rest
Day 5	30 squats 15 2x/day	Day 15	44 squats 22 2x/day	Day 25	52 squats 26 2x/day
Day 6	30 squats 15 2x/day	Day 16	44 squats 22 2x/day	Day 26	52 squats 26 2x/day
Day 7	30 squats 15 2x/day	Day 17	44 squats 22 2x/day	Day 27	52 squats 26 2x/day
Day 8	30 squats 15 2x/day	Day 18	44 squats 22 2x/day	Day 28	52 squats 26 2x/day
Day 9	Rest	Day 19	Rest	Day 29	Rest
Day 10	40 squats 20 2x/day	Day 20	48 squats 24 2x/day	Day 30	54 squats 27 2x/day

3. Full body challenge

The goal here is to strengthen your entire body and get motivated to start being more active on a regular basis. You could:

Do a squat and push up challenge by doing a certain number of push-ups followed by a predetermined number of squats. Or you could alternate exercises: one push-up followed by one squat, 10 or 20 times in a row. This would imply getting up and going back down onto the floor after each repetition, which will get your heart rate really pumping!

Do spider push-ups: you start standing up and bend down forward placing your hands on the ground. Slowly you crawl forward until you are in a push-up position. You do your push-up and then crawl backwards and come back into a standing position.

Burpees: There are different ways of doing burpees that can either make them easier or harder, depending upon your goal.

A normal burpee: start in a standing position and come down, place hands on the floor and make your legs jump back, in order to find yourself in a plank position. Then jump back until you find yourself in a crouched position. You then return to the initial standing position.

Second level burpee: do a normal burpee but add a jump once you have reached the standing position.

Third level burpee: same as the second level but this time add a push up once you are in a plank position. You could, of course, start out with a normal burpee routine to move on to a level two or three burpee routine.

Full body challenge: Below you will find a table which you can follow that proposes a full body challenge over a week.

FULL BODY CHALLENGE		WORK SPACE
☐ Monday	☐ Do Push-ups for one minute (eventually, go down on your knees), followed by 30 seconds of jumping jacks (cardio) Rest 30 seconds. Do seven times for a total of 14 minutes and finish with two stretching exercises one for the upper and lower body.	
☐ Tuesday	☐ Do abs for one minute and then jump rope for one minute. Do seven times for a total of 14 minutes and finish with two stretching exercises one for the upper and lower body.	
☐ Wednesday	☐ Do 10 to 20 Lunges (or squats or step-ups) followed by 1 minute elliptical trainer. Do seven times for a total of 14 minutes and finish with two stretching exercises one for the upper and lower body.	
☐ Thursday	☐ Rest day	
☐ Friday	☐ Distance challenge: alternate walking one minute and running one minute. Do seven times for a total of 14 minutes and finish with two stretching exercises one for the lower body.	
☐ Saturday	☐ Do 10 pull-ups (eventually with elastic or assisted) followed by 1 minute of cycling. Do seven times for a total of 14 minutes and finish with two stretching exercises one for the upper and lower body.	
☐ Sunday	☐ Do 10 push-up + 10 Jumping jacks + 10 abs + 1 minute jump rope + 10 to 20 lunges + 1 minute walk + 1 minute run + 10 pull-ups + 1 minute cycling. End with a nice stretch session.	

You could also do 10 Sun salutations. This exercise is complete as it requires strength and flexibility, and it is also challenging. Why not film yourself to keep track of your progression. I do highly recommend that you get help and advice from a qualified professional to make sure you do the exercises properly.

The exercise is complete and challenging. It requires strength and improves your flexibility. Remember to film yourself to follow your improvements. I do highly recommend that you take a session with a professional yoga instructor every once in a while, just to make sure that you are doing the series of exercises properly.

Alternating upper and lower body challenge
- 1 push-up followed by 10 squats
- 2 push-ups followed by 9 squats
- 3 push-ups followed by 8 squats etc.
- until you reach 10 push-ups followed by 1 squat

Or

Lateral lunge / push-ups
- Start off by doing 10 lateral lunges, alternating between left and right and then do10 push-ups.
- Next set, do 8 lateral lunges followed by 8 push-ups
- Then 6 lateral lunges / 6 push-ups and so on until you reach a count of 2 lateral lunge / 2 push-ups.

You will have completed 30 lunges, left and right and 30 push-ups!

If you have a higher level of fitness, you could repeat the whole process once, twice… and why not 10 times for a total of 300 lunges and 300 push-ups!

High Intensity Interval Training (HIIT): This type of training will have you pushing yourself at about 90 percent of your maximum for one minute and then resting for one minute. You then repeat these two minutes 10 times for a total of 20 minutes. It's short and will get you sweating. If you are short for time or not up to doing one-hour sessions, this could be what you need. Make sure however to warm up a little before you start and to end the session with a few stretches.

TABATA. This type of exercise is for trained individuals: do a TABATA program 6 times a week that works your entire body! For those of you who do not know what TABATA is: it is a high intensity workout, that has strength and cardiovascular benefits. For this reason, I do not recommend it for beginners. It was invented by a Japanese physician, Dr. IZUMI TABATA. Basically, what you have to do is:

Choose 4 different exercises that make up a cycle, concentrating on alternating upper and lower body. For example:
1. push ups
2. step ups
3. medicine ball slams
4. burpees

You do exercise 1 for 20 seconds and then rest 10 seconds before moving on to exercise 2 for 20 seconds and so on until you have completed the 4 exercises. And then you repeat the whole cycle 7 times, for a total of 8. Each cycle should take you about 2 minutes which means that the entire workout would only take 16 minutes!

I recommend a warm up before, one balance exercise, then adding two to three minutes to work your abdominals or core, and a few simple stretches at the end for a perfect workout. That would take it to a total of 25 to 35 minutes maximum. If you have a busy schedule, TABATA training is for you. And don't be fooled by the numbers: since this training is performed at high intensity, you will be burning lots of calories even after the session is over. To avoid monotony try changing your exercises. Here is a whole list of options to choose from:

TABATA WORKOUT EXERCISES

☐ Squats	☐ Sit-ups	☐ Biceps Curls
☐ Deadlifts	☐ Crunches	☐ Chin-ups
☐ Jump Rope	☐ Lunges	☐ Side Lunges
☐ Leg Raises	☐ Triceps Dips	☐ Stairs
☐ Jump Squats	☐ Sprints	☐ Mountain Climbers
☐ Lateral Raises	☐ Calf Raises	☐ Leg Press
☐ Other………………..	☐ Other…………….	☐ Other…………….

Select four different exercises. You do exercise 1 for 20 seconds and then rest 10 seconds before moving on to exercise 2 for 20 seconds and so on until you have completed the 4 exercises. And then you repeat the whole cycle 7 times, for a total of 8.

You can also run or walk up a hill as fast as you can and then walk back down, and repeat. Like H.I.I.T., you can integrate this into pretty much any workout.

4. Time challenge

- In this case, the goal is to reach a certain amount of time: you could choose to exercise daily for 20, 30, 40, 60 minutes. For example, you could take up a 20-minute cardio challenge: you simply do 20 minutes of regular cardio. If you want to notch it up a bit, you could alternate doing your exercise for 1 minute at a low level of intensity and then move on to do the activity at a more intense rhythm for a whole minute. Repeat the process 10 times. Try to vary the activities each day to work different muscle groups and for added variety.

- Do the 20/20/20 Challenge. In this challenge you will alternate 20 minutes of strengthening exercises on Day 1, 20 minutes of endurance on Day 2 and 20 minutes of stretch on Day 3. Day 4 could be a rest day or you could come back to Day 1 again.

Day 1: 20 minutes of strengthening exercises:

Try to do a full body routine:

- Lunges 10 repetitions left and right followed by
- Spider push-ups 10 repetitions
- 10 double crunches to work your abs
- 30 second planks to work your core

Repeat the routine 4 to 5 times until you have reached the 20 minutes.

Please remember to do a few stretches at the end

Day 2: 20 minutes of cardio

Simply do 20 minutes of steady endurance or interval training in which you would alternate regular pace (you can talk) with a higher pace (you can no longer talk).

You could also choose to do 4 different cardio exercises for 5 minutes each:

- Run for 5 minutes
- Walk fast for 5 minutes
- Walk up hill for 5 minutes
- Walk up and down the stairs for 5 minutes

Or you could use the Rowing machine followed by the elliptical, treadmill and the bike.

Day 3: 20 minutes of stretching

Find at least 5 exercises to get your entire body stretched, put on some nice music, breathe deeply and relax into every exercise for a nice deep stretch. No bouncing: try to maintain each position for at least 30 seconds in a steady state. Each time you exhale, try to move further just a little notch. You should feel a good stretch but it should never be painful. Release and then repeat once or twice before moving on to another exercise.

Finish off the session by closing your eyes for a few minutes and letting your body fully relax. Enjoy!

5. Training for a specific challenge

Have you always wanted to be able to do something specific, such as climbing up a rope, doing 10 pull ups, rock climbing up to the top of the wall, doing double-unders with a jump rope? You name it!

This challenge would require that you lay out a plan of action and think things out to get the results you are looking for. In this case, it might be a good idea to get a personal trainer: you could hire them once a week and ask them to lay out a plan of action for the remaining days of the week in order to reach your goal by D day. The good thing about hiring a trainer is that they will help you set up a realistic challenge – set it out for success - *and* you will be accountable to them.

Examples:

Jump rope. Your goal could be to jump rope 100, 200 or 300 times in a row. Of course, this goal depends on your initial level, but if you already know how to jump, start off by seeing how many times you can jump in one go and work your way up from there, by trying to add a few more reps each time.

If you can't seem to go past a certain point, it probably means that your technique needs some minor corrections.

At one point, I wanted to master double-unders and just couldn't seem to progress anymore. Frustrated after trying time and again, I went to a cross fit training center and hired a trainer. He watched me jump for a few minutes, took the time to film me and then told me what needed to be adjusted. He gave me lots of little tips and some visual cues to improve my technique. We created a full body checklist that I would go over regularly while jumping: on the balls of the feet, knees slightly bent, both elbows in same position and open, only the wrists moving, chin up and so on. At the end of the first session, I was already doing an additional 10 reps! One session was all it took: I avoided stagnation and it got me really boosted again!

6. Hula hoop: Do 10 minutes each day. Have fun doing the challenge with your kids and see who can stay the longest without the hoop falling! Learn to let it go down and have it come back up again.

7. 10 minutes of Stretching a day Challenge. It may not seem a lot, but the benefits are endless. Choosing to do it for 10 minutes isn't time consuming, which means you will more likely stick with it. You could do it first thing in the morning or while watching TV at night. Remember to prepare this 10-minute goal. Take the time to do some research or learn from a professional. I suggest creating two or three different stretch routines and alternating them. Or you could do the same routine every day and at the end of your session add in one brand new exercise. If you have decided to create your own little routine, I would suggest stretching the major parts of your body: arms, chest, hips, back, legs and calves.

Why not take a stretching class once a week to learn proper technique and get some ideas or hire a personal trainer to create these sessions for you. You could do it several times with your trainer just to make sure you are doing the exercises properly and then do them on your own. Or you could do one session a week with your trainer and two without. Stretching benefits are countless: feeling much better, being less prone to injury and correcting your posture are only three of them. So why not start your stretch routine challenge today!

8. Walk more and Stair Challenge! That seems like an easy goal! Well it all depends on where you live. If you live in the city you will be getting a heck of a workout, especially if you live on the 10th floor! All jokes aside, if you choose this goal, you will be surprised to see what impact these short bouts of exercise, while spread out throughout the day, can actually have on your general level of fitness! You will get your blood circulating and give your heart and muscles a great workout! Remember, everything counts!

9. Yoga Challenge. Are you one of those people who have always wanted to practice yoga? Why don't you schedule 15 minutes every day just for yourself and create a little ritual? The best way to do this is to attend a yoga class once or twice a week and make sure that you do15-minute mini-sessions the remaining days of the week.

Going to class will allow you to discover new poses, the ones that are relatively easy and that you can integrate into your home routine. After your initial introduction to yoga with a professional, you could continue with exercising with an online instructor. I would suggest that you do poses for 10 minutes and keep the remaining 5 minutes for nothingness. You could, for example, do 5 sun salutations followed by 5 minutes of relaxation. Just lie down on the floor or relax in a chair, shut your eyes and spend a few minutes doing absolutely nothing. You deserve it!

10. Walk Tall Challenge

This is one of my favorites! Just get outdoors, walk and concentrate on your posture: pull those shoulders back, tuck in your tummy and contract your abs! And if you can't pull that tummy in because there is a little too much there to tuck in, that's ok; simply focus on standing tall. Be proud! You know when they say: "act as if you were already there, as if you had already succeeded", Well this is the time to put it into practice. Walk out those doors thinking "The world is mine to embrace!"

I can't stress enough the importance of good posture. Most of your pains are directly related to poor postural habits: sitting too many hours at your desk, slouching during the day, carrying a heavy handbag on the same shoulder… sounds familiar? Why not invest yourself in this project for a whole month? There are thousands of good books to choose from. Check out a few from my "Recommended book selection". Do some research. See what feels good for you. Check if there is a postural class near you or take an appointment with your chiropractor. See what exercises he recommends and stick to them for one month. The benefits are considerable!

11. A Number of Steps Challenge

Pretty basic: get yourself a pedometer and decide to walk a certain number of steps each day. 10000 is a recommended amount but it might be a good idea, the first few days, to see how many you actually do on average and start from there. If you walk an average of 5000 steps you could increase the number of steps by 1 or 2000, for example. This way you are pretty sure to reach the programmed number of steps. Doubling it might be signing up for failure.

12. A Calorie Challenge

In a calorie challenge, you could decide to burn a certain number of calories every day, for example 300 or 500 calories. All you have to do is check out how many calories each activity burns, and then calculate how many minutes of exercise you need, to reach your goal.

As with any other goal, be sure to map out your entire week ahead of time and don't start thinking "I can eat more since I exercised". That's a total miscalculation. Don't add anything extra to your diet, as it just doesn't make sense.
A reminder: to lose 1 pound you need to burn 3,500 calories.
If you burn 300 calories a day, you will lose one pound in 12 days
If you burn 500 calories a day, you will lose one pound in 7 days

Ideas on how to burn 300 calories:

Note: The number of calories burned is according to weight/size and intensity. It goes without saying that a 200 pound person will burn more calories per hour than a person with a weight of 150 pounds. A work out done vigorously will burn more calories than a less intense work out:

TO LOSE ONE POUND YOU NEED TO BURN 3 500 CALORIES

If you burn 300 calories a day, you will need 12 days to lose one pound

IDEAS TO BURN 300 CALORIES

☐ 30 Minutes Biking/Spinning	☐ 30 Minutes Rock Climbing	☐ 30 Minutes of Rowing
☐ 15 Minutes of intense Jump Rope	☐ 30 Minutes of Jump Roping	☐ 30 Minutes on Stairclimber
☐ H.I.I.T. Workout	☐ 30 Minutes of Running	☐ 30 Minutes of High Energy Dancing (DVD)
☐ 30 Minutes of Power Swim	☐ 45 Minutes of Weight Training	☐ Other........................... .

☐ 30 Minutes of Roller Skating (If you weigh 200 pounds, you burn 340 Calories. If you weigh 160 pounds, you would need to roller skate 35 minutes to burn 300 calories)

☐ Walk (A rule of thumb : 180 pound person will burn 100 calories per mile and a 120 pound person will burn approximately 65 calories per mile. Walk accordingly)

☐ Other...................	☐ Other...............	☐ Other.................

IDEAS TO BURN 500 CALORIES

☐ 1 Hour 1/2 walk	☐ 1 Hour of Rowing	☐ 50 Minutes of Cross Country Skiing
☐ 45 Minutes of Jogging	☐ 1 Hour of Swimming Laps	☐ 1 hour of Zumba
☐ Other...................	☐ Other.................	☐ Other........................... .

13. A "something you have always wanted to be able to do" Challenge

Is there something you have always wanted to be able to do? I know I dream of doing a great number of things: to rope climb breezily all the way up to the ceiling, do a pancake… not the one you are thinking of: I'm talking about the one where you are seated on the ground, legs open and then you put your chest flat on the ground, doing 10 perfect pull-ups, to name only a few.

What have you always dreamed of doing? Or what were you able to do in the past and would love to be able to do again today? Chin-ups? Pull-ups? A marathon? Jumping off a plane with a parachute? Jump roping? Reaching the summit of a certain mountain? Trekking? Signing up for a boot camp? Boxing in a ring? Competing?

You name it. It could very well be anything. But if you want to give it your best shot, it would probably be more reasonable to begin prepared. What component does your challenge require? What can you do to achieve your goal? Once you know what it is, set a date, plan ahead and start reaching it.

14. A Distance Challenge

Why not decide to reach a certain number of miles this month? Plan a specific distance ahead of time, break it down into increments and program your monthly training accordingly.
You could also walk, run, row, hike, swim between two set points.

15. Get ready for a specific event challenge

Do you have a specific event coming up: a wedding, a high-school reunion, a special birthday, such as turning 20, 30 or 40? Does your city organize an annual event such as a 10k, a mud race, a marathon, a biathlon, a tennis, golf or beach volley tournament, or cross-country ski race?

Why not decide ahead of time to sign up for this event and then train your best, really give it your all, in order to be ready. Get your focus off the weight loss and 100% on achieving that specific goal.

What if there are no events? You can always create one:
A few years back, I booked a photo shoot, 5 months ahead of time. Once the date was set and the session paid for, I only had one thing left to do: work my ass off to look my best! Having a specific date marked on your calendar can have an incredible effect on your motivation and get you moving like never before! And when your goal is reached, all you have to do is plan a new one for the upcoming months. Make it completely different and with new challenges to tackle. Turn each new challenge into a growing process.

B. How to stick to your challenge

a. Plan ahead

Once you have decided upon a challenge it's important to get organized and plan ahead: when will you be doing it? How can you make your challenge attainable? You don't want to get injured in the process either, so what can you do to ensure that you are doing it properly? Some challenges require only one short 20-minute session, whereas others might necessitate several short 5 minute bouts scheduled throughout the day. Try to assess, the night before, when you are most likely to have the time to do it. Planning ahead is probably *the* most important factor if you want to succeed in your challenge.

b. Set an alarm

A good way to make sure you get things done is to set an alarm. Most of us are busy. It's not necessarily that you didn't want to do it, most often it's because you let time slip by. Setting the alarm is a good way to remind yourself about your next scheduled session.

c. Take "before and after" pictures

I was really surprised once, after watching a video on YouTube where two young men decided to take up a push-up challenge. *"We did 100 push-ups every day for 30 days"*
The results were really visible and it made me think… what if they had done 100 push-ups – 100 abs – 100 lunges or squats? A few more minutes and they would have challenged their entire body. They weren't really convinced any transformation would occur, but once they saw the before and after photos, they were impressed and so was I!
So, make sure you take a photo from different planes: from the front, the side and the back, with your arms flexed and then relaxed by your side.

d. Chart it

I find that creating charts and recording your progress really helps you keep track of what you have accomplished. If you choose to record things down on paper, it will only require you to prepare a chart ahead of time which will take you approximately 5 minutes. Each day, you simply take your highlighter and draw a thick line representing the number of reps that you have accomplished.

You could also choose to use an app to chart things out for you. You download the app on your phone, you wear the watch and it basically keeps track of all your activity throughout the day and it allows you instant access to your stats: what activity you have done with the intensity, the duration, the number of steps you have reached and your heart rate.

e. Become accountable and do the challenge with a friend

Doing a challenge with a friend can be a great source of motivation: Which one of you will be a quitter? Or, will you both be able to finish it? Who has the most willpower? You could send your daily stats to one another or call each other up for motivation to see how you are doing. "I have done my 50 pushups today? Did you?" And you won't feel alone on this ride. If the challenge requires going to the gym or doing an outdoor workout, knowing you are going to meet up with a friend also makes you less likely to cancel.

f. Find your "why", your reason for doing it, and post it

When you feel your motivation going downhill, remind yourself why you decided to tackle this challenge in the first place and what it is contributing to. Write it down and post it somewhere you are sure to see all the time. Consistently remind yourself what you're working towards. This can really help to keep you on track.

g. Install a habit tracker app

There are many apps that keep track of how many times you engaged in a new habit such as drinking water, doing push-ups. You name your new habit and log in the number of times/reps you have done or not done it, for example, if you are trying to cut down on cigarettes or coffee. The good thing about some apps is that some have an integrated alarm to remind you to do your "habit".

h. Ask if your gym is hosting a challenge

Many clubs and gyms offer short term packages such as 3 classes a week for a certain price. Other clubs also propose specific challenges open to all members. Why not decide to commit to 3 classes every week or register for this month's best before and after picture, to show your results?

i. Get a movement tracker and keep track of how many steps you do

Get a movement tracker or a free pedometer app. These devices allow you to keep track of your progress. Decide upon a set point (for example, 10,000 steps) and make sure you do it every day. Let the app do the work for you.

j. Sign a contract with yourself and tell others you are doing a challenge

Prepare a contract in which you detail your challenge and sign it. It can be a great source of motivation. Make sure your contract looks real and paste it somewhere visible: it will greatly increase your chances of committing to what you have signed for. Let others know about your challenge as well. You could, for example, ask one or more friends to witness the signature: it will most definitely make you more accountable.

So, grab a piece of paper and prepare a contract or why not use the Letter of Commitment that you can find at the end of Chapter One. If you make your own, simply make sure to make it look like a real contract.

k. Avoiding things and situations that might distract you

Most of these challenges are short and require little time. Make sure you do them 200% in mind and body and do your best to avoid being distracted by technology and social media. Turn off all of your devices, leave them in your locker or bag so you are not tempted to engage. As a rule, try to do things with your full attention, give it your all. The added benefits and results will be visible.

1. Avoid adding components to your challenge

Many people make the mistake of doing a challenge that contains too many components. So, instead of making sure they simply get their 20 minute workout done, they tend to add on some other more drastic measures, such as going on a strict diet as well. This, however, is not a good idea, unless you want to fail your challenge. Instead, make sure to stick to your challenge this week or month and to do it 200%, fully committed. Your next challenge could be a nutrition challenge, such as eating fruit and vegetables at every meal, or drinking more water. Do your challenges one at a time. If your workout has become a habit, then that's another story: you are of course welcome to add on new components and start your journey.

Keep in mind, no matter what challenge you have decided to tackle, to do it correctly and with intent. No cheating or quitting things half way. Stick with it! Complete your challenge, accumulate your successes and strengthen your inner pride. Wishing you the best of luck!

CASHING YOUR DAILY CHECK

What is your relationship with money?
Do you feel that having a comfortable bank account
is something only accessible to certain people?
Why not decide to change the way you think?

To help you shift your mindset, why not start cashing daily checks?

To start with, decide upon a certain amount of money
you will be receiving on a daily basis.
It's entirely up to you: $20, $50, $100, $500, $1000.
Then ask yourself:
"Am I going to spend or save it?
If I spend it, what for?

There are no right or wrong answers.
You can spend your daily allowance on whatever makes you happy.
You can be totally selfish or generous.
You can splurge on shopping, or save up to buy something
you have always dreamed of.
It's all up to you.

Keep in mind that every day, you will be cashing in that same amount of money.
To keep track of your daily income, write everything down in a little notebook:
those are all of your savings and expenditures.

This moment should be pleasurable and fun.
Keep at it for several weeks and start seeing your relationship with money change.
See yourself prosper.

B&B UNIVERSAL BANK

DATE_____

PAY TO
THE ORDER OF_____ $_____

_____DOLLARS

FOR_____

⑆12345⑈6789⑆   ⑆12345⑈6789⑆

MY NOTES

CHAPTER FOUR

CHANGE THE WAY
YOU WORK AND PLAY

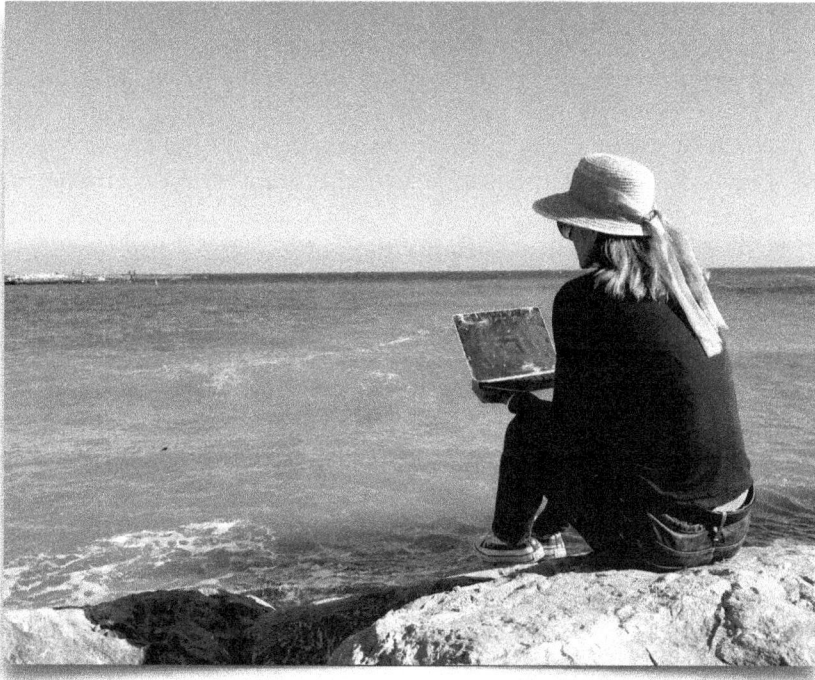

They were just thoughts
that danced through my little head...
life's challenges, could they be Gifts?

When I look back upon my life, I can't help but be amazed at the way certain events have occurred and I can't help but question myself: isn't it incredible how life seems to put on your path precisely what you most need to work on? Have you noticed this in your life? Take a few minutes to reflect upon this. What are your flaws? What are your fears? What, for you, would be really challenging to tackle? Have there not been moments when life knocked at your door to challenge you or offer you opportunities to find yourself face to face with them? How did you react: fight or flight response? Maybe you saw it as a threat, but could it have been that life was offering you a gift, the possibility to grow?

As a child, I was homeschooled. But with my mother's work that took us on the road I wasn't able to study regularly and often found myself reading instead of doing my academic work such as math, science, history or geography. When I went back to school, in 9th grade, I quickly realized the gap between me and the other students and how deficient I was in numerous fields.

I remember clearly my very first day back in 9th grade... school had already started a few weeks before and the day I arrived there was a math test. I stared blankly at the sheet of paper and at all the different questions and exercises. I was totally clueless to what it was all about. So, as I sat there uncomfortably not knowing what to do, I decided to copy the test so that it looked as though I was at least doing something and that I would have something to hand in. The next day, the math teacher came in and returned our copies. At one point, I saw her at her desk folding a piece of paper as if it were a paper plane. She then grabbed it and made it fly through the class in my direction and said: "As for you, Miss Ratkoff. You have nothing to do in my class. You may go to the principal's office." I left the classroom feeling mortified with shame and not being able to utter a single word. The school principle was far more comprehensive and suggested that although they thought the best option was to put me back into 6th grade, they were willing to give me a chance if, and only if, one of the math teachers accepted the challenge to get me up to the mark. I was lucky that one thought it was worth a try. Thank you Monsieur Girault, I still haven't forgotten your name! Somehow, the other math teacher's name seems to have slipped out of my mind!

Still, for years, I often found myself in situations where I had no clue what my friends or teachers were talking about. At first, I would ask questions spontaneously to help me understand, but the mocking and concerned looks on people's faces rapidly taught me to know better. I ended clamming up and became a passive listener not daring to partake in any conversation, fearing that people would see my deficiencies. The library also ended up being my favorite place, since there was no internet at the time! I would look everything up and voraciously study and research in order to fill out the gaps and cross out all the question marks that were buzzing through my head, one at a time.

But how does one fill up years of non-learning? I kept telling myself that as I was catching up on the past, others were learning new things and that I would always be behind. In French there is an expression "toujours avoir un train en retard", translated literally, you are always "catching the next train" I like this expression because it really translates how I felt. I would always be running to try to catch the train: I would be happy to make it on time, but when I would get on board, I couldn't help but notice that the others were already one train ahead. It was so frustrating.

But there is a good thing in all this as it gave me an insatiable thirst to learn and as of today it hasn't been quenched yet. The way I see it, every moment is an opportunity to learn something new. When I hop out of bed every morning I immediately see what little learning challenges lay ahead. What will help me succeed in doing 30 double-unders? I have to check out one or two videos before I head out to the gym. Oh, and I am going to have to do some researching for that idea I am developing in my book? That article I started reading yesterday is really interesting, when can I set a little bit of time to read it today? Oh, that thing I read to clear my mind of negativity, I really have to keep at it, I really feel like it works! I have to make sure that I keep an eye on those insidious thoughts that want to take a control of my mind throughout the day.

Knowing what I have been through, imagine how I felt the day my husband told me he wanted to homeschool *our* children. I looked at him and felt as if time had stopped. I thought he must be out of his mind. After everything I went through, how can he possibly want our kids to live through the same thing?" But even though I had told him about my experience, it was evident that he had no clue of what I had endured. Life is like that. Haven't you noticed? Sometimes I find it easier to feel empathy towards someone when you read what they have gone through. I don't know exactly why it is so. Maybe the lack of dialogue. When we talk to someone, we often have an urge to cut in and give our own experience, whereas when we read we are fully attentive to the writer. My husband was all excited about this idea and all the opportunities, travelling and discovering we were going to offer our kids that we couldn't if they went to regular school. When my husband decided something, there was no way of saying no, because he would go on and on about it, until I quit resisting. And so, we took our kids out of school and started a new adventure. After what I had been through, I saw to it that my boys were studying every day. I had signed them up for a homeschooling program and believe me, if there were 256 pages in the school manual, we did the 256 pages. We homeschooled our boys, eight years our youngest and seven years our eldest, and I made sure they completed the entire program every year.

But when I look at it now, I realize that I did the entire program from kindergarten all the way up to 9th grade almost twice. Life gave me the opportunity to make up for all those years I had not been able to do as a child. Now how strange is that?

Change n°37
GET READY
TO CHANGE JOBS

37.

Embracing change in your life can mean packing your bags and moving to a new city, discovering a new place or going around the world. Embracing change can mean putting your foot down and leaving a useless relationship and finding the strength to start anew. But embracing change can also be changing jobs. Do you like what you are doing? Do you feel you have pretty much learned all there was to learn and it's become a bit of a routine? Do you aspire to take up more challenges, more responsibilities? Do you want to earn more? Do you have a dream job?

What's holding you back? Fear? Security? Lack of self-confidence?
Whatever the reason, if you chose to read change n°37, chances are that this idea has been bubbling up in your mind for a while now. No need to jump into this cold turkey or handing in your resignation without thinking it through. You can very well do this at your own pace and take one step at a time. It all may seem very daunting and you might be wondering "where do I start?" To be able to move forward, you need to know exactly what it is you want. I can't really help you on this one, but once you've decided the direction you wish to take, there are a certain number of things you can do to get things moving. You might want to check out Chapter 1, *Improve Your Self-Esteem,* to find ways to boost yourself up. In this point we will have a look into a very important aspect of changing jobs: preparing your resume or CV and getting ready for your job interview.

A. Getting started

When you really want something, there are different phases you must follow through in order to succeed.

a. Phase ONE: Know what you want

The very first thing to do is to precisely decide what it is that you want. When job searching, start off by writing down exactly what type of job you want. Do you need to take a course to improve certain notions or to become more qualified? In this case, do some research and start exploring what your options are. If you are not sure what you want but aspire to change your job, take the time to write down on a piece of paper what you are good at and what you enjoy doing. Sometimes getting things down on paper can be a real eye opener.
You could start by searching for job openings to see what is on the market. Don't start panicking about the list of qualifications that are required. Look at the job descriptions and start seeing where you qualify. By reading these you will also get ideas for your resume. If this all feels terrifying for you, why not ask a friend to help you look through job search and both of you go over your qualities and qualifications together. When you read adds, many times they use big terms to describe the responsibility a job holds, and they are often difficult to decipher. Research online what these terms mean.

For instance, if a company is searching for a "detail-oriented person" it most likely implies that the person that is hiring is not only looking for someone capable of sending an email without typos, they also want someone capable of managing the details of a complicated event. Indeed, detail-oriented people check, and then double-check their work to ensure flawless execution, meaning that their task is error-free.

If you are applying for a job that requires you to be "detailed-oriented", make sure you manage all the details of your application and are prepared for your interview as both provide a firsthand demonstration of your ability to manage details. Follow all application instructions carefully; have a flawless, typo-free resume and cover letter; it goes without saying that you should show up on time for your interview, with adequate copies of your resume and a professional demeanor.

If you don't really understand what an add is requiring, then research further. It can only help you to be better prepared for the day of the job interview.

b. Phase TWO: Get moving!

The second step to reaching a goal is to actually start moving, literally get up off the couch, to reach this goal.

To clear things up for you: the first phase *"knowing what you want"* means having a clear idea of what you want and getting your resume ready is a great way to start. Phase two implies that you get up and move: you want to start improving your appearance, researching for jobs on line and actually go to job interviews. Because, once your resume is done and you start booking appointments, you know your door is opening to change!

B. Why is your resume important? What's the purpose of a resume anyway?

When you are getting a resume ready, you have to view it as a way of promoting yourself, as if you were sending off your very own advertisement. That's right, in a way you are selling yourself. Don't forget that a professional recruiter can tell within seconds whether your resume is worth looking at or not. So, your goal is to be able to capture the recruiter's attention and convince them that they should definitely call you for an interview.

So, in order to stand out, read below and see what you can do to make sure that 1) you send the best resume and 2) that you are ready for your interviews.

a. Getting your resume ready

The first impression is of utmost importance: your resume must look professional, spotless and must be easy to read. This goes without saying but unfortunately, I have to mention it since I have received resumes that were stained, or a little crumpled. You want your future employer to be able to glean the information they are looking for in a few quick glances. For this reason, it is important to put some effort into it. Here are a few tips to help you:

1. Importance of the consistency of your presentation:

- **Fonts**: use the same font for your entire resume and choose amid the most popular choices: such as, Times new roman or Arial. If you want to showcase certain parts use italics, boldface, capital letters or different font size, but stick to the same font. For the major part of your resume use size 12.

You don't want it to be too small making it hard to read or too big making it look like you don't have much to offer and that you are just trying to fill out the space. Avoid putting too much color, smart art or shapes. Your goal is to attract the employer's attention.

- **Photo**: No need for it and I would avoid it unless it is required. Statistics show that it diminishes your chances of getting the job. If you do however choose to put one, make sure you look professional and confident.

- **Headlining**: make sure you use the same headline presentation for each section, for importance of consistency, and that each one of them is to the point and puts emphasis on what needs to be featured.

- **Length**: importance of being concise and succinct. Normally one page should be enough but if you have more than 10 to 15 years experience, two pages might be necessary.

- **Spelling/grammar** errors are unacceptable: If you are not sure about the spelling or grammar, have it corrected. Reread your resume several times to avoid typos.

- **Format:** you want to have the same spacing all around the resume, for example a 1-inch margin all around the edges looks nice.

- **Personal information:** Write down your name, address, phone number and email. Please note that your age, religion, marital status and political affiliation should not be included and are illegal questions for an employer to ask.

- **Order:** List your most recent experiences first and work your way down. Write your current or last job at the top and finish your resume with your very first job. It is not necessary to write every single job that you have done. Your goal is to highlight the jobs that are relevant to the one you are applying to.

- **Make it airy:** if you want your resume to look professional it needs to be airy and pleasant to read. I know it contains a lot of information but it's really important to leave a little bit of white space. If your resume looks crammed, it is challenging to read through.

- **Bullets vs paragraphs:** Bullets make your resume a lot easier to browse through then reading through a thick paragraph. Break it down and put only what's essential.

- **Acronyms**: Make sure your employer knows what they stand for. Save them time having to look them up. If in doubt, and even if it takes up quite some space, write out the whole name.

- **Dates**: don't put them on the forefront. Most resumes start with the date and then have the company name or position. Write down what is really important first: your Title/position, then your employer's name/name of company, followed up with the city and finally the date. Concerning your education, write the name of your degrees, what schools and university you attended and where, by adding the city/country.

If you are not sure, get some help, and have your resume done professionally. You can also check out software or apps that offer pre-formatted designs.

2. What to include and what not

Compose a general resume that has all of your job experiences, a detailed description of your education, your life experiences as well as qualifications. Once you want to apply for a particular job, simply delete what is not relevant and try to modify or add elements that will match the job description. The goal is to demonstrate that your past experiences will help you in your future job. Make sure you do your research online about the company and its competition. Really take the time to look at the job description in detail: understand precisely what they are looking for and how you could show them that you are qualified to do it.

- What to include:
Copies of diplomas and certifications, to prove your level of education, past employment experiences, documents proving any skills acquired in domains relevant to job you are applying for such as language, computer skills, accounting etc.

One of the most important things is to tailor your resume to the job you are applying to. Some people tend to think that a resume is a "one fits all" document but it is far from being the case. Take the time to scrutinize the job add you are responding to and highlight keywords as they might help you understand exactly what they are looking for. If the job requires certain skills, make sure you add them into your resume. Next, write these words down and see what you have done in the past that shows you have the qualities and qualifications they are looking for. Make sure to present your resume in a way to make them want to read on and call you for an interview.
An idea could be to look up the qualities that are needed in your area of expertise whether it is marketing, finance, music, acting. Have a look online and then explore ways to show that you have these qualities.
Ask yourself the right questions: What is your employer looking for? What can you bring to the company? How you can contribute? Find the answers to these questions and showcase them in your resume. Let your future employer know that you are the one they are looking for! Impress them with your achievements and qualities.

- Remember to add the following:
Your CCAs, co-curricular activities. No need to write a whole paragraph; one line is enough. Show how this activity can be of help for the job you are applying to.
Your skills: can you speak several languages, do you excel at something in particular, such as presentations, computers, writing articles, translation. Let your future employer know.
Computer: one line is enough to let them know which programs you master.
Life experiences are as important as any job experience! Have you done something out of the ordinary, that required your personal investment, willpower, determination, courage. Let them know!

- What if your resume is a little too long?
So, your resume is finished and you notice that it takes up 1 whole page and 2 or 3 lines on the second page. If this is your case, then you have to find a way to make it fit on a single page. Read below to find a few tips to achieve just that:
• Reduce the font size by 0,5 or 1
• Reduce the margins
• Reduce the space between lines
• Don't skip as many lines
• Cut out elements such as meaningless jobs, personal information, too much information but also jobs that are not relevant to position
• Remove unnecessary words such as "a", "and", "the" etc.

- What words to use and which ones not to:
Look online to see what words are best suited for a resume, such as achieved, managed, resolved... and which ones need to be avoided.

C. Getting ready for your job interview

Below you will find a list of things you can do to be ready and more self-confident for your job interview:

a. Pamper yourself

Prior to the job interview, take some time to exercise, relax, do yoga, meditate, walk, visit a spa, get your hair done, have a facial, get enough sleep, see your fun friends, watch a funny movie, go to your favorite restaurant, visit places you love, see or call your parents if they are supportive. Some people might like the idea of a friend coming along in order to help keep a calm mind or ease the whole process. Others will prefer some alone time to help center themselves. I have done both. I have a preference for going alone but have to admit that having my friend waiting for me outside after a job interview was really helpful. Afterwards, we went for a coffee and talked about the interview, laughed and it really helped me put things back into perspective. It's not something I would have done naturally, but I have to admit that I felt a confidence boost and had fewer questions flowing through my mind since I had discussed them with my friend.

b. Do your research

Before going to your interview, it's important that you do your research. The first thing to do is to check out the company's website, but, clearly, that is not enough. You want to be on top of the latest information regarding their current situation, their competitors. You want to know what the market is like and how exactly you can contribute. How can your past experiences, your KSAs - knowledge, skills and abilities- help you land this job?

c. Dress appropriately

Make sure you dress according to the company you are applying to. Try to find out beforehand what the dress code is. If you do not know what to wear, your best bet is to stick with a classical look: avoid too many colors (I call it the Christmas tree look), too much makeup, wearing too much jewelry, revealing too much cleavage or heals that are too high. What's important is to look professional, confident and comfortable in your own shoes.

d. Posture

It is essential, when you walk in, that you stand tall, maintain eye contact and give a firm handshake. In my case, I always give a firm handshake, but some people think it's a good idea to try to match your employer's grip. Whatever you choose to do, don't make it too soft, you want to show that you are interested and happy to be there. Once you are seated, sit tall, have an open posture, believe in yourself, maintain eye contact to show that you are interested and keep a firm attitude. What you really want to avoid is slumping down in the chair, fidgeting, playing with something and looking around the room while your interlocutor is speaking. If you feel stressed or are feeling uncomfortable, remember to BREATHE and sit up straight: these two simple adjustments in your attitude can help you feel stronger and appear more self-confident.

e. Language

Remember, it's the whole attitude that is essential: your posture of course, but also what you say and how you say it, your intonation, your facial expressions. In regards to your voice, make sure you speak loud enough to be heard and that you articulate properly. Sitting tall and talking distinctly can really help convey an image of confidence to your interlocutor. Be careful not to use any slang words and that you speak appropriately and with consideration, which means NO racial, religious or sexist comments.

It's important to speak, but it is just as important to know when to listen and to pay attention to what your interviewer is saying. And please, don't interrupt! As much as possible, try to see the interview as a dialogue which means that both of you should be able to speak and have a real exchange. Let the interviewer express himself, and when it's your turn just make sure you stay low profile and don't talk too much so as to drown the interview with unnecessary blabber. Try to keep the conversation going.

Another important issue is when talking about your previous employer: don't bad mouth them and avoid telling any lies, especially if you were fired or left under bad circumstances. You are not here to settle accounts, but to sell yourself. Criticizing your previous employer will only make you lose credibility.

f. Remember

Your interviewer is a human being just like you, so put yourself in their shoes. How would you feel if you were interviewing people all day? What kind of person would YOU like to have in front of you? Do you want a frightened, nervous, anxious, jittery person or would you rather have an open, natural, smiling, positive person that looks comfortable and at ease? Would you like to meet someone who is boasting and bragging about everything they have accomplished or would you rather have someone who is interested and attentive? It's important to build rapport with the person in front of you.

g. Be prepared

One thing I believe that you should take the time to look into are the top job interview questions. Even if they don't come up, taking the time to answer them before, might really help you situate yourself and get prepared for the job interview.

h. Meditate

Interviews are stressful, so it might be a good idea to take the time beforehand to relax. What better way to de-stress than to meditate or visualize. Meditating will help you achieve a relaxed state of mind. Visualizing will allow you to see yourself in a successful situation: reach a relaxed state and imagine the interview going smoothly.

List of most common questions:

1. **Tell me about yourself.** This question is *very* vague and could take hours to answer. That's why it's a good idea to prepare your answer beforehand. For this type of question, you want to focus on your professional background and experience and not your personal life. How did you get into the business? Are you passionate about what you do? Explain why and then bring the conversation to why you have applied for this job and how you believe you can contribute to the company.

2. **Why should we hire you?** Tell them how your experience and knowledge can contribute to the company.

3. **What are your greatest strengths and weaknesses?** Don't enumerate them. Choose one strength and one weakness and explain how your strength has helped you in the past and how you overcame your weakness or what lesson you learned from it.

4. **Why do you want to work for us?** This is where you can show you have done a bit of   research. Don't spill everything you know about the company, but sparkle your answer with what you know.

5. **Why did you leave your last job?** Just remember that they can call you ex-employer, so stick as close as possible to the truth. If things went wrong, it's not the time or the place to start complaining about it. Prepare your answer ahead of time and try to turn it to your advantage. Perhaps it became a bit of a routine and you weren't learning or growing anymore. You really saw this as a sign that you had to move on.

6. **What is your biggest accomplishment?** This is precisely the type of question that is really necessary to prepare for beforehand. The last thing you want is to find yourself with no answer at all. Not everyone has accomplished something. If you have, perfect! But if you haven't, try to remember a time when you were going through a challenging moment and tell them how you overcame it.

7. **Where do you see yourself in 5 or 10 years from now?** Where *DO* you want to see yourself in 5 or 10 years? Take the time to think it through and write it down. If you really want this job and hope to stay there for a while, try to find ways to match what you want with what the company has to offer.

8. **Do you have any questions?** This question usually comes at the end of the interview. Most people seem to automatically reply that they have no questions which is not a good idea because it will seem as though you are not interested. Avoid asking about bonuses, advantages, holidays at this point. Your goal here is to show the interviewer that the job interests you. You need to ask some relevant questions about the position, such as what do they expect from you and what can you expect to attain in the years to come.

i. Believe

If you are good at what you do, or if you feel you are a trustworthy person, that your future employer can count on, and if you are proud of everything you have achieved, then there is no reason why you shouldn't feel confident during the interview. Try to act as if your life doesn't depend on this job, so you don't appear desperate. If this doesn't work out, well something else will. Not everything is within your control. And even if you are not hired, it doesn't mean you were not competent. It simply means that somebody else had a little extra something. If you know what was lacking, try to make sure you work on that aspect before the next interview. Make each interview a moment that allows you to grow and enrich your life for the future.

After the interview, it might be a good idea to thank the company and interviewer for their time by sending them a follow up letter and seize the opportunity to tell them how interested you are in getting this job. The idea is to go over the interview and tell them what you think the job consists of, and how you believe you can be a positive contributor to the company.

Be 200% present. If you want to succeed you have to learn to invest yourself completely. You are going to a job interview. This event could change your life around, so give it your all: be fully present, prepare for it, arrive with a determined mind and the conviction that you too can do it. Face your interviewer and show them with your positive and strong attitude that you want this job, and you believe that you have what it takes. Try to keep in mind that no one is superior to you, or inferior for that matter and that the person in front of you is your equal. The outcome of this appointment is greatly determined by what you are going to say and do.

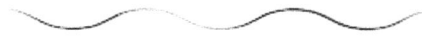

Change n°38
BACK TO SCHOOL

38.

So, what's your story? What is your dream? Did you quit high school or college? Is your lack of diplomas impeding you from moving forward? Going back to school isn't as complicated as it may seem, it just requires a little bit of research and some programming. As the saying goes:

> ### How do you eat an elephant?
> ### One bite at a time...

Don't look at the whole picture or it will just frighten or even terrorize you. It's better to break this goal into small achievable goals and begin tackling them one at a time.

Just like when I started writing this book and was researching for what needed to be done. I found an online course on how to get a book published. As I followed this course and started realizing what publishing really required, I would sometimes stop and look at the list of things required and tell myself: "This is impossible. I can't do it all!" To name only a few: writing a book proposal which required a lot of research, finding someone to edit the book…where would I start? Getting the cover of my book done by a professional… who do I turn to for this? Creating a platform? Publishing houses require you to have a certain number of social media followers that could potentially buy your book. I needed a minimum of 5000 followers and I had 160!!!! The list seemed endless and impossible to attain and when I really stopped to think about it, the whole thing would throw me into a panic. But, I would take one look at my book and would tell myself: "All the way. I am doing this no matter what. It might not lead to anything, but I am going to give it my best shot." I followed through the whole course taking notes. I started asking around for book editors and found three different ones! The online course proposed solutions for my book cover and my son took control of my Instagram account: within one month I already had 1000 followers. One step at a time, things that seemed insurmountable, were slowly finding their way and I started seeing that the impossible was something I could achieve. Let me tell you something: I don't have any super powers and I most certainly am not smarter than most. If *I* can do it, then, believe me, you can too. If my book can help some of you reach your dreams then I will have achieved my ultimate purpose.

In this change I propose to go back to school. I chose nutrition as an example, but you can very well choose any other subject of interest. What are you passionate about? What have you always dreamed of becoming? What are you waiting for? Come on, grab my hand, let's take a few steps together and then off you go, take the leap.

A. Start with a little leap
a. Webinars, seminars, retreats and conferences
Maybe you are hesitating and are wondering if this is for you. In that case, *the first step*, before getting started, might be to **get away for a few days and take a** *short* **course**. There are many different choices. You could also look into food and nutrition seminars that are coming to your city. There are also a variety of Webinars - online seminars - that you could look into as well.

I live in Monaco and there are several weekly retreats nearby where you can learn how to choose foods, cook them, and eat them mindfully. The retreat proposes yoga, long walks in nature, meditation and some alone time. Of course, this might be something totally impossible if you have children, but if you research a bit you can also find some retreats that accept children and propose healthy activities for them as well, so you know they are busy while you are taking your course. If budget and time are your concern, there are weekend or one day getaways. You often have to share a room so it might be a good idea to get away with a good friend unless you enjoy meeting new people and are not worried about sharing a room with a complete stranger!

These getaways, seminars and webinars are amazing for getting you all revved up and motivated. After completion, you will be boosted and in the mood to learn more about nutrition and health, or whatever topic you are interested in.

b. Take a home study course
If time is an issue, you can also take a home study course. There are numerous options to choose from. For your first challenge, it might be best to find a relatively easy and short course. It's important to do things gradually and not to set yourself up for failure. Make this goal fun and interesting but also a little bit challenging. If this experience is positive, set yourself a new one later on that is a little more difficult. Baby steps is the key. So, start easy and move forward gradually.

What's great about this goal is that if you take it seriously, at the end, you get a diploma proving that you are more knowledgeable in this field. Now that's a wonderful way to reward yourself for all your hard work!

c. A college course
That's a great idea! If you are interested in food and healthy eating and wish to become more knowledgeable in this domain, you will find many courses out there and it might be interesting to meet new people who share the same interest as you. It may seem daunting at first, but taking a course as an adult is completely different from when you were back in high school or University. The most important thing is to remember that you are doing this for yourself with only one objective: to expand your knowledge and learn. You will not be accountable to anybody, no results are really required: this is between you and yourself. So, if you fail the test, no stress, no worries… but then go for it a second time.

d. Ready for the big leap!

<u>1. Choose a course:</u>

Do it wisely and see what works best for you depending on:

- the time you have
- your level of education
- what you really are interested in. For example, is it learning about healthy foods and making healthy choices or is it more the psychology behind eating and how to manage weight?
- the money you are willing to invest

<u>2. Set a date!</u>

Make sure you choose a test date that will give you a reasonable amount of time to study all the material. Don't put too much pressure on yourself. What I normally do is count the total amount of pages from the different books I am required to read. I see how many pages I am able to read in one day. Then, I simply divide the total number of pages by the number of pages I can read in one day to obtain the number of days that will be necessary to complete the whole course… then I double that time to be able to read it all a second time. When calculating, remember, that you might only be able to study 2, 3 or 4 times a week. I highly recommend to put in less time, but work at it every day - the ideal being 1 h – 1h ½ a day on most days of the week – however, we all know that "life" very often gets in the way…

If you only have a few time slots available to study, don't let it discourage you: that's fine as well. What really counts is consistency. If you work regularly, in the long run, it will all add up and can only lead to success.

<u>3. Get organized and plan your way to success!</u>

The biggest part in attaining a goal is to make a plan. It's very important to take the time to sit down and see when you are available throughout the week. Write down all the time slots even if it there are only a few. Draw a time schedule of your entire week or month and add in some study slots…and stick to it. If you have an agenda or if you keep your appointments on your phone, cross those slots out. If you are still dubious about planning ahead, please read the following two reasons why you should:

- First you are creating intent. By blocking out these time slots, you're getting your mind ready to sit down and study.
- Second, if you don't block these slots out, once you are back to your usual routine, there is a likely chance that you will forget about your resolution. Give yourself the opportunity to succeed: believe me, planning ahead is by far the most important one!

Try to establish a time schedule that works for you, write or print it out and post it somewhere so you can see it, as a reminder. And don't be too hard on yourself: if at one point you don't study for a few days, just get back on track. There *will* be ups and downs and it's totally normal. Accept it and get back to it.

People tend to think that the path to success is a straight line where you go from point A to point B. But that's not the case at all: it's a line that may be straight at first when you are highly motivated but then life gets in the way.

You may get busy with spouse, kids, daily chores, moods, lack in motivation… and the line starts to get crocked and bumpy. That's when it's important to know that this happens to everyone. It's at this point, that you decide whether that line will keep going, or come to a stop. Just hang in there! Who cares if it's "zig-zaggy", or even turns into a dotted line! What matters is that it's still a line that's going somewhere. And I promise you that if you keep at it, you will no longer be going to some random place, you will be making your way towards SUCCESS.

4. Prioritize

If you want to reach a goal, you must set some priorities. What this usually implies is that you are going to be saying "no" more often to friends, family and to certain activities. It might be a good thing to start off talking to your family and friends and letting them know about your new goal and that they can really help you by being supportive. They can also alleviate the burden by doing some of the chores you normally do or simply by respecting the time slot you have set aside to study. For example, you can't be disturbed, interrupted or called within a certain time frame, and they won't make you feel guilty if you do not partake in certain activities or are not available.

5. My story
Blaming the outside world

While writing this book, getting organized and prioritizing turned out to be the most challenging aspect of it all. I was mentally highly motivated, but it seemed as though the people around me had no respect whatsoever for the new goal I had set myself. I had to beg over and over again not to be disturbed. Despite the fact that I made it clear to everyone that my mornings were reserved for my book, my spouse, kids and friends always interrupted me for one matter or another or called and texted me proposing activities exactly at that time. It was really annoying and I found myself repeatedly saying "no" and constantly feeling guilty about it. Even after really putting my foot down several times, things were not getting any better. I tried working my way around it, turning off my phone, getting up earlier in the morning, organizing appointments after 12:30, but somehow something always seemed to challenge me.

Cancer : the wake up call and learning to let go

It's at this very moment in time, as I was struggling to write my book, that I was diagnosed with cancer, which was a big blow, and that my husband and I filed for divorce. It seemed as though I was going in and out of doctor's and lawyer's appointments all the time. And as if that wasn't enough, all these thoughts started to gather in my head making it really, *really* challenging to sit down and work on my book. At this point, I couldn't help thinking that it was a sign trying to tell me that I was wasting my time and that I should quit. I wondered "Why is everything going against me?" But deep down inside, I never stopped believing; I felt that my book could help a lot of people and that I *had* to write it. In a way, it was as if I had been assigned a mission and I had to go through with it, all the way.
It dawned upon me that these challenges were there for a purpose: maybe in fact they weren't there to bring me down, but on the contrary, to strengthen my willpower and determination, and prove to me that I could move forward with my writing no matter what. One thing became clear: this book meant the world to me and no one was going to stop me.

Although being diagnosed with cancer may seem the worst possible thing that could have happened to me, it ended up being just what I needed. Everyone around me was concerned about my well-being and started offering help. I was sincerely touched by how much people really cared and were willing to make an effort for me. I decided to focus on "quietness", "me time", long walks, laughing with my friends and meditation. When I needed to be alone, I took the time and went off to Planet Café, where you can get the best ristretto doppio coffee in Monte-Carlo. And so, when things started to settle down in my head and I felt able to concentrate once again, it seemed quite clear that what could really help me get my mind off my cancer, would be writing my book. I found so much joy in the whole writing process and each day, one paragraph at a time, I felt a sense of accomplishment that was so gratifying!

And so, I decided to stop making excuses and blaming others for not being able to move forward. I actually opted to go with the flow and accepted to let them interrupt and text me. By now my determination was undeterrable. I accepted the fact that it was going to be a longer process than I had previously expected, but you know what? That wasn't such a big deal after all. Cancer had given me one important lesson: to stop fighting and let go.

Observing others: finding a role model
After my last radiotherapy session and my divorce underway, it was urgent to get a job. I was fortunate enough to get hired by an important businessman in Monaco. Working for him and observing him was an eye opener for me, as well. To see, day in and day out, the amount of work he could pull off by the hour was a real lesson to me: he didn't find any excuses, he just went right down to business!
And so, I questioned my own ability to get things done and at one point I told myself: BB, stop the bullshit and just get to work! He is often a good reminder to stop beating about the bush and to simply get things done. Is there someone near you who could be a source of inspiration? Observe them. And remember something: if they can do it, well then you are more than likely capable of doing it too!

Going back to school will most definitely be challenging, and there *will* be some ups and downs. That's when Belief and Persistency are the best empowering tools to have around: they will both keep you going and pull you forward.

Change n°39
TALK AND LISTEN

39.

You are probably wondering: why would anyone want to change the way they talk? You may not be aware of it, but the words you use and the way you talk are essential and can make a big difference on how people perceive you.

A. Increasing and Improving Your Vocabulary

The first thing that might be interesting to look into, when it comes to the way you speak, is enriching your vocabulary. Did you know that the average person knows approximately 10,000 words but typically only uses around 2000 on a daily basis?

Just to compare, a college educated English teacher uses approximately 15,000 to 20,000 words! Now, your goal might not be to reach that many, but you could gain a lot by making your sentences more to the point.

Your purpose is not to learn very complicated words and show them off; if your interlocutor doesn't understand you, you will only come across as being pompous and this simply doesn't make any sense… Why do we talk in the first place? We talk in order to communicate and for others to understand us.

It would, however, make a world of a difference if you could express *exactly* what you are trying to say. People will perceive you as smart and witty. So why not try to increase the number of words you use thus improving the quality of your speech.

To expand the number of words you use, there are quite a few things you can do. Below, you will find a few suggestions:

a. Read More

Get into the habit of reading every opportunity you get. You could start off reading the newspaper every day. It is a good idea to write down not only the new words you have learned, but also words that you already know, but seldom use. In this way you create a kind of "bank of words", a rich vocabulary. The best way to understand a word is to use it in a sentence. Try to write two sentences using your new word and then find opportunities throughout the day to use them.

b. Try exercise books

There are also exercise books that can really help you to increase your "word bank". I really recommend the books listed in my References section of the book. I have personally used them with my son. It was fun and creative and taught us how to decompose a word in order to understand it. These books also taught us the origins – etymology - of each word.

c. Take lessons: Find a Voice and Speech Coach!

Learn how to talk. Why don't you make an appointment with a **"Voice and Speech Coach."** This professional will teach you how to develop your vocal strength, breathe properly for an improved flow of speech and help you find added confidence when you are interacting with others.

d. How-to or self-help books

If the cost is an issue, there are amazing books that can really explain to you what to do in order to be more confident while speaking. Once again check the References section of the book for recommended readings. Indeed, speaking goes hand in hand with listening. If you want to get people to like you, listen to what they have to say with real interest and they will be telling everyone what a fantastic person you are!

You could also make a list of all the topics you are interested in and improve the way you talk about them. This requires you to practice by choosing one topic or a related word and to talk about it for 60 seconds.

Have fun practicing regularly and each time try to add more vocabulary: add new words that are more precise and to the point.

e. Use Images To help Express What You Have To Say

Ever heard of the expression "a picture is worth 1000 words"? Try using more vivid imagery to express what you have to say as people relate more to images than to words.

For example: "When I spoke in public I really wanted to be at ease and communicate my enthusiasm to the people that were around me. Instead, I felt lost. I like to use the image of a pebble. I was a pebble lost in the midst of thousands of other pebbles. That's really how I felt. And then one day, life, like a wave, hit me in the face and it got me rolling, thinking and wondering. It was my wake-up call. I realized then that I had so much potential, so much to look forward to. Today I can say that I *ROCK* in life!"

I could also have simply said it the following way: "I wanted to succeed, but I was scared. One day it hit me that I had so much potential."

I believe using imagery livens the whole picture I am trying to convey! What do you think?

B. Improve the way you speak in public
a. Take a course or look online to learn how to speak in public.

Now, this might not be your goal and let's make things clear, sharing a conversation with a few people is not at all the same thing as taking up the floor and speaking in front of a big crowd. However, you might learn from watching videos or watching other people give speeches in real time: keep your eyes open for attitude, hand and arm gestures, and the way they talk: Do they articulate? Do they speak loud and clear? Is their voice warm? Are they smiling? What makes you want to keep on listening to them?

As you may have understood, talking isn't just talking. You have to BE present. When talking, make sure the person in front of you understands you, speak loud enough and articulate. Equally important is to know when to pause. Every once in a while, take a moment to breathe and then go on. Some people are hesitant to pause, because they fear their interlocutor will interrupt them and not allow them to finish what they were trying to say.

I have a tendency to speak too fast. However, it is not because I fear being interrupted. I tend to speak quickly because I want to hand over the conversation. I do not like being the center of attention, so I will literally pour out everything I have to say, to give the floor to somebody else.

Whether you believe it or not, the way you speak tells a lot about you. Someone shy might speak in a low imperceptible tone of voice, and someone who is knowledgeable, on the contrary, will have a more passionate, vivid way of speaking. Someone who speaks in a slow and articulate way, with clarity and a smile on their face, will come off as confident, there is no doubt about that! So, observe yourself: How do you talk? What is the way you speak, telling others about you?

b. Take acting lessons

There is so much more to acting, than just simply standing up on stage and reciting your lines. Check out below a list of the many benefits of attending an acting class:

- Build your self-confidence in ways you cannot even imagine
- Get to know yourself better and how you react in different situations, what you are capable of doing or where your limit stands
- Through teamwork, learn to be more supportive of others and see how your or someone else's attitude, can affect an entire group
- Learn to accept having other people look at you and probably judge you
- Learn how to express things that you have been holding on to, inside. Many of us tend to bottle up what we feel. When acting, you are forced to express these emotions. It might help you in the future to find the courage to express how YOU feel in your own personal life
- Overcome your fear of taking the floor. This can help you in a number of areas: job interviews, oral exams, talking to a stranger, when you wish to go up to someone you like, going to an audition…
- Learn about your body language and how it expresses itself. See how an incline of the head can mean one thing and silence can mean another. See how crossing your arms can come across as aggressive or defensive and standing very close to someone you are talking to, can be invasive and uncomfortable.
- Notice how people understand you better and discover different ways of getting your message through to others thanks to repetition, diction exercises, working on your intonation and discovering the use of your body language

c. Film Yourself

A good idea would be to have someone film you while you are talking in order to listen to yourself afterwards. You probably won't like your voice and many other things, but just keep practicing and you will get past this awkwardness. Try to focus on your ability to talk about a certain subject. And why not ask the person filming you what they are passionate about and listen to what they have to say about it. First of all, you would be taking the focus off yourself so you will eliminate the stress and you might just learn something new and increase your knowledge about a topic you know nothing about.
You might want to look online and view various videos of people talking. Observe them, scrutinize their attitudes, listen to their intonations, pay attention to their vocabulary and learn!

d. Visualizing and Affirming

Visualize yourself in public, speaking in a confident way. Affirm throughout the day, how confident you are speaking in front of other people. Indeed, visualizing and the use of affirmations can do wonders to prepare you. It's a good idea to take the time, quietly in your own home, to practice visualization and see yourself feeling comfortable, talking nonchalantly amid a crowd of people. This will help you the day you actually find yourself in such a situation. I love a technique in which you visualize yourself successfully doing or having what you wish. Simply place the image inside a dandelion seed or on a cloud and watch your wish fly away and trust the Universe to make things happen. Then during the day, if you have created a P.E.T., a Personal Empowering Tape listen to it or else repeat an affirmation. Both are real boosters when it comes to improving your self-confidence. Check out Change n° 05: *Create Your Very Own* P.E.T. for more details. You can either download one from my website or create your very own from scratch. You might want to check out Change n° 18, *Visualize*.

Below are a few affirmations you might want to try, but remember that an affirmation is something personal so try as much as possible to create your very own that reflects what YOU think, need and believe.

"When I speak, my words flow out easily and I radiate self-confidence."
"I speak with confidence and ease!"
"I listen attentively and I speak with ease!"
"I take my time. I stop, breathe and choose my words wisely."

e. Quit swear words, or what my son, Diego calls "Rage words", for good!

There is nothing worse than seeing someone who looks charming, but whose language is vulgar. Decide, this very instant, to never, ever say a swear word again! Observe yourself and make a list of the words you habitually use and try to find substitutes for them that you can quickly replace with, in case your tongue twitches. A classical example is to replace "shit" with "shoot" and "f***" with "fudge". But in the long run it would be better to get rid of these substitutes as well. Try to find one line that manifests your anger or the fact that you are aggravated, and use it. Make it your signature and decide that from now on, not one single swear word will come out of that mouth of yours. Examples: what or where on Earth…? How is that even possible? This cannot be happening to me? Incredible! Instead of saying "f*** you" just say: "I refuse to put up with this", or "Oh please!"

Here you will find a list of common swear words and some alternatives! Ok! I have to admit some are hilarious!
- **Asshole:** Ashcan, ashcake, hasbeen,
- **Bastard:** Bogus! Bad Word!
- **Bullocks:** bullfrog!
- **Bloody hell:** Bad word! Blimey!
- **Bullshit:** baloney! bull spit! bullfrog! Bb Sanders!
- **Cunt:** kitty whiskers!
- **Damn:** Darn! Drat! Dang!
- **Dickhead:** Dead hick!

- **F***:** Freak! Fudge! Fiddlesticks! Phooey!
- **F*** you!:** Yuck Fou! Pluck it!
- **God damn:** Good night! (not sure about this one!)
- **Holy shit:** Holy cow! Holy guacamole! Hot Diggity!
- **Jesus:** Gee whiz! Golly! Jinkies! Cheese Whiz! Chiz!
- **Mother F*****:** Milk and Cookies! (really???) Mother smucker!
- **Oh my god!** Oh my goodness! oh my gosh! Golly! Gee whiz! Oh my Stars! Oh Man! Oh dear!
- **Piss off:** get lost! Sip off!
- **Shit:** shoot! shaitz! Six and two is eight! Shucks! Sugar! Sweet peas! Sugar puffs! Chiz!
- **Shut up!:** Shut the front door!
- **Son of a bitch:** Son of a gun! Son of a bucket! Son of a biscuit! Son of a monkey! Sufferin' Soketash!

Other alternatives: for crying out loud! Peanut butter and Jelly! For Pete's sake!

C. Improve your listening skills

In order to improve the way you talk, it's important to understand that a big part of talking involves listening. Sometimes our conversations are casual and we are there just to chat and exchange anecdotes, but at other times a friend, a co-worker, our special someone, our children have something that's weighing them down and are in need of a kind ear and some advice or a form of comfort. It's often like a confession and just by being there and listening relieves them of the burden that is weighing on their chest. The fact that someone who cares is there, willing to listen and allowing them to express their sadness, their anger, to admit their mistakes or simply to express their opinion, can go a long way in helping them feel really good about themselves. You can, without expressing a single word, simply with your presence and sincerity make someone feel understood. So, read on as I explain to you the importance of listening and also how to become a good listener.

a. Why improve your listening skills?

Just to get you motivated, I am listing a few reasons why you should improve your listening skills:

- You will allow the speaker to express everything they have to say
- You will make fewer mistakes.
- You will get higher grades and will need less time to study because you will actually remember more
- People will appreciate you more if you let them have the spotlight. You will come out as being a sensitive person, someone who authentically cares
- You will make the speaker feel like they are important
- Your overall understanding of what people are saying will improve
- It can be really annoying to have someone constantly interrupting you or speaking to someone who isn't really listening or is fidgety

b. How to become a good listener

Most people can be classified as "average listeners" but you can develop this skill to become an "amazing listener." Decide that from now on, that's how you are going to be. Below are a few tips to help you. Keep in mind that nothing beats sincerity, an honest and true desire to listen to what others have to say.

- **Be more present**. This means you will have to turn off your phone, ignore everything and the people around you and give your interlocutor your undivided attention.
- **Check your attitude:** are you looking the other person in the eyes? How are you holding your arms? Are they crossed in front of you or are they relaxed? What about your body, is it turned in their direction or turned away? And finally, your legs, are they crossed in the direction of your interlocutor or away from them? You want to show that you are open to listening and that you care. So, as much as possible, face them.
- **Please don't interrupt.** Let the person finish their sentence and while they are talking, focus on what they are saying, and not on what *you* have to say next.
- **Empathize.** Listening means empathizing and putting yourself in the other person's shoes. Try to really understand what they are going through as much as possible and without judging.
- **Become an observer.** Throughout the day, spend some time silently observing what is going on around you. Observe people, their attitudes, the way they talk, and their facial expressions. Learn to read between the lines. Observe your interlocutor's body language as well. What is their face and body expressing? And what about their tone. A person can be saying one thing, while their body is revealing the complete opposite. With practice you will see that a lot of information will come from the body parts that don't do the talking.

c. Be real. It's not an easy task to stay silent and focus all your attention on one person. At first, you might feel impatient or fidgety. This is normal but just remember, the speaker sees these signs as well. Try to have a reassuring and interested look on your face.
- If you do partake in the conversation, make sure you **don't bring everything back to you**. Why is it that we systematically need to share our own experience all the time? Let the speaker have his moment and allow them to be the center of attention.
- Once you got the speaker talking, **encourage** them to go on and say everything they have to say. You can achieve this by using certain words like: "go on", "yes", "uh huh".
- **No moralizing please** or trying to show that you know what's best or worse for them, as if you know it all. Sometimes people simply need to be heard. And remember we are all different: what may seem daunting to someone, might not be for you; if they are devastated, you both haven't had the same life, so there is no way you can know for sure what they are feeling exactly.
- **Accept blanks.** If your interlocutor has stopped talking and you see they are collecting their thoughts or searching for the correct word, allow this moment of silence between the two of you. You might want to encourage your interlocutor with a smile or an encouraging attitude.
- **Don't be defensive.** The speaker is talking about what THEY feel. You don't necessarily see eye to eye. But they don't have to see things YOUR way. Put your weapons down, breathe and accept the fact that this person in front of you is not you.
- To finish, you might want to **call and check on the person** in the next few days just to see how they are doing and to show that you really care.

Talking and listening go hand in hand. If I had to sum this change up in a few words, I would tell you to slow down, take your time when you speak, but also make some time to really listen to others as well. In this fast-paced world, it's essential to step back a bit and learn to focus, observe, calm down and be present.

Change n°40
YOUR CONVERSATION 40.

Are you the type of person that always feels awkward or out of place in a crowd? I know I always have and still do. I have often watched other people and admired how at ease they were amidst a crowd: it looked like second nature to them. Is it innate or is it something that one can learn? Although I am sure some people are naturally gifted, there are things that you can do to improve your social qualities. And although I will always consider myself as a quiet, reserved, and private kind of person, over time I have learned different little tools that have enabled me to open up a bit more and feel more confident when surrounded by people.

Find a list of things that you too can do to open yourself up to the world and get your conversation going.

1. Practice Makes Perfect

The most important way is probably to get out there and start talking. Practice, practice, practice, because practice makes perfect. If you are alone, start going out and observing others. Observation is a great way to learn. Look at people's attitude while talking, listen to what they are saying and how they express themselves. Compare them, those who look ill at ease and those who look like they are rocking it. What makes one look awkward and what elements make another come out as being so self-confident?

If you are going out with a friend, which will probably be easier, since your goal is to open up, try to choose someone that you love to be with and that has an open and outgoing personality. You are more likely to attract other people if you are open to a conversation or already in one, as opposed to sitting alone in a corner. From now on, every time you get out there, see each person you meet as an opportunity to practice small talk, casual conversation or hold a real discussion.

2. Be Prepared

The second most important thing to improve your conversational skills is probably to have something to talk about.

As much as possible, try to stay abreast of current issues. Take the time to watch the news or read the paper. Watch documentaries, read books that just came out about topics of interest, go out more to the theatre, movies, museums and conferences. It's important to open up and embrace different areas of interest. When you learn something new, you often feel like sharing it. And although it's tempting to watch your favorite soap opera, try to take the time to focus on other interesting topics.

And if you are in a conversation and someone talks about something you know nothing about, don't pretend you do. On the contrary, admit it. You could formulate the following: "You seem to know a lot about this topic.

And I find it really interesting. I, myself, don't know much about it, do you mind if I ask you a few questions?" Most people will feel flattered and will be happy to give details or explanations. There is no shame in not knowing...but I do believe there is shame in not trying to understand. With today's technology and possibilities, it's easy to research and get some information. If someone spoke to you about something you don't know much about, make a note to search the topic up a bit later. No need to become an expert, simply read and try to grasp the important aspects of if.

3. Read out loud

When reading out loud you get used to hearing your voice and speech. Try to read at a slow even speed, articulating each word and pronouncing loud and clear. I am not asking you to yell or overly articulate, but to read with a voice that is audible and comprehensible to listeners that could be in your room.

Being shy by nature, I have a tendency to speak very fast to get it over with and I often gladly pass the conversation to my interlocutor.

Taking the time to read out loud, helped me get used to hearing myself speak at a normal speed. I find it interesting to read stories and put emotion into it. Reading is also a good idea to learn how to express emotions and make facial expressions and physical gestures. You can learn to express joy, anger, relief, impatience and many other emotions that you experience throughout your daily life, emotions that you might not dare to express clearly. Expressing them through reading and reciting can actually help you when you find yourself in a similar emotional state. So relax, breathe and take your time to express what you have to say. Learning to choose the right words is also of utmost importance. Taking the time to speak will give you the time to think things through and carefully choose your words, so that you express exactly what you wish to say. You can eventually take acting lessons. They will greatly improve your diction and how you express emotions.

4. Learn Key Phrases

When having difficulty expressing yourself it is a good idea, to **prepare several key phrases** that you can learn by heart ahead of time and place them in order to gain some time to structure your actual thoughts. Here are a few examples to help you find what seems natural to you:

Oh! I see...and pause
So, what you are saying basically is...rephrase it
Interesting...and pause
That's a good point...and pause
Can you run that by me again...when you don't understand
And you know this from...and pause

5. Learn to listen and have presence.

When in a conversation, being a good listener is essential. There is nothing more annoying than having someone who interrupts you constantly or that isn't listening.

A lot of people feel like they can pretend they are listening and get away with it, but it's usually easy to know when this happens because they end up revealing themselves afterwards by asking, for example, a question that you have already answered. Let's face it, you cannot pretend to be listening or pretend to have presence. At one moment or another your body language or what you are saying are going to expose you one way or another. Practice giving your undivided attention.

And please, never make the conversation all about you. This is definitely a big no no.

6. Stay abreast of current issues.

Participate in more interesting activities. If you want to improve your conversation, you need to have something to talk about. Try to get out of the house and visit new places, go to the cinema, take a class and learn something new, visit the library and browse through the different sections, explore festivals and conferences.

There are also things you can do in your own home, such as discovering new places online, reading books, watching documentaries and so on.

7. Speak slowly.

When in a conversation, articulate. If you speak slowly you will present yourself as being more in control. It will give you the time to search for new words as you are speaking, but also convey the idea that you are more self-assured.

8. Be and Act confident.

If worst comes to worst, fake it. Your body language is of utmost importance. The message your body is conveying to others is as important as the words coming out of your mouth. Check your posture: stand tall with your head high, and a relaxed torso, keep eye contact, keep your arms and hands relaxed, no fidgeting and smile. No need to make a huge fake smile, keep it natural and real. I find that simply straightening up already boosts my self-confidence. If you don't know much about the topic at hand, maintain eye contact, listen and be attentive about what the other is saying. Don't hesitate to ask questions and admit you don't know much about the topic. If you are sincerely attentive, your interlocutor will appreciate your attention and interest.

9. Get your Interlocutor Talking

If you want to keep the conversation going, take the habit of asking questions and getting the other one talking. I am not talking about prying or being inquisitive, but simply asking questions about the topic to show interest in the subject.

10. Get into the Habit of Researching What You Don't Know

When you don't know something, look up the information immediately or make a note to look it up later. Several times a day, I find myself in a situation where I don't know something either after a question someone has asked me, but mostly from personal interrogations regarding the news, my work, an event, or something I have read. I can't always look it up but at least 80% of the time, I grab my phone and google it. So next time someone mentions a country and you realize you can't exactly situate it, or you read a word and you don't really grasp the meaning, take the time to look it up. The way I see it, life is an opportunity to learn and grow.

So, instead of seeing your lack of knowledge as incompetence, see it as an ongoing process.
I don't know,
I learn,
I don't know
I learn
This scheme goes on until your very last day.
That's what makes our life so much more fascinating!

11. Develop empathy.

When discussing with someone, it's of course OK to have your own opinion and disagree. Avoid being obtuse however. Why not practice empathy by putting yourself in other people's shoes and trying to understand how *they* feel? Life is not square. I often think that there are almost 8 billion people on earth, 7.6 Billion to be exact and that means there are 8 billion different life paths. What can hold true for one, might not be an option for another, and we all make decisions in accordance to what we have been through and what we are going through at the moment. We might make a mistake, but we don't need other people's judgment, nor to be condemned. Next time you disagree with someone's viewpoint, practice empathy and try to see that maybe, if this person is acting a certain way and saying certain things, it's because that's where they are in their life's path, and just maybe it's the very best they can do to cope with their situation for the moment.

12. Stop putting yourself down.

Aren't we good at this one!! It's a natural process, our mind loves to ask questions. Why would someone be interested in what I have to say? Can I do that? Am I good enough? If I say that, I am going to make a fool of myself, right? I wonder what they thought about me after our conversation... Did they like me? The questions go on endlessly. Just remember you can't please everybody and some people are out there just to criticize. Start small. Start by doing small things that boost your self-confidence.
Check out Chapter 1: *Improve your Self-Esteem,* and every time your mind puts you down, see it happening, grab it by the neck and tell yourself you are not going down this path any more. And if you put yourself in a humiliating position, hurry up and get back on the saddle. Don't let a single failure determine your entire future. Soon you will be laughing about it!

13. Improve Your English.

You might be wondering why, but in fact when communicating it is really important, to use the appropriate words to express what you want to say. Reading can help you a lot especially if you take the time to look up some words in the dictionary. Another interesting option is to take a writing course. What level of conversation are you using: colloquial, common, or formal language? Make sure you use the appropriate form depending on the people you are talking to.

14. Try mimicking the one in front of you.

Many sales people learn that in order to come through to a customer, one has to mimic their ways. People feel comfortable being around people that are similar. The key, however, here is not to overdo it. All you have to do is mimic the person's manner, either relaxed or on the contrary, businesslike and as mentioned in the point above, use the same level of conversation.

15. Flatter people.

Let's face it: everyone loves a compliment. If your interlocutor says something interesting, tell them how interesting this discussion was for you. If your interlocutor expresses their emotions well, tell them. You could say, for example, "You expressed it in such a way that I really understand how you felt." Or, if you like the way a person is dressed, give them a sincere compliment. Flattering someone is quite easy, there are numerous ways to make someone feel better about themselves.

Flattering people usually makes them open up and be less defensive. And if you also manage to make them smile, you will be one step closer to creating a connection and engaging into a pleasurable conversation

They were just thoughts
that danced through my little head…
…about becoming a Woman.

When I was 16, I recall thinking: "Wow, in two years I will be 18. I will be an adult. I will be a woman."
But when I reached 18, nothing happened. Nothing changed. I was still the same girl inside.

And so, I wondered when it would happen and it got me thinking… It's probably a question of feeling self-sufficient. Most certainly, the day I have a job and pay my own rent, *that* day, I will feel like an adult. I will become a woman.
When I went to University I had to work to pay for tuition and rent, but I still had the same feeling inside me, as though nothing had changed. I was still the same girl.

I then thought, without a doubt, this profound change will most certainly occur the day I get married and give birth to my first child.
But, although I was 34 when I had my first son, and was overcome with joy, while aware of this great new responsibility, discovering a totally new kind of love, when I turned inside to see how I felt, I was still that same girl I was at 16.

The years thus passed and I often wondered about it. It was strange for me: Adulthood. Womanhood. Maybe they were just words.

But one day it happened. It hit me: I had become a woman! It was a subtle feeling, but it was clear to me that I had changed. I understood at that moment that it had something to do with my femininity. Age, being self-sufficient, giving birth had nothing to do with it. It had to do with the awakening of my sensuality that came one day in the arms of a man. I blossomed with his touch, his passionate kisses and his love. His special ways made me feel beautiful and complete…. And so, it was then and there, as I lost myself in his manhood, that I became a *Woman*.

This is all very personal, and I am sure that many of you will contest my words, saying that you have experienced your passage to womanhood in a different way, at a different moment. It would be an interesting discussion to see when each and every one of us experienced this profound change within themselves…. The path that leads to womanhood isn't a common path; we won't all experience it at the same time or in the same way. I wanted to share my experience to invite you to take a minute and reflect upon yours:

Note: I was going to name this page "about becoming a man or a woman" and apply it to men and women alike. However, being a woman and not having the necessary depth of perspective to talk in the name of men, I thought it best to leave them out. I would find it interesting, however, to know whether men experience this same kind of feeling and if so, what event in their life enabled them to feel like they had become a Man.

When did you get your rite of passage to womanhood?

Change n°41
EMBRACE ROMANCE AND SEX

41.

What place does *sex* have in your life? Is it your main preoccupation or are you one of those people, who wonder what all the fuss is about and claim that you could easily live without it? Has it become a routine or is it a moment you look forward to? Is it conventional or is it hot?

I mean let's face it: while it is great to share moments with your kids, to have a coffee or a good laugh with your best friend, dedicate yourself to a job you love, or watch a ball game… nothing beats an eye gazing passionate kiss, the feeling of being loved and held… and being able to just let go!

Sex allows you to float in time. It's a moment in space. It's also a moment of giving and taking… of simply sharing. What can be more fulfilling than receiving love, being kissed and touched with passion and desire or looking at that special someone you love, letting go of all resistance, abandoning himself in your arms? What can be more satisfying than knowing that your hands, your mouth, your sex are procuring him great pleasure?

Where else, when else do you experience this feeling that nothing else matters or exists but the two of you?

I know, I know, life just seems to get in your way and one must be realistic: it's not a "loveboat" ride. Many of you will even say that if feels more like the movie "Tully" in which Marlo, alias Charlize Theron, is literally crushed by all of her obligations and spends most of her days hanging in there doing the best she can, struggling to get it all done, before collapsing into bed, right? By then, the last thing on her mind is more the word "sleep" than "sex." Indeed, with our hectic lives and the years going by, it's not always easy to keep that flame going.

In "Change n° 41: Embrace Romance and Sex", I would just like to take a few minutes of your time: let's go for a stroll together and chat about "sex". You are too busy and have more important things to do? Before putting this book down to rush off to complete more chores, I would like you to take a minute or two, close your eyes, breathe deeply and ask yourself: wouldn't you rather be on a soft bed, with that special someone holding you passionately and making you feel like you are not only beautiful but the most important person on Earth at this very moment?
I heard that sigh…

A. Kissing

a. Why you absolutely need to kiss more

Seeing how many copies of *50 Shades of Grey* were sold can only prove one thing: there are a lot of people out there who are craving for MORE.

The goal here is not really to give you tips and ideas on how to have better sex, I just want to take a bit of your time to make you step back and think about your sex life. Does it need a boost? What could get you motivated to bring it back into your life? Or maybe your sex life is fantastic and you want to make sure you keep that flame going. To get things started, I thought I would remind you about the pleasures of kissing. Think about it? Could it be that you are missing out on something? Read on…and let these words carry you away.

"There was fire in his kiss and he left every part of me was melting."

"I don't know which part of the kiss I love the best: right before when we slowly move closer and look into each other eyes, during the kiss as the alchemy happens with its illusion of suspended time or right after as he leaves me feeling breathless."

His eyes were saying: "Don't you want to kiss me?"
And I was thinking "More than I want to breathe."

"He had a way. A kiss for him was never taken for granted. It was never just a simple kiss. He made me feel as though it was a gift. Every time, he would gaze into my eyes in silence, slowly building upon the moment. He enjoyed making me long for him. I loved that we had all the time in the world and that he would wait until I would look at him with begging eyes."

"When he kissed he gave me everything he had. I could feel his power, his passion, his hunger and his love. He wasn't holding anything back, he was giving himself totally, revealing everything."

"I had loved the others - the other guys, that is - and they had been, at the time, my reason to live. But as this man kissed me, I knew it was different. I knew I was in the arms of LOVE. Even as the weeks, months, years passed by the kissing, the need for his touch became a drug and he became my oxygen. No one had ever touched me the way he did. No one had ever left me breathless. I just wanted one thing: for him to lock me in his arms and to be able to feel his skin against mine, his gaze stare back into mine and for him to kiss me ever so gently, ever so passionately and for it to last forever."

"There's a moment between a glance and a kiss where the world stops, for the briefest of times, when the only thing left between you and me is the anticipation of your lips on mine. The moment is so intense and perfect, that when it comes to an end, a simple gaze and we realize, this is just beginning."

b. What are the benefits of kissing?

The first and most important reason of all, kissing feels good and it makes you feel great! But did you know that…

- It improves your mood?
- It boosts your self-esteem?
- It lowers anxiety and blood pressure?
- It stimulates saliva… which is good because it helps to clean your mouth by getting rid of bacteria that cause cavities?
- It increases oxytocin… which is your soothing and calming hormone?
- It involves 29 muscles to French kiss?
- The longest kiss ever recorded lasted 33 hours?
- Passionate kissing burns 6.4 calories a minute? So, why don't you go ask that special someone if he or she wants to "workout?"

c. Make him/her want to kiss you

- Make sure you smell good and that you have good breath. It seems rather obvious, but it can't hurt to say it.
- Be really there: give yourself. I recall one man… when he kissed, he made me feel like there was only me and that nothing else mattered. He wasn't preoccupied with the rest of his day or the things that needed to be done. He was mine: his eyes, his gaze, his lips were all mine. As the months went by, the magic was still there, and I told him: "You make each and every kiss feel like the very first time." His answer only left me begging for more: "You are my drug, it just seems as though I never seem to get enough." C.B. Stella
- Look into each other's eyes.
- Be flirty. Play around a bit before trying to kiss or play a little hard to get.
- You can write a text message before coming home to let your special someone know that once you get home they are going to get a passionate kiss.
- Be generous with compliments. Forget the other one's flaws in these particular moments and focus on their lovely qualities. I have had numerous friends complain about the fact that their special someone chooses this moment to pinch the fat on their tummy or hips. This can only damage someone's self-esteem and turn a pleasurable moment into an uncomfortable one. This is not the time to mention the few extra pounds or to criticize.

B. Touching, Hugging and Massaging

a. The pleasures of touching, receiving and giving a massage

"Honey, let's turn the lights out tonight. You won't be able to see me but you will be able to feel me."

"I want to make love to you like you have never been loved before. I want time to stop, all your thoughts to stop… and for you to only feel, to lose yourself in the moment and reach heights like never before while never letting me go."

"I can't remember wanting something or someone so badly. It's as if everything about her is enchanting: the way she moves, her eyes, her smile, her laugh. I would so wish for her to be mine."

b. Why you absolutely need to touch more, hug more and massage more

- Hugging makes you feel good and can improve your mood
- A hug can bring joy, warmth, pleasure and literally recharge your batteries
- You release all the tensions you have cumulated throughout the day and you find yourself in a more relaxed state. Have you ever noticed, how when being massaged, certain parts of your body feel tense and you only become aware of it when the massage starts? Let yourself go and feel how those massaging hands are actually helping you to release all that tension you have built up inside.
- It makes you or your partner feel special. Taking the time to massage or caress someone, really shows that you care.
- Receiving a massage can help restore your emotional balance
- Massaging improves your blood circulation
- It makes you feel less lonely
- When you are down or feeling troubled it can lower your level of anxiety
- When you are scared a nice hug can alleviate your apprehensiveness
- Receiving a massage can greatly improve the quality of your sleep and your capacity to fall asleep
- It boosts your immune system, so it's good for your health
- Touching is another form of language, a non-verbal one. Why not learn it?
- If you are suffering, it can alleviate pain and bring comfort
- If you are depressed it can help promote happy feelings
- If you are ill and being cared for, receiving a gentle or invigorating massage can actually help you heal faster
- It shows that someone cares for you and is understanding
- It can bring a smile to your face
- In massaging each other you will not only find pleasure in giving, you will also be more open to receive. Feel how the energy emanating from both of your bodies mingle and intertwine
- A hand gesture can express many different things: it can be reassuring by placing your hand on someone's shoulder it can be sexually arousing with a light touch and sliding of the hand on the thigh, it can express sympathy with a pat on the arm or shoulder.
- It can make someone cry and sometimes it also feels good to have a shoulder to cry on
- Massaging yourself is a great way to get to know yourself. Massaging a partner is a great way to get to know them. Receiving a massage is a great way to get to know yourself. Massaging in general is a great way to bond with your special someone or to reconnect yourself with your body.
- It can be a good way to initiate sex

- It can revamp your sex life. If you have been in a rut lately, taking the time to massage each other is a great way to light the spark up for action.
- Massaging each other or taking turns to massage each other is a great way to maintain that special bond you both share.
- It enables you to be in harmony. Your energy vibes transmit this state of inner peace.

Although most people would agree that the act of touching is extremely important, many couples seldom do. For babies, massage is fundamental: they need it to thrive. For most couples it's natural at the beginning of their relationship, but most often, after 18 to 25 months the touching withers away. All those moments of holding hands, the gentle gestures when we approach each other such as caressing the others arm, shoulder or hair, and the kissing are what maintains that special connection between the two of you.

This is why I find massaging essential. The kids are in bed and your wife can finally lie down on the couch? Grab her feet and give her a nice gentle massage. Your special someone has just come home from work after and exhausting day? Reach for their shoulders and give them a relaxing massage. Take turns or better yet, massage each other at the same time: something just seems to happen when you receive one that makes you stop and relax: you feel relief and inner-peace and you can finally surrender.

Touching is an act of giving. So, remember, when administering a massage, do it with conviction, put your heart into it and really share a part of yourself. And when receiving one, close your eyes, breathe deeply, let go, feel all your bodily sensations and be thankful for this gift.

A final few words about touching… do both of you ever take the time to look into each others eyes? I mean really look into his or her eyes while talking, or to simply do a bit of eye gazing. It's the same as hugging each other, but without the touching. As you both gaze at each other, something strong and powerful happens. Many couples seldom take the time for this intimate interaction after a while. Become aware of this fact, talk about it and reconnect. Recreate intimacy by bringing back these little moments of touching and eye gazing into your love life and watch as your relationship deepens.

Change n°42
LOVE,
SEX AND COMMUNICATION

42.

As I reflect on couples, love, sex and relationships it seems essential to write about communication and the importance of having intimate and meaningful conversations. And so, as I sit here writing I can't help but wonder: how many times, in the past, have I actually open-heartedly expressed to a man I was with how I felt, what I really liked, wanted and secretly desired: *Never*. And then, it also hit me that not many of my partners - if any- had ever really dared to express how they felt and what *they* liked, wanted or secretly desired. There is kind of an invisible line that we never dare to cross. I thought about that, and it got me wondering: "why?"

The answer is: "*because it's not easy*". In fact, it's quite difficult to open up and lay it all out. I mean, let's face it, when is it the right time to talk about sex issues, for example? Most certainly not in the middle of sex. Before? Will it not then feel like an obligation? And what about after? Couldn't it be interpreted the wrong way, as though you were disappointed or come out as a critique? And then with the hectic lives that we lead, especially once we have kids, it gets complicated to have any intimacy. I mean the kids have to be occupied or asleep, you have to hush so they don't hear anything or be quick before one of them barges in. It's already not easy to find time to have sex or a quiet moment alone, how do we find the time to talk about each-others wants and needs? Should we schedule an appointment? Uuurghhh! That sounds like we are already set up for failure….

No, it's really not easy to express sexual issues or any other topic couples have to deal with for that matter, especially where the ego is concerned and you have to consider the other person's susceptibility and sensitivity. First of all, you can't help but ask yourself how will my partner take it? And then, how will *I* take it? Am I ready to hear it all?

Shouldn't I be able to express myself freely, if our goal is to obtain a fulfilling relationship? Before I do, I had better think things through and find the right words to avoid hurting, shocking, getting a testy remark, getting scorned or misunderstood? How do I reach out and have my special someone hear me out, without being defensive? I really wouldn't want us to start settling scores or pushing each other apart because I honestly have our well-being at heart and am really open to listening as well. I wonder…should I initiate the first step?
Maybe I could buy a book about couples, intimacy and communication and suggest that we both read it together, this way we can share our perspectives.

1° Communicating in writing

If you are trying to open a door for deeper connectedness, it might help you to write it all down on paper; take the time to question yourself so you will know for sure what it is that you want. Have you ever given it any thought, do you know what you actually want?

Why not take a few minutes to write in the form of a letter, what it is you are really looking for in your relationship, regardless of whether you are involved with someone.

You are free to approach this on your own, or you can ask your special someone to write their special wants and needs as well. Once the letters are written, you could either read them together, or on your own.

To help you, here is a list of questions you can ask yourself:

What do I want in a relationship?
What do I have to offer? Let's face it, many people are very demanding about what they want, but are they equally demanding of themselves? Do you really have something worthwhile to offer? Now is the time for a little bit of introspection and to think this through. Do you really deserve what you are asking for? Maybe you need to address a few issues about yourself first.
What do I like the most about sex? Explain why.
What makes me feel uncomfortable about sex? Explain why.
What ticks me off or infuriates me? Stick to what's really important for you. Avoid making a list or being overly critical.
What do I love? Express something that happened to you that made you utterly happy.
I want more….
I want less…..
What do you feel you desire the most in a relationship? Express it. Maybe give examples of when you did receive it and how it really had a positive effect on you.
How do you function? Are there any clues you could give to help your partner understand how you operate?
As an example: when something upsets me, I tend to bottle it up and not say anything. I hate explosive discussions: I think about it for a few hours or maybe a day or two, and then get back to my partner about it when I am calm and have taken the time to think it through and put things back into perspective. Although it may be interpreted as though I am backing off or refusing to dialog, I am in fact trying to find a way to handle the issue calmly. Having my partner pressure me for an answer and go on and on about the situation, is not the right way to go about it with me. And so, you might ask, what do you do if your partner prefers to settle things immediately? It's not necessarily insurmountable, but it certainly helps to know how we both function to better handle any given situation that could arise in the future.
Objectively now: **Do I shut down opportunities for a deeper relationship by automatically being defensive or overly sensitive? Is there something that my partner could do to make me feel safe, to maybe reassure me, before we tackle any issue?**

My fiancé and I have both written such letters to each other when we were about eight months into our relationship. It's a good thing to do it early on when a couple is enthusiastic and willing to do what it takes to make the relationship really work. Indeed, we never argued about anything and we were open to hear what the other had to say. It's easier to hear and laugh about certain issues after a few months into a relationship, than when you are completely settled down.

If you have settled into a relationship, however, make sure that both of you decide not to be overly sensitive about this and read each-other's letters with an open mind and with your special someone's interest at heart.

For us, writing these letters ended up becoming a moment of sharing, learning, surprise, as in "Really?? You would like this??" or "I didn't know that! It made us laugh, connect and get even closer. Something happens when you finally dare to reveal your true self. I mean, if you can say these things to each other, it means you could pretty much share anything. No more taboos, which comes as a great relief.

2° Engage in a conversation

If you are not much of a writer, then talking might be a better option for you although it isn't all that easy either. Here are a few helpful tips to think about and apply when engaging in that next, delicate conversation.

- The first thing I suggest, is that you both get into the habit of discussing less important issues from time to time. Start off by having little debates about various topics or about couple problems that your friends might be going through. Take turns expressing what you think, without interrupting each other. Be open-minded and make it clear that you both have to express what you really think. The goal is to have these discussions without one of you clamming up, or getting upset.
- On a day to day basis, get into the habit of asking how your partner feels about various things that do not necessarily have to do with couple issues, and learn to express your feelings as well.
- Take turns listening, which doesn't only imply not interrupting. Listening means really being attentive. If you are silent, but you let your mind wander off to prepare for an answer or counter argument, then it cannot be qualified as true listening. It's time to practice empathy and really understand how your interlocutor feels.
- Choose the appropriate moment to talk. It goes without saying, but it needs to be mentioned.
- Remember that when deciding to talk about a delicate subject, it's usually because you have a desire to improve a situation that isn't quite right. So, make this goal clear and start off by saying that you do not wish to hurt, offend or argue, but something is troubling you, and you have to get it off your chest. It's not a good thing for either of you to keep things bottled up, as it can only build up over time and lead to a major argument.
- Make sure you address only one issue at a time. Make it clear that you wish to discuss one specific topic and stick to it. If you start tackling them all, things will probably get out of hand.

- It's important that you are able to express what you really have to say. Speak the truth. Let's be honest here, many times these discussions turn into power struggles. At first, we want to improve a situation and then insidiously the dynamics shift and we are both trying to win a battle. If this is often the case, I would recommend you both write on a piece of paper: "A winning conversation is one in which our couple becomes stronger and we both come out happy". If you both try to impose your point of view or to win a battle, it defeats the purpose.
- Commit to sticking with the conversation and doing everything to solve the problem *before* engaging in a discussion.
- Even if you disagree with what your partner is saying, understand that you are different and that although you might be convinced to be right, there are different ways of being "right". This depends on a multitude of factors, such as what a person has experienced in the past, what someone is capable of admitting at that specific moment, and how many problems a person is tackling at the same time.
- Don't resort to nagging, making insidious remarks, blaming, insulting or badmouthing, as this type of behavior can only worsen the situation.
- You are trying to be honest with your partner but remember to be ABSOLUTELY honest with yourself. It's not easy to do, but learn to admit if you are feeling jealous, selfish, have a bad temper and if it's necessary, sincerely apologize. Now this is not the time to win a conversation: your goal is to win back your relationship, and restore a dialog between the two of you.
- If you see your partner clamming up, wanting to leave or raising their voice then the conversation is not going the right way. Even if you feel that you are in your right, this is obviously not the case for your partner. You must immediately recognize that the situation is drifting in the wrong direction and quickly find a remedy. Either say you are sorry, if you are, or say something that shows you wish to restore the conversation. Make them feel respected and demonstrate that they are allowed to express their own opinion. They have to feel your sincerity and that you care about what they have to say. Let them know that even if you do not share the same opinion, you are on the same side.
- Words can hurt or slowly make two people drift apart, but they can also be food for each-others souls. If you really love the person you are with, then feed their soul with loving and encouraging words. Observe how your partner's attitude towards you changes, because let's face it, all we ever really want is to feel loved and supported.

3° How to sustain a harmonious and happy relationship

A relationship is an equation: "Relationship = me + you" and it starts with "me"
If you want to be happy, then the first thing to do is to stop believing in "fairytales", that someone is going to come into your life and make you happy. It doesn't work that way. All of those beautiful fairytales, such as Cinderella and Snow White are not about a handsome Prince coming to the rescue. Each story, in fact, withholds a secret message. Unfortunately, we are taught to take them literally, without giving them any thought whatsoever, never taking the time to decipher their true meaning. And so, we plant unrealistic dreams in our minds in which we unfortunately end up believing. Once we get into a real relationship, they become a great source of disappointment.

Cinderella stands for the "ray under the ashes". Each and every one of us is a mineral in its raw state, a rough stone. Once purified and washed, we transform ourselves into a pure beautiful mineral, a gem. The fairy godmother is in fact that guiding spark within, that we must listen to. The mean step-sisters are there to show us, that our inner beauty is not necessarily seen by others and we don't need their approval or help to thrive and turn into someone beautiful. You will note that Cinderella meets her Prince charming only once she has done all the hard work on herself and turned into a beautiful person inside and out. Only then can they live happily ever after.

Fairytales are in fact ancestral stories that have been handed down century after century. You must learn to read between the lines. It is up to each and every one of us to open ourselves up, uncover the hidden truths and apply them to our lives. We must live in faith that there will come a day when we are capable of receiving. It's up to each and every one of us to choose: You can either take these stories literally and live a lost life just like the step-sisters, or you can get down on your knees and work hard and turn into a Cinderella. This young girl was reduced to doing all the unwanted and degrading chores and yet still managed to thrive in a difficult environment deprived of love and respect. Nothing waivered her faith and she continued to spread love and kindness all around her, never expecting anything in return. That love and faith made her blossom into a beautiful wise woman, who was finally ready to receive love and meet someone worthy of her.

You have to understand that YOU and only YOU have the power to make yourself happy and that it all starts within. You cannot be happy if you harbor mean or negative thoughts, are envious or have feelings of jealousy throughout the day. In order to have a fulfilling relationship, you have to work on yourself which begins with learning to be happy on your own. Once you find that inner happiness, you will know that no matter what the outcome is of any relationship, you will always be ok. When you start feeling that your happiness depends on someone else or their actions, then you know for sure that something is not right.

One day, my 16 year-old son came home crying because he knew that his relationship with his first love was coming to an end. He told me that he couldn't imagine living his life without her. It can be truly heart-wrenching to see your child suffering and at that moment you wish only one thing: to find the right words to ease their pain. This is what I told him: "Although this love story was beautiful, and you feel that your world is coming to an end, keep in mind that you did not come to Earth only to meet this one special person. You have a mission to accomplish. You have something greater to do that involves only you. You will meet many people, some will change your life, some will disappoint you, but none of them are the reason why you are here today. Who knows, maybe your life path is to be a singer and composer and you will write a beautiful song one day that will touch thousands of people's hearts. I know you are in great pain and it's going to take a while, but remember you are not here for "her", you are here for "you"." He looked at me and said that he never thought of it that way.

A few months later, as I was driving around town with him, he made me listen to his latest songs. I couldn't believe my ears when I heard the lyrics from one of them: "spread the message, spread your wings, you won't be here long: You've got a purpose on this planet, kid get up, get going."

Just goes to say: don't make another person your only reason to live. Don't put your happiness into someone else's hands. Start creating your own.

A relationship is an equation: "Relationship = me + you". Let's move on to "you"
If you are happy on your own, you know deep down inside, that even if the person you love ends up leaving you, you will be ok. This allows you to set them free and become the very best of who they are. You are happy and you want the same for that special someone. You have no wish to control them.
If you really love someone then setting them free is the most beautiful proof of love you can offer. Help them thrive, encourage them to bring out the best of themselves and you will see that they will never want to leave you.

Understand that there is no room for jealousy and possessiveness here: seeing the other one grow, blossom and being fulfilled is your reward and it can actually bring you a lot of happiness.

Of course, this works both ways: in a loving relationship, your special someone has to be supportive of your dreams as well.
In many relationships, I find that it is seldom the case. Often enough, both partners are selfish and don't want the other to reach their full potential. Indeed, they fear that their partner might succeed and then move on to something or someone better, which will supersede the love they feel for them. There are also couples in which one of them is allowed to thrive, to the detriment of the other. This often happens when one has an important career, or is striving for one, which takes up a lot of their time, and leaves the other partner on standby or completely left out. Although both couples may end up staying together their entire life, I would not qualify them as "happy and harmonious".

It goes without saying that you have to wish the best for your partner… but also for yourself. You cannot accept to be with someone who depreciates or controls you. It has always made me wonder why, when the situation is toxic, we still persist in staying in the relationship.

Indeed, this idea of freedom and well-being has to be mutual and utterly sincere: There has to be a strong desire to help each other thrive and become a better person. It's important that you both feel FREE, which means no reprimands or guilt.

A good relationship is based on respect: without it you will never, ever, be happy together and you will know it's time to move on. If you accept the unacceptable, it might go on for years and all you will end up with is a toxic relationship.

A little note about children here, as the same holds true for them as well. You must help them find what makes them happy and encourage them to thrive in that direction without imposing your hopes and ambitions. What better gift than watching them thrive and do something they are passionate about. Sure, they will make their mistakes and you will feel like telling them they are wrong sometimes: just keep in mind that these life lessons are necessary for their growth.

4° Something to reflect upon

I would like to end this thought with a special note, to draw your attention on the spiritual significance of making love. A lot of young men and women have sex simply for the pleasure of having sex and that's fine, but when you dig down a bit deeper, you will come to realize that most people, men and women alike, are simply filling a void. They actually crave more intimacy, something deeper, and more profound. It's hard to reach that state when true feelings are not involved.

Indeed, sex for some of you is an opportunity that allows you to let go and enables you to be relieved from all that pressure that has built up inside of you. For others, it's an act of love in which they take the time to share and show that special someone that they love them.

But sex also carries a spiritual meaning. Did you know that you are composed of 50 trillion individual cells and that each one of them is alive, vibrating and full of energy? Each and every one of them is independently controlled by your brain! I am emitting a certain vibration and so are you. Our emotions and thoughts influence our cells and the way they vibrate. Our aura reflects how we feel and reveals our wounds, our fears and our lack of trust in many different areas, depending on what we have experienced in life. When two bodies come together and make love, their vibrations interact as well. It's a moment that allows us to vibrate in unison. When we make love, if we really are in osmosis, with the desire to express and give love to one another, then our vibes, by intertwining with each other, contribute to healing each-others auras. And so, as we make love, we are both stronger and capable of rising together and literally healing each other. That is why it is so important to choose your partner wisely and understand that trust and complicity are the basis of every strong relationship. When you manage to reach this level of maturity in a relationship, sex becomes a mixture of pleasure, well-being, healing and strength and it regularly allows both of your inner lights and souls to mingle and intertwine.

So, take the time to think about your relationship or the type of relationship you would like to have and do something about it. Remember that it starts with you: if you are happy and thriving, you will most likely attract someone who has the same frame of mind. Once you understand how attraction works, it becomes clear that you have to begin by working on your very own personal happiness.

Change n°43
YOUR LIFETIME BUCKETLIST

43.

This goal has several parts to it but each one of them is a lot of fun. The idea is to write down 100 things you would love to do in your life: it should go from the simple things to the downright crazy ones. Since it might not be all that easy to find 100 things you would like to do, it would be a good idea to write down 8 categories to cover the different aspects of your life and start filling out each one with different ideas. Feel free to add new categories: this is your bucket list, so tailor it to match your personality. Remember that a bucket list doesn't necessarily have to be all about you... you can include ways of making other people happy too!

- **Love and Friendship**: things to do with spouse, loved one or with your friends.
- **Work**: things you wish to accomplish at work
- **Leisure/hobby**: something that you would like to do or that you are good at, but want to improve
- **Travel**: the places you would like to visit
- **Sports**: the goals you wish to reach or sports you would like to try out
- **Money**: how much you wish to earn or put aside, how much you would like to donate or collect for a certain cause.
- **Lifestyle and possessions**: what would you like to own or buy?
- **Fairytale fantasies or making your dreams come true**: what is your dream?
- **The exciting, crazy stuff or those things you should have done at least once in your life...**
- **Just for you**: do something just for you and the way you want to do it

Here is a whole list of ideas that might inspire you and help you create your very own bucket list.

A. Love and friendship

- Say "I love you" to someone. Many people have a hard time saying these 3 little words. Gather up a bit of courage and call your mom and dad, a special friend who has always been there for you, your child and let them know
- Fill a room with flowers for the one you love and / or sprinkle petals in the house that lead to the bedroom
- Rent a place out in the woods and go with your best friends and all the kids
- Save up and get them a special piece of jewelry, a trip, or an object of their desire
- Save up and get him the motorcycle of his dreams or sports equipment, or electronic device etc.
- Go on a road trip with your all-time friend

- Find what your special someone is dreaming of and make their dream come true
- Get your kid the puppy he has been dreaming of
- Why not have as many people as possible "walk for a wish"? The idea is to walk a certain distance with a wish written on your t-shirt or on a piece of paper in your pocket. The message? If you want your wish to come true, you have to get up and make it come true.
- Ask your special someone to marry you in a special way
- If you have a cleaning lady or someone who helps you around the house or garden, find out their birthday: do the work yourself, give them their day off and pay them anyway. Be grateful for the work they do for you every week: what better way to thank them!
- Get married or renew your vows
- If your kids are all grown up, organize a "two or three" day trip with only them to spend some time together!

B. Work
- Quit your job! Perhaps we could add, "finally"
- Do a presentation in front of your co-workers
- Find and commit to reading 10 to 20 books to become knowledgeable and excellent at what you do!
- Go back to "school" and learn something new to be more efficient at work

C. Sports
- Go to the Olympics!
- Get tickets to see the super bowl!
- Go see your favorite tennis, golf, soccer, football, ice skating sports star for real!
- Run a marathon!
- Run a marathon in 5 different capitals (starting with New-York)
- Try a new sport. I have always dreamed of doing a bi-athlon: that's cross-country skiing and shooting or swimming and running
- Participate in a competition or a sports tournament in fitness, boxing, beach volley, cross fit. Do it!
- Set a specific sports goal such as doing a handstand, the splits or 10 chin ups

D. Leisure and hobby
- Write a book or a novel and get it published
- Learn how to drive a motorcycle and then buy one!
- Get your boat license
- Read every single book and watch every single video that exists about your hobby. For example, become really good at playing pool, chess, crossword puzzles, you name it!
- Sign up to do something artistic or creative, such as a painting, an artistic project, or pottery
- Get 1000 or any specific amount of followers on Instagram
- Do a time capsule and program to open it in 10, 20, 30 or 40 years!
- Organize a huge bonfire and cook hotdogs and marshmallows with some friends and family
- Take a picture of you every single day for one year or every month for 10 years. Set a date ahead of time and stick to it!

- Book a table at the restaurant you love…alone
- Learn how to play your favorite guitar piece
- Learn how to swim
- Learn how to survive alone in nature, start a fire from scratch with sticks and stones, find your way with a compass and explore interesting plants
- Get your pilot license and learn how to fly!
- Invent something and patent it!
- Write an article and send it out to get published.
- Go see an opera… and if you are into opera, go see a country music or rock concert.

E. Travel

- Travel on your own and discover the pleasure of doing exactly what you want, when you want
- Go on a cruise. Why not do one that crosses one of the major oceans
- Visit Easter Island. This one's on my bucket list!
- Fly in a hot air balloon
- Visit Alaska
- Visit the Fjords in Norway
- Go to Brazil
- Visit Paris and sleep in a "peniche"
- Go to Vegas
- Go to Hawaii and take surfing lessons
- Go on a safari
- Go to the North Pole
- Go on a gondola in Venice (Italy)
- Go inside the crater of a volcano, and soak up the energy by meditating while you are there
- Sleep in an igloo
- Search for gold in Australia, near Perth
- Do route 66 with your family or a friend
- Save up, take a leave from your job and drive around the USA for several months
- Go party in Ibiza
- Next time you have a few days off, don't organize anything and book the night before, at the very last minute
- Decide to visit one country from every continent. For example, Brazil, Namibia, Italy, China, New Zealand
- Watch the sunrise from a hot air balloon
- Do the GR20, the great hike that crosses the island of Corsica from North to South
- Go on a Pilgrimage to Lourdes or Compostelle
- Go see the Wall of Lamentations in Israel
- Take the Trans-Siberian train
- Go scuba diving at the Great Barrier Reef
- Throw a coin over your shoulder at the Trevi fountain (Italy)
- Place a lover's padlock in a special spot
- Go on a wine tasting and discovering trip
- Go around the world

- Sail across the Atlantic, take the route Christophe Columbus took
- Do a humanitarian trip, and help a family build a house
- Cross the longest hanging bridge in Switzerland

F. Money
- Make a 100, 1.000, 10.000, 100.000 or million dollars
- Save up 5 to 10% of everything you earn
- Find a way to generate more income and put the money aside for a project
- Donate some money to an association you believe in
- Calculate the cost of a trip around the world and save up for it

G. Lifestyle and Possessions
- Buy the house or apartment of your dreams
- Get a pool
- Redecorate your home one room at a time
- Change that old piece of furniture such as your couch or bed
- Sell all that stuff you never use and get something your home really needs such as getting the rooms repainted, creating a vegetable garden or flowering your balcony
- Sell some of your clothes and get some new ones
- Buy the car of your dreams.
- Buy a boat
- Quit smoking and decide to put all of the money you would be spending on cigarettes aside until you manage to buy something specific that really makes you happy
- Get a surf board or windsurf

H. Fairytale dreams or making dreams come true
- Fall in love, get married and live happily ever after. You can' t really program this one but you can put intent, be receptive, open yourself up completely and accept that the universe will give you exactly what you want. If you can dream it, you can have it!
- Go on a honeymoon or a second one!
- Have a baby. Have you been hesitating because it's not the right time? It never will be. Do it and you will find a way!
- Swim with dolphins
- Have a limousine come and pick you up and go for a ride around New-York or other favorite great big city
- Go meet Santa Klaus or bring your kids to meet him
- Do something artistic and present it on stage
- Participate in a play
- Attend several film castings

I. The exciting and crazy stuff or those things you should have done at least once in your life...
- Do what it takes to be on the cover of a magazine
- Ride a tandem
- Ride an elephant

- Get yourself a dog
- Go see a striptease
- Have a sleepless night in Vegas
- Jump into a puddle, pool, lake, the ocean all dressed and who cares!
- Write your name somewhere special and maybe add someone else's name
- Rent a sign for a day or a week to post a message
- Go see a Broadway show in New York
- Go skydiving
- Try target shooting
- Do a bungee jump
- Train and climb one of the highest mountains
- Do one of the longest ziplines
- Do something that terrifies you
- Try to organize a meeting between you and a famous person you admire
- Go on a helicopter ride
- See a fortune teller
- Enter the Guinness book of world records
- Go in a submarine
- Organize a crazy party
- Drive a race car
- Be on TV
- Go on a nudist beach. I could never do this one!!! One must never say never!
- Go on the biggest roller coaster in the world
- Milk a cow
- Swim in the nude
- Play a feature role in a movie
- Eat an insect
- Sleep outside under a starry sky

J. Just for you
- Talk on stage in front of a crowd, do a presentation
- Get a trainer and get in the shape of your life!
- Write your life story, your memoirs
- Organize a photoshoot. Be in the limelight for a few hours
- Do something you said you would never do
- Decide to say "no" more often, decide you don't care what people think
- Eat 5 fruit and vegetables every day
- Get your house in order

Making your wish a reality.
Is there such a thing as a "good" wish?

The most important thing when deciding on a wish or goal is to make sure that it is something you love doing or have always really dreamed of doing. You have to feel motivated in your gut. It has to thrill and even scare you a little. If it's too easy, you won't get much satisfaction, so it has to challenge you somewhat.

As an example, I always dreamed of doing a photo shoot but never felt confident enough. In March 2016, I knew I was going to Florida in August, so I started looking online for fitness photographers and I found one close by. After doing a bit of research and making sure that he was recommended and that I really liked the quality of his photos, I booked ahead of time. Once I had paid part of the service, I knew there was no turning back and so the countdown started. I trained with determination and conviction. I looked for poses that I would like to use. I found a makeup artist and booked an appointment with her the morning before the shoot. I told my friends about the photo shoot so they were expecting to see the photos which sure put more pressure on me! At one point, I just had to focus on the training part, but believe me, I kept at it conscientiously and I also paid attention to my diet, making sure I was drinking a lot of water and eating very healthy. When D day arrived, I knew I had done my utmost to feel picture perfect. Perfection doesn't exist, but I knew that I had given it my all. The photographer turned out to be amazing: he understood the reason behind my decision, he was reassuring and helped me feel comfortable and at ease at all times. The cherry on top of the ice cream: his shots were AMAZING! I couldn't believe my eyes. It turned out to be one of the best life experiences I had ever done for myself and it really helped to boost my self-confidence. I highly recommend it! Thank you, Luis. I look forward to working with you again!

When deciding upon a goal, it's important to know yourself. Don't set yourself up for failure. Don't decide to take a challenge you know you will not be able to handle. As an example, I know for sure there are certain things I cannot do: dancing makes me feel terribly uncomfortable so why set myself up for failure by reaching for a goal that would push me way too far out of my comfort zone. There are other things, however, that terrify me, but that I know I must do: such as standing in front of a crowd and giving a speech. I wouldn't do it cold turkey, but I did find ways to challenge myself progressively such as talking about my book in front of a class of middle school kids, for example.

Don't over pressure yourself by setting a drastic goal such as losing 30 pounds AND having a photo shoot. It would be a lot smarter to first fit in my size 10 dress again in 6 months and then get ready for a photo shoot. When choosing a goal, it has to be S.M.A.R.T., which means you have to keep the following words in mind: specific, measurable, attainable, relevant and time.

Specific means that your goal should be clear as opposed to vague. For example, the goals "being in shape" or "save more money" are too vague.

If you want to turn into a more specific goal you could decide to "lose 1 pound per week for the next 10 weeks" or you could "save 2000 dollars in the following 12 months by putting 10% of everything you earn aside and making a bit more money by offering private tutoring lessons." Understand that if your goal is too vague, you will have no way of knowing whether you have truly reached your goal or not.

Measurable means that you have a number in mind: reach 5000 followers by a certain date, write 100 pages per month, lose 10 pounds in ten weeks, save 2000 dollars this year or do 10 chin ups by June 5th.

Attainable means that the goal isn't unrealistic. If you have 100 followers, deciding to reach 1 million of them is completely farfetched. However, if you set out to get 25 followers every week or 5000 in a year depending on your commitment, your goal seems far more attainable.

Relevant means that it is YOUR goal and not someone else's. Your goal has to be aligned with who you are, what you want and your principles in life and not what your family and friends think is good for you. Make sure you are not setting this goal because you are trying to fit in or because you want your family or other half to be proud of you.

Time: as mentioned above, your goals must have a deadline. Decide upon a date and commit to it. When you choose a date, you know where you are going and how much time you have to reach your goal. It might be a good idea to sit down and define a plan of action. In sports, we time our training, but the same thing can be applied to any goal in life. What can you do this week and the following weeks to achieve this goal? Who can you contact that can help you? Who can motivate you? Research everything you can about your goal and read it all. Write everything down, program appointments, set increments and cross each one out once they are completed.

While writing this book, I signed up for a book contest which had a deadline. It really helped me, because I knew that my book had to be written to meet that due date no matter what. It was a big challenge, but I refused to waiver and managed to get it done on time. I was so proud!

Going all the way

Why write a bucket list if you are not going to knock them down? See your life as an opportunity to make your dreams and as many of your wishes possible come true. Remember: the sky is the limit. The most important thing to remember is that once you have decided upon reaching a goal, you must go all the way and give it your all, 200%. Your mind must be willing to give 100% and you have to get up and get your body moving 100% in that direction as well.

When I decided to write this book, I knew it was going to take up a lot of my time. I decided to quit watching TV, quit social media, learn to switch off my phone and say "no" to invitations. I posted a picture of the front cover of my book on the wall in front of my desk and placed it as the backscreen of my phone. I made sure to tote around a book or an article relevant to what I was writing about, in my bag at all times.

And although I somehow never seemed to be moving forward as much and as fast as I wanted to, I didn't give up. I would usually set aside a certain amount of time each day to write and did my best to get down to business, but it wasn't always easy. But my commitment was at a rate of 200% and, slowly but surely, I knocked down each stumbling block one at a time.

So, why not start embracing change: see your life as a bucket list with the possibility to knock down goals on a daily or weekly basis. Don't let all of those days just slip by. Make the most of each and every one of them by deciding to become the creator of your life. It's not about the money. Make your life exciting. Tackling little accomplishments, achieving little successes can be extremely rewarding. Read more, get your home in order, get moving… Understand that it's basically all up to you. *You* decide. So, start off by being curious and a little bold, add determination and a smile and never waiver, just keep moving forward with resilience.

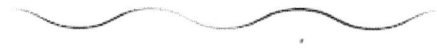

Change n°44
COMPLETING THINGS

44.

As a child, it was almost impossible to live up to my mother's expectations: although I was pugnacious and kept on trying, no matter what I did, it seemed as though I was never quite good enough. But that didn't stop me from trying. When I think about it, I don't really know what it is exactly that kept me going: even though I could tell that I was a constant source of disappointment, I would get back up and try again. The downside of this situation evidently was the ravaging effect it had on my self-esteem - which later required years of hard work to overcome – but there definitely was an upside to it: it has taught me, no matter what, to never quit trying and to keep on believing.

I don't know how things are for you, but I can tell you one thing, I have always had this faith within me, and as I ponder about it today, I realize that all those years that found me craving for recognition, have made me who I am today: someone who just keeps on trying!

As Steve Maraboli, an author I enjoy reading says: We have to stop seeing ourselves as victims. No matter what we have been through, whether we have been hurt, betrayed or even beaten, we are still here, which, in the end, means that nothing has managed to defeat us. Take a moment to think about this: Start seeing challenges you faced as victories you managed to overcome. Stop seeing yourself as defeated. The opposite is true: you have grown and learned from what has happened to you. It's time now to see yourself as a *Victor!*

The years have gone by now and, having reached my fifties, I can't help looking back, surprised by the number of goals I have accomplished, goals most of which I have done to completion. Some of them were supposed to be only temporary, but as it turned out, ended up becoming a way of life. It has also become a habit for me to regularly decide upon a goal and then to set out to accomplish it.

What about you, take a look at *your* life's challenges. What events have made you suffer, while forcing you to adapt? Ask yourself in what way they have transformed you into who you are today…. Those events of the past, whether you acknowledge it or not, could probably explain most of your flaws, but they are also the source of most of your qualities. Today they are the reason why you are so determined, patient, loyal, tolerant, understanding, open-minded, unselfish, responsible, warm-hearted, reasonable, imaginative, self-disciplined, original, ambitious, conscientious, courageous, constructive, ingenious, sensible, generous, tender, independent, frank, realistic, adventurous, modest, calm, careful, self-critical, disciplined, and perfectionistic. I am sure you can find yourself in some of these qualities.
So, instead of wasting your time dwelling on past disappointments why not try to see in what way those hardships helped you grow and turned you into the beautiful person you are today.

But let's get back to what brings us here today: doing things to completion…

This week, why don't you decide to stop procrastinating, finish everything you start and get things done, not later, but right now. Remember that phone call you need to make, call now! You see that pile of documents on your desk? Go file them and from now on, put things away immediately and systematically. Do you have things that need fixing and mending? Decide to tackle them all, this week. Structure this week to getting things done. If you are not up to working on this all day long, choose a topic of interest or find an educational method and commit to completion.

A. Getting things done

To help you reach this new goal I am suggesting a few tips on how to get things done:

One thing at a time. Give your project undivided attention. Stop the multitasking and stick with one thing at a time: there is a high probability that you will get things done properly and a lot faster than you think. Sometimes, we believe that we will save time by doing several things at once, but in fact, it makes us waste a lot of energy and there is a high risk that things, in the end, will not be done optimally.

Keep a writing pad handy at all times or use your phone and when something is troubling you or an idea pops up, write it down. This way you can quickly refocus on what you were doing and later on, once you have finished the present task at hand, you can tackle these other issues.

Keep track. Have a calendar and get into the habit of writing down everything you have completed. Be proud of yourself! You could choose to place a star in it every time you complete a task. Keeping track can keep you motivated and the increasing amount of stars will give you an added sense of pride.

Make it your priority. When something is important, try doing it first thing in the morning. For most people morning time is the optimal time to get things done. Of course, we all are different. If you are not much a morning person, try to find out when *your* optimal time is and then make sure to block this time to do what needs to be done.

Keep your desk and home tidy. To think clearly, the place you live in needs to be clear of all clutter. Keep on your desk only what you really need, right now, to get your job done. Your environment needs to suggest clarity, freedom of movement and openness. Stick to what is essential.

Slow down and do less. To get things done, you have to start making sure that you have fewer things to do throughout the day. This means that you are going to have to start using the "no" word more often, refusing invitations and or solicitations. You have to start focusing on what really counts.

B. Reaching "The Zone": entering your magic bubble

What magic bubble? I am sure you have all witnessed the fact that when you are completely absorbed by what you are doing, whether it be reading, writing or any other activity for that matter, you are capable of abstracting the outside world completely. When you are in this specific state of mind, nothing can perturb you. Decide to sit down and do what it is you have to do in a set amount of time and don't allow anything or anyone disturb you.

It goes without saying that if you want to stay focused you have to make sure you won't get interrupted. Put your phone on plane mode, turn the T.V. and radio off and inform the people around you that you do not wish to be interrupted for the next half-hour or so.

Before you start to create this bubble, take the time to intentionally and consciously establish a specific state of mind to get your task done. Close your eyes, breathe deeply and try to slow things down. It's impossible to fully concentrate on what you are doing if you are jittery and your mind is wandering all over the place. Take one or two minutes to center your attention on the now and prepare to embrace the task you have decided to tackle.

Now is the time to put intent and to get down to business. The goal you are trying to reach is called "The Zone" and as your concentration and focus deepen, you will feel a sort of wall, or a bubble, building up all around you, shielding you from any type of distraction.

You will see that in this zone you will be at peace and when you come out of it, you will feel a sense of accomplishment, so much stronger, and more in control of your life.

Why not practice in "15 to 20-minute" increments and slowly increase the duration of these practice sessions. One thing is for sure, if you want to get things done to completion, improving your concentration could prove your greatest ally.

C. Choosing an educational method and doing it to completion

You can decide to do every little thing throughout the day to completion or you could choose to find an educational method, something you have always wanted to learn, master or improve and get down to business.

There are hundreds of educational methods out there that will teach you just about anything: from sewing to singing, learning a language to fully mastering your computer, knowing how to fix your car to learning how to master the basic DIYs - do it yourself - in your very own home. Choose something you have always wanted to acquire knowledge about and commit to learning the ins and outs of the trade. No pressure here: the goal is not to become a professional, but to learn something new, enjoy the process while doing it and get in the habit of doing something to completion. You don't need to do it every day, but make sure you plan ahead of time: you could count how many chapters you have and schedule accordingly to get it done in one week or one month. Think of it, in the matter of only a few weeks, you could master how to sew, cook, fix, read faster, clean, or type. It's all up to you to decide!

a. Let's get Started!

The first step is to decide what you wish to learn and then to choose what educational method is best suited for you:

- You could take a course, private lessons or even go back to school
- Purchase an educational method, in which you can break down into increments what needs to be learned
- Enroll into online education program

A good idea is to use all three of these methods. I think that when it comes to learning it's always best to study the basics with a professional, that way if you have any questions, you have someone to ask directly. You will also want to buy a book so you have a step by step guide or a set number of days to get through the method. And finally, you might want to complement what you are learning by participating in an online course. Indeed, sometimes, visual video study can make the whole process a lot easier.

b. Examples of educational methods you could choose from

Think about it: What's 10 to 15 minutes in a 24-hour day? It's really nothing, but when you add it all up, you can become knowledgeable in any domain that you want.

• Train better

At one point, as I was trying to improve my workouts, I had the opportunity to meet an amazing coach who had taken the time to produce hundreds of videos about weight training, each one better than the last and giving great advice, based upon scientific proof, anatomical structure, research and logic. I made a point of watching one of his videos every single day for an entire month. I would take notes, try out all the moves to get a better grip on what he was saying and sometimes watch the video again to make sure I had grasped everything he said. After only a few sessions, I clearly understood the importance of posture, anatomy and being more knowledgeable about the different muscles involved to execute each exercise properly. You can very well decide to view one video every day or you could get a book and commit to reading 10 pages or one chapter every day. Set a specific goal and do it to completion.

• Read faster

A few years ago, I tried a method to **read faster:** There are books out there that actually show you different ways to increase the speed at which you read. I gave it a try and although at the end of the 10-day long method, I did not greatly improve my speed-reading skills. I did find some helpful ideas and tools to work on what I needed to improve and when constantly applying the method over time, I managed to double the number of words I could read in a minute. The method also taught me how to grasp the essential elements of an article or book by reading "diagonally". This turned out to be a fundamental tool while I was writing my book, as I had a lot of research to do.

• Following an online course

I also had the opportunity to follow a course on how to **get my book published**. Believe me, it sure isn't easy to juggle work, family, chores, exercising AND studying, but I managed to go through the entire course, simply by making sure that I took the time every day to view one or two lessons. I also made the commitment to sit down at least one to preferably three hours a day to write my book. So, I ask you: What are you into? What have you always wanted to master? Research and find ways through courses and reading to make.

• Increase your vocabulary

There are many books available to help you increase your vocabulary, improve your spelling or grammar. When my kids were homeschooled, we had lots of fun doing these types of books as well as methods to improve mental math skills. My children still talk to me about how fun the exercises were, how much they have improved those specific skills and how these books still have an impact on them today, more so than any of the academic books they had!

• Improve your knowledge of History, Geography, Math…

Do you fall into the category of those people who are really bad at history? Geography? Math? Why don't you choose one and commit to reading a few pages each day to learn more about it.

When it comes to learning something new, I find that nothing beats children's books. So, when I decide to acquire more knowledge in a certain domain, whenever possible, I go and search the children's section. It may seem strange at first, but if you are not very good at something, reading the simplified version of it first, will greatly help you understand the situation prior to reading something a little more complex. In a way, it allows you to roughen the subject out to get a basic picture of the whole story. You can then move on to reading something more complex afterward, to finetune the details.

Another idea to learn history is to buy games. The one I particularly like is Timeline. You have a whole series of cards with events that took place from the beginning of time to our current year. You are dealt a certain number of cards and the goal is, while taking turns with the other players, to place your cards out in front of you in chronological order on a common timeline. It's lots of fun and interesting too!

You could even play this game alone by simply dealing yourself twenty cards and then by trying to put them in order. Once it starts getting too easy, add 10 more cards and so forth and so on.

Learning new things doesn't have to be a burden and doesn't necessarily have to come from a book. Be imaginative. Remember: the more fun you have, the more it will stick with you!

• Become more knowledgeable about wine

Are you tired of going out and never knowing which wine to choose? As with anything, if you start to look into the details, learning about wine can be a never-ending process. Believe me! So, at the beginning, start with the basics and slowly move your way up. An idea might be to take a photo of your favorite restaurant's wine list, find out about their different wines and see which ones go with the different dishes you normally eat. You could also buy a book to learn the basics of wine. Why not also check out your local wine shop: many organize wine tasting events and you might just learn something in the process.

• DIY – Do it yourself!

How to improve your home. There are thousands of videos out there to show you how to do things on your own at home, from changing a lightbulb to putting up wallpaper, checking your washing machine, cleaning the filter, getting rid of and changing moldy tile grout. Most of these videos take only a couple of minutes, so no more excuses for not getting things done.

But DIY could also be about **redecorating, reorganizing** your living space or **putting some more order** in it as well.

A few more ideas:
• Improve your knowledge about car mechanics
• Improve your sewing
• Learn the basics of playing an instrument
• Learn the basics of ice skating, roller skating, surfing or windsurfing
• Learn how to master your keyboard, typewriting skills - without looking
• Become an expert at Excel, Word, PowerPoint
• Improve your general cooking skills and add a specific area of expertise such as vegan, smoothies, French cuisine
• Learn…………………………….. I will let you fill this one out yourself!

And why not **create your very own method** to learn something. Let's say you decide to learn all the different countries of the world, their location and capital. Knowing that there are about 200 countries, go get 200 flash cards, print out from the internet the list of these countries and set about to learn 5 new countries, their capital and location every day. On each flashcard you will write the country and capital and it might be a good idea to print out its location, but also a small typical photo of a famous place to visit. Once you have done all 200 flash cards, you could invent a game. You could, for example, take turns, with a friend or your children, picking up a random card and trying to situate the country on a map.

These flashcards could very well be made to learn pretty much anything: so, why not be creative and start your very own set of cards today.

The purpose of this change is to get you into the habit of starting and completing a "challenge." Start off by finding an easy one that you can finish over a matter of weeks. Keep in mind that you will not retain everything and that it's ok. Then, once it's completed, just make sure to keep setting new goals over and over again. Define each one of them clearly, so that you know when you have completed it. It might not happen the very first time but, little by little, as you reach more and more goals, you will get a real sense of pride: it will be so gratifying when you look back to see everything you have accomplished and also knowing that you did them all on your own incentive.

One day, you will realize that all this practice has a purpose. Indeed, there will come a day when a major challenge comes your way, and you will see that all that practicing will kick in and you will be able to tackle it just fine.

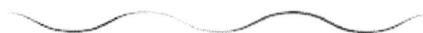

Change n°45
NEWNESS

Are you tired of going through the same old routine? Do you feel bored with the monotony of your life? Why don't you spice things up a bit? Some of us basically live the very same day, every day, until the end of their lives. But remember one thing: a big part of your life is within your hands and it's up to you to go on living a bland life or to turn it into an adventurous one.

No need to do something drastic to bring a little bit of change into your life as there are thousands of things you can do to add variety, diversity, creativity, fun, and adventure.

When you start bringing more "new" into your life, you get into the habit of accepting change. If you do it regularly and willingly, it becomes easier to accept and adapt to difficult situations when something unplanned arises. Indeed, by challenging yourself when everything is going well in your life, you will develop strength to face problems when they pop-up unexpectedly.

It is important to view change as something positive and ask yourself what positive change you can bring into your life, right now. Then, set out to do it. When life lays a serious problem on your plate, remember to ask yourself "What's positive in all this? What life lesson do I need to learn? How can this situation help me grow?"

Ask yourself what you really want from your life at this moment, and then break your goal down into little increments, setting out how you can accomplish them all. Take a good look at what needs to be changed in your life and see what you can do to make it happen. Become the creator of your life.

Start asking yourself what you really want: a happy relationship? A new job? Do you have a desire to be fit? Put your fear of failure aside and go get it. Although some things are not within your control, there is always something that can be done at your level. So, saddle up, take control of your life and embrace change. Remember, if you want new things to happen, you are going to have to get up and get moving. Visualize your success to reinforce your determination, write your goal down on a piece of paper to make it real, and then start taking decisive steps to make your dream come true.

To help you prepare for success, you will find below a list of new things that you can do. Try to make it fun and tackle changes you have always wanted to.

A. Why add something new into your life?

- Doing new things gets you out of your comfort zone: it's an opportunity to practice finding yourself in an unfamiliar situation. Every time you do something new, whether it's milking a cow, daring to ask for something, tasting food you never ate before, you have to adapt. At first it may be a little challenging, **but soon you will be looking forward to the sensation, it will become fun** and you will want to start engaging in things that challenge you even more.

- When you try something new, at first, it may seem uncomfortable, or even disagreeable. But when you think about it, most "habits" we have today did not stem from a "love at first try" situation. Let's take, as examples, cigarettes and coffee: most people don't have a pleasant first experience, indeed, pleasure comes only after a while. When I first met my fiancé, he encouraged me to join him in his morning ritual that consisted of eating lemon slices accompanied with raw turmeric, raw ginger, pepper grains and a bit of coconut oil. There was no need for him to give me an explanation or to list the benefits of all these ingredients, I instantly knew that it would be good for my health. This reason alone was a great source of motivation. It didn't happen overnight but at one point, I realized that I was longing for the experience: the bitterness of the lemon with the rind, the spicy, somewhat fruity taste of raw ginger, the earthy-sweet taste of turmeric, the tongue-tingling effect of pepper grinds, the cocktail of which would create a characteristic explosive sensation inside my mouth. Today, I look forward to it and it is clear that **trying new things can create long lasting habits that are healthy or good for you.**

- **Doing new things will forge your character** into believing that you are a "do-er", that you can handle situations and are in control of your life.

- **Trying new things will make you proud of yourself.** Who cares if you make a strange face while eating your first oyster, it doesn't matter if you scream the first time you take a cold shower, let others laugh at you while attempting your first dive into the swimming pool... hey! *YOU* at least tried! So, stand up tall, smile and be proud!

- **You will be more appreciative of other people's efforts.** When you start doing new things, you realize that you need to have the guts to do it. It's not easy to be a beginner. Notice how you start observing other people around you as they try new or difficult things. That guy at the gym attempting to jump rope, that woman returning to college, you name it! You will start to see things with a new eye, criticize less, become more open to change and more appreciative of other people's efforts.

- **You will develop a more daring personality.** As you gain more confidence, you will boost your self-esteem and start doing and saying things you never thought possible.

- **People will look up to you.** While they might at first laugh at you, you will see that over time many people will start looking at what you do and even attempt a dialog with you: they will want to become more like you and ask you for advice.

B. Ideas to spice up your life

- Try new food you normally wouldn't buy
- Attempt something you thought was too late do to
- Check out some isles at the supermarket you normally don't
- Try a different restaurant or commit to trying foreign food restaurants. This month go to Asia, try Moroccan or French. If you love Italian food and don't wish to change, then try something new on the menu. Take your time to savor this new food and discover its flavors.
- Go around the world in your kitchen. With your family embark on an adventure to discover a new meal every week, coming from a different country. Just before eating, enjoy watching a short documentary on the country. You want this experience to be fun. No need to turn it into a chore. Have a look online how to say hello, goodbye and thank you in that country's language and turn this meal into an experience.
- Look up a recipe in a cookbook or online and enjoy cooking with your family. Preparing food together is actually a good way of bonding. Why not have the entire dinner homemade and do it all from scratch.
- Dance or go dancing more often. Why not take up tango, rock 'n roll, line dance or jazz?
- Rearrange all the furniture in your home, redecorate it by changing some elements of decoration: new cushions, new curtains, a new vase, or a new rug. See how one thing can change the whole atmosphere! Or you could simply clean and clear things up
- Change the color of your hair, your hairstyle, get bangs, get your hair straightened or curled. Change your makeup, try a new look
- Wear different colors or change styles. Be feminine one day and boyish another, wear a classic dress or suit one day and then more modern the next. Have fun wearing different hats and playing around a little bit with your look.
- Have a switch around day and change your routine: examine what you do on a daily basis and see where you can implement changes with things you eat, places you usually go to, how you commute to work or what time you exercise. Try changing radio stations, have your coffee somewhere else, share lunch with someone different. Make this a special day. And then let the kids in on the fun by asking them to bring some ideas too. Propose a "switch around night" and see what they can come up with.
- Volunteer: be a part of an organization. For example, give your time and energy to help the Red Cross
- Try a new hobby: something you have always wanted to explore, such as playing an instrument, taking pictures or pottery or sewing and commit to doing it!
- Visit all the museums in your city, even the ones you are not really interested in
- Listen to music you normally wouldn't listen to and go to a variety of different concerts featuring jazz, rap, or classical
- If you are a man, try growing a little beard or let your hair grow longer or on the contrary, shave it off
- If you like sleeping in, try getting up early for a change and make the most of your day. If you are like me and you jump out of bed early every morning, stay in bed and take your time enjoying breakfast in bed!
- Decide to start studying a subject of your choice. Take up a course or better yet graduate!
- Stop watching TV
- Try a new recreational activity: have you ever tried paddle boarding?

- Try something artistic such as singing, playing a part in a play or painting?
- Be more creative. Make things with your hands.
- Find out what conferences are coming to your town and sign up
- Decide to meditate every day or take the time to relax
- Smile more
- If you haven't started yet, go green. Start little by recycling and then add more things every once in a while to help our Mother Earth
- Take your showers cold instead of hot
- Have sex differently
- Do an Escape game and get your neurons working
- Give compliments to people more often
- Surprise people by doing something out of the usual: buy a lottery ticket for you and your colleagues to share, buy coffee for the people behind you at a drive through.
- If eating in front of the TV is out of the question for you, why not turn it on tonight and watch a good movie during dinner, or if you always have it on, why not turn it off and enjoy your family's company
- If someone asks you for a favor and you don't feel like it, say "no" for a change.
- If you are the type that likes to workout after work, why not call a friend and go out to enjoy a drink for a change and if you always go out for a drink, sign up for a biking or yoga class.
- Take up a new sport even for a day. Have you ever played golf or tennis or tried boot camp training? Sign up for a lesson today
- Don't talk for a whole day, be an observer and a listener. Be attentive to what is going on around you
- If on your day off you planned to do the usual cleaning up, instead, leave the mess behind and pack up a little bag for the day and get away. Take a drive to the beach or countryside
- Or, do you always do the same thing on weekends, such as lunch with the in-laws? Say hello to change! If it's impossible to change a family tradition bring some change by proposing, to eat something different in a new location, or go for a picnic. Have everyone, including kids participate in making the meal by bringing something they baked or cooked themselves.
- Change neighborhoods to do your shopping today: see new faces, different shops
- Play with your children today. Take the time to be there for them and watch them play their video game, play a game together, and then go ride your bikes
- Bring your dog to the park and play fetch with a frisbee. Someone is going to be really happy!
- Have your coffee differently today: maybe a cappuccino, a tall latte, black coffee
- Get something done that you have been wanting to do for a while: wash your car, get your finances and all your papers in order
- In the same line, finish something you have started and then left aside. Did you start a project and never completed it like knitting, sewing, painting, drawing, writing a poem, a book, or interior decorating? Just do it and get it done
- Go out for a long walk after dinner tonight
- Take a look all your stuff and see what you no longer use and put it up for sale

- Visit the store and try a new perfume. if you find a scent you really like, ask the saleslady to spray it on you and try it for the day, before buying it
- Get that pet you have always dreamed of getting
- Change your name. I know that this is something that has been lingering on in my mind for a long time ever since I stopped living in the past and started to look ahead
- Move. Have you been wanting to move, but just haven't had the courage to look. Start today!
- Call someone you haven't talked to in a long time
- Switch off your phone today
- Go learn how to milk a cow
- Book your next vacation on a ranch or find a place that allows you to go back in time
- Visit the library. When was the last time you went? Go for a browse and just enjoy. Remember to bring the kids along too!
- Give some of your time to help out a neighbor or a friend

b. My experience
• Finally mastering the Rubik's Cube
Learn something new: I am sure that there are a lot of things that you have always wanted to master. You know, the things you say you will do someday, when you have the time. Well *now* is the time. Have you ever wanted to know how to cook a specific dish? Have you ever wanted to learn how to draw? Each and every one of us is different and enjoys different things. For example, I have always wanted to know how to solve the Rubik's cube and one day I set out to accomplish this challenge. It took a little bit of commitment, a lot of trial and error, some research on internet…but I did it. Then I challenged myself to do it in a certain amount of time. It was lots of fun and I was proud of myself when I finally understood how it worked.

• Finally getting things done
If you are like most people, then you probably have a to-do list. You know, all those things you say that need to be done and that you really believe you are going to do, such as: putting those frames up on the walls, changing pictures, clearing and cleaning the cellar, fixing something that is broken, mending socks or certain clothes, repainting an old piece of furniture, getting yourself off all of those emails you don't wish to receive. Write this to-do list and decide to knock each and every single item off. An immense satisfaction is guaranteed! You are going to ask me: "In what way is this something new?" It's new because you never got things done before, and now you did!

c. Why not go all the way
Why not take this point to its extreme by deciding to seize every opportunity you get and do things you normally wouldn't? Why not push yourself completely out of your comfort zone and become someone adventurous? Why not decide, this week to say "yes" to all or many different aspects of your life?

Why not decide to live dangerously and do all of those things you have always said you would love to do or the ones you said you would never do: have you ever ziplined? Tried Bungy jumping? Hang gliding? Swimming with sharks? You name it. Push yourself out of your comfort zone, make your life thrilling and decide that you too can do it!

Here are a few Ideas of things that you could do:
- Sleep outdoors
- Eat a worm, an insect, alligator or shark meat, oysters or a fresh vegetable juice? What scares you the most?
- Go shark cage diving
- Have sex in a daring place
- Be in a cemetery at midnight
- Watch a serial killer movie alone or read a serial killer book with your flash light under a tent in your backyard
- Jump off a cliff (into water)
- Do a mud race
- Go audition for a part in a movie
- Go sing on stage
- Sip a glass of wine under the Eiffel Tower
- Do a presentation
- Create your very own piece of art
- Go on a huge Ferris wheel
- Dare to kiss her (or him)
- Do the scariest roller coaster ever
- Do the San Francisco bay escape race
- Go rafting down some crazy rapids
- Ask him or her to marry you
- Organize a flash mob
- Smoke a joint
- Do a wheelie
- Tell a guy or a girl you are crazy in love with him/her.
- Live without your cellphone for a week
- Cross America with your backpack
- Go skinny dipping
- Skip work today
- Go Quad racing
- Drive a Ferrari or a Rolls Royce
- Handbrake and twist your car

You might want to check out Change n°43: Your Lifetime Bucket List for more ideas.

A few years ago, I had the opportunity to watch a T.V. program called *"50 ways to kill your mother"*. I really had a great time watching this show in which a son, Baz Ashmawy decides to make his mother do the craziest things he could imagine. Not only was the idea a great one, but the mother was fantastic. The son would call his mother up every week and take her on a new adventure. She would of course have her say whether she felt capable or not of doing what had been proposed. She accepted every single challenge, including skydiving, crocodile wrestling, rafting rapids, ziplining, eating insects, participating in a drag queen show, being a co-pilot in a desert race, and riding an ostrich. You name it, she did it. The only thing she ended up refusing was the bungee jump.

That for her was an absolute "no."

She explains that she was surprised by the things she did which she never thought she could do. She learned new things about herself and how important it was to push yourself out of your comfort zone, no matter how old you are. These adventures created excitement in her life and her positive attitude towards change encouraged many viewers to take up challenges as well.

I love life and feel privileged to be here. It's a sacrilege not to make the most of it so, I am always seeking opportunities to discover new things, new flavors, and new places. Open up to the world around you and see all of its possibilities. Start embracing life to its fullest.

Change n°46
CONCENTRATION

46.

Many of you might be wondering why have a specific *Change* about concentration. As surprising as it might be, you may need it a lot more than you think.

Think about it: What would happen if we lived our lives totally focused on the present moment, completely attentive to others and to what is going on, while being 100 % concentrated on what we are doing…our life would have more meaning and so much more depth to it.

This is probably unrealistic and impossible to do, but what if we tried to open up more and give our undivided attention to every aspect of our lives as much as possible, throughout the day. I know that when I train, I give it my all. What's great about that is that I always feel amazingly strong and in control of my life afterwards. When I am fully attentive at work, I get so much more done. And when I slow down and take the time to really listen to someone, I feel more alive, more present and I know that I make the other person feel special.

So, whether it be at work, leisure, while you study, meditate or simply getting things done, you will see that concentration is of utmost importance in all areas of life.

You are going to say: but today's world is a busy one and it seems as though we never get a chance to slow down. When we finally get a short break, our phone "dings" with a text message or we feel the need to check out our social media accounts. We are constantly solicited. When I was younger and would walk out the door, no one had any way of contacting me. I would walk in silence without music from my Ipod in my ears. I would train at the gym without being solicited by anyone via text message and if something was urgent, well, it would have to wait until I listened to my messages on my answering machine once I got home at the end of the day. When I watched TV, I watched TV. And when I went to bed, I did so without the company of my cellphone and my followers. Remember, our brains need to rest a little. They need to simply be.

So, make a point of turning off your Ipod to be more in the moment, turning off the radio and phone while driving, to give your brain a break and don't bring your phone to bed with you so you are not tempted to check it out. Finally, when something is really important, give it your all. If you want to make the most of life, you need to do as many things as possible with undivided attention. Don't you find that most of the time we are always doing two things at the same time? Such as:

• Watching a movie and social networking
• Driving and talking on the phone
• Being with the kids at the park and worrying about everything we have to do
• Working, but instead of focusing on the task we are thinking about everything else we have to do

And what about the noise and interruptions when you are working? When do we ever get to do things in total silence anymore? There no need to fight against the way things are, however, we have to learn to accommodate and adapt ourselves to our ever-changing environment.

So, this point is about trying to find ways to improve your concentration in order to be more productive at work and also in your life.

In the first part, we will learn about the importance of concentration and in a second part, we will find different ways to improve it.

Part 1.
Defining concentration

Concentration is the ability to hold the awareness of your mind on one point, without wavering, while excluding everything else from the field of awareness.

Why improve my concentration?

I am sure it has already happened to you: you are at work, but your mind is constantly wandering off somewhere else or is open to every single possible distraction. Maybe you are thinking about how you would much rather be somewhere else. An hour has gone by and you have made several silly mistakes and are feeling increasingly annoyed with yourself and the task you have to finish. Your morning appears to be endless, it seems as though lunchtime is still hours away, and the job you have been assigned is never ending.

Other times, on the contrary, you are capable of turning a blind eye to distraction and can manage to funnel your entire attention on what you are doing, while time flies and you get most of your work done.

It's all a question of concentration. When your mind is concentrated it becomes POWERFUL and can achieve great things: it becomes sharp and to the point, it marshals facts and arguments, it is more efficient…in other words, you get things done.

The benefits of sharp concentration may seem obvious, but let's have a look at them as some may surprise you:

Give your mind a break. Concentrating means you no longer waste time with all those restless thoughts and problems that normally keep popping up. You also don't waste time procrastinating. When your mind is fully focused on one thing, you are actually keeping your problems and negativity at bay, thus becoming a much more positive person.

Get better at what you are doing. By practicing to concentrate during the day with the use of various techniques, you will progressively improve, for longer periods of time. This will actually help you become a better meditator, a better student, a better employee…you name it.

Be able to do more. As you get better at concentrating, you will see how the quality of your work greatly improves and you are getting more done whether working or studying for an exam. You are determined to sit down for one hour, concentrate and complete the project.

Gain more free time. By allotting a certain amount of time to get things done, you will consequently have more time off!

Save a lot of energy. Letting your mind run wild from one idea to another is comparable to having a wild horse: You can't do anything if your horse is going buck wild: you need to break it, keep it under your control. The same holds true with your mind, you need to break the habit of letting your mind run incessantly and freely from one idea to another. By concentrating on what you are doing, you are actually channeling your energy, funneling it in one direction. When you are in this state of concentration, your entire thinking process is clearer, target thoughts come flowing in, and it feels as though a shield keeps you protected from all exterior distractions. When you start mastering mind focus there will be a point when you reach a certain calmness. As you feel that you have reached a greater sense of inner wellbeing, the importance of structure and keeping things under control become really clear.

You give importance to others. If you concentrate on your interlocutor during a conversation, you actually make the other person feel more important. It's a very pleasant feeling when you see that someone is listening to what you have to say.

Remember things faster and for longer periods. When you are in the moment, I mean *"really here",* you learn a lot faster and will remember things more clearly, compared to when you simply learn something in a distracted manner.

You will feel more motivated. When you see that you are making progress learning more, getting things done because you are concentrating, you will be even more motivated to complete your tasks.

Your capacity to focus on one thing without being distracted by your thoughts or what is going on around you, is something worth working on, if you wish to improve the quality of your work. Here you will find different techniques and ideas that can be applied, to help you achieve greater concentration skills. Sharpening your mind will bring more clarity, peace, and will enhance your overall wellbeing.

Part 2.
Tips and ideas to improve your concentration
Concentration is like a muscle: you can train it, to make it stronger.
- After taking years to learn how to juggle and master the art of multitasking, now is the time to practice doing **one thing at a time** and staying focused while doing it. Once you are settled in your activity, get into the habit of giving it your undivided attention.

- It's not always possible but try to **do things to completion** before starting something else and avoid delaying. Get things done before they pile up, adding more clutter to your desk and mind.

- **Slow down and do it right**. When you have too much going on, your mind will have a hard time focusing on what you are doing. You will also have a tendency to do things in a rushed manner, which leads to mistakes and seldom to a job well done. When you start slowing things down and relaxing, you accept the fact that you only have two hands and can only truly handle one thing at a time. You will see that your focus will slowly shift on trying to get things done properly and on enjoying the process, rather than simply getting things done.
- **Create interest**. It is a proven fact that if you add pleasure to the learning process, you will retain more and far better. Many times, when we sit down and "have to" do something, we find it irrelevant and boring. Instead of complaining, why not apply yourself and change your approach by finding ways to make your task more enjoyable and interesting. This is a technique I often use when helping my kids with their homework. After a day's work, it's the last thing I feel like doing but many times, I manage to shift from a negative mindset to a "ok, let's see what's interesting here," type of attitude.
- **Shut out distractions.** Did you know that once you are interrupted, it can take you up to 15 minutes to return to the same point of concentration? So, before you set out to do anything: turn off your phone or any other device or T.V. and shut the door. If possible, **create time slots** when you are no longer available under any circumstances. Once your door is shut it means "do not disturb".
- **Get to know yourself.**

What is your <u>When?</u> Take the time to find out when you work best: are you a night owl or an early bird? Observe yourself over a period of five days and see when you are able to concentrate best. See if there are any recurring patterns and then plan accordingly: if you tend to be alert around 10 a.m. every morning, then make sure you put this time slot aside to address what most requires you to concentrate. If you tend to feel drowsy around 2 p.m., plan for a ten minute nap or try to see if a brisk five minute walk or a cold shower are helpful and then tackle some easy chores at work. Of course, when we have a job, we don't always get to choose when we do certain tasks but it is a good idea to get to know yourself and if you can, plan your work schedule accordingly.

What is your <u>Where?</u> Do you work better at home or do you need to get away? I know I work a lot better at the library or in a café. At home there are way too many chores and things to do. It seems as though every time I look up or get up, I find something to do. Either create a concentration friendly atmosphere or find a place where you know you will not be distracted.

What are your <u>How's?</u>

Do you need to be surrounded by your books, your sticky notes, your mess? Or do you need to have everything all nice and tidy?

Do you need silence? If so, you might want to try using earplugs. Do you need a background noise? You might want to consider playing "white noise". It's a steady sound such as ocean waves and rainfall. You can easily find apps that offer this kind of steady background.

Little by little or full on? Some people feel they get more work done by setting aside a couple of hours every day, while others might be more productive getting away for three whole days of intensive work. Observe yourself and find out how you function.

- **Practice.** Practice doing one thing at a time while doing it with 100% of your undivided attention. Start with a timer and try to stay completely focused for 10 to 20 minutes and work your way up.

- **Train your brain.** Why not take up activities that stimulate your brain such as Sudoku, Rubik's cube or any other type of mental challenge. These activities literally open new wire connections to the brain.

- **Start taking responsibility.** Many times, we tend to find excuses and procrastinate. When you have something that needs to be done, sit down and get it done. Period. Decide that you will no longer be distracted by noise, colleagues, or phones. Stop putting the blame on others or exterior factors and quit delaying.

Concentration is that powerful state you can reach
that shields you from the outside world,
making obstacles magically disappear
and allowing you to open certain channels
to receive the inspiration
and attract the opportunities you need
to get things done....

- **Practice meditation** to slow things down and achieve stillness of mind

- Remember: it's important t**o lead a healthy lifestyle,** which means to sleep enough, eat healthy, eat the right amount and exercise. This will improve your concentrate.

- **Set a goal before you start** to read or write: decide to get a certain number of pages read or done, do a specific task to completion, finish a report, and answer all of your emails

- **Commit** to working for a certain number of hours, an allotted amount of time.

- Don't forget, your **bed is for sleep not work.** If you want to have a high level of concentration, it is important to stick with a work environment.

- **Keep a writing pad beside you.** Do you constantly have ideas popping up or remember things that need to be addressed? Make sure you have a pad close by on which you can quickly jot down a few lines. This way you are sure you won't forget your ideas and can quickly get back to work.

- **Need to memorize?** Take notes, write things down or tape them and then reread your notes or listen to the tapes occasionally.

- **Remember to move.** When sitting down for a long period of time, although your blood is still flowing, getting up and walking gets the whole system pumping. So, move. Keep your machine active to keep your brain active as well.

- **Say a prayer.** Take the time to sit quietly right before you start working and close your eyes just for a few minutes. Prepare your mind by slowing things down, calming the flow of thoughts, and being receptive to receiving inspiration, ideas, focus and everything else you might need to make this a great working session. Imagine that everything you need is channeled towards you and you are ready to receive.

By taking the time to fully concentrate on what you are doing, what people are saying and observing life more attentively, you will see that you will live more intensely. Think about it: what's better? A day of multitasking, of rushing and stress, or a life in which you slow down, are able to be more attentive and enjoy each moment. Realistically, we all know it's not always possible, but you can make a conscious effort, you can choose to lighten up your days and take the time to be more present. And what a surprise it will be when you realize, that slowing things down and concentrating more on what you are doing will actually enable you to get more things done!

Change n°47
TRAVELING

47.

While it can be relatively easy to bring a little bit of change in our everyday lives and "day to day" routine, it may seem a little daunting to accomplish that while we are travelling. But what if next time you went away on vacation, you turned your trip into more than just another destination: Why not create an unforgettable experience by soaking up the local culture and trying to feel the heart of this new place that you are discovering? If the idea seduces you, then next time you hit the road, whether it be for leisure or work, turn your future trip into a meaningful experience.

Most of the time, when we travel, we tend to visit the top 10 tourist spots that each country or city has to offer such as the Eiffel Tower, the Arc de Triomphe, the Champs Elysées, The Louvre, The Notre Dame Cathedral if you are visiting Paris. Although it would be a shame not to visit these monuments, why not take the time to visit some unbeaten paths or, as Robert Frost would put it, choose the ones" less travelled by"?

The first thing you need in order to create a memorable experience is to do your homework… homework meaning that you must prepare your trip ahead of time. If you are not an adept of choosing your destination at the last minute, then try to start preparing your journey a month before you go. The good thing about planning ahead is that the whole process will get you all excited about leaving, it will enrich your experience and make it seem a lot longer than it actually was.

A. Making the most of your trip before you go
a. Read ! Read ! And do your Research
The first thing to do is to take in as much information as you possibly can about your destination. You can, of course go to your local bookstore and buy a guide or flip through books at your library, but in today's modern world it's just so much easier to turn on your computer and browse on the net. Check out the following points:
• Find short videos about your destination and discover the local colors, typical arts and crafts, and music
• Research a short history and the major facts about the place
• Search for any photos that will help you discover the sites but also the different landscapes
Gathering all this information will allow you to get a good idea of where you are headed and the best places to visit.

So, what can you do prior to departure?

b. Learn the language!

It's pure courtesy to learn the basic words such as "Hello, Good-bye, thank you and please", but making the extra effort to learn the language can really help you immerse yourself and feel a part of the place. There is no need to become fluent, but learning the basic words, a few simple phrases and local expressions will allow you to have a simple conversation. The locals will appreciate the effort you put into learning their language and chances are your accent or mistakes will make them laugh or create an entertaining misunderstanding. That's a great way to get the conversation going and create a relaxing atmosphere. There are many ways to learn a language ranging from books that teach you the basics in 20 lessons, or apps on your phone, videos on YouTube and why not opt for private or group lessons. The options are there to grab and today, you can pretty much learn a language without spending a dime. Go to your local news stand and see if they have a magazine in the language you need to learn and keep it with you, in your bag or briefcase, to pop open when you have a few minutes to relax.

c. Discover the flavors before you go! Why not check out if there are any restaurants that serve typical dishes from the country you are planning to visit, such as Moussaka if you are going to Russia, Trippa alla Romana if you are going to Italy, Cassoulet, Choucroute or Crèpes if you are going to France. If you can't find one or if it's out of your budget, why not look online for an easy recipe and create the ambiance at home. You could add a little bit of local music and chances are it will already feel like you're travelling, although you are in your very own home!

d. Plan events ahead of time

A month before you go, check out the local town's website to see what's happening, what there is to visit, if there are any festivals or concerts that you could attend. Where are the local clubs? Where can you get a drink and mingle with the local crowd? If you love dancing, try to discover which ones are close by to where you will be staying.

e. Make a list of the "Musties"

The "musties" are the places you absolutely want to visit. There is nothing wrong with visiting the typical touristy spots, but it would be a shame to limit yourself, so leave room for the unexpected, for some "farniente". Plan whole afternoons just to stroll around the city streets or country side, sit at a café with a local magazine and just relax while taking your time. Maybe if you are brave you can try to strike up a conversation.

f. Decide where you are going to stay

When booking for your next vacation, why not try a homestay experience by staying with a local family: there is no better way to be a part of a place than by immersing yourself completely. If, going on vacation means for you "zero obligations" and the idea of living with other people is already stressful, you could opt to rent an apartment or studio in a typical neighborhood. This way, you would be in the middle of the action and mingling with the local population every day.

You could also split half / half: in other words, spend half of your trip living with a local family and the other half in a hotel or a rented apartment. The good thing about living with the locals is that you have someone to talk to that will give you many tips about what and what not to do, as well as to know where to go and which places to avoid. It is definitely a convincing option when you want to really get to know a place. I won't insist too much about the downsides but there are some, of course, and you should take them into consideration: what if you don't get along, hosts can be invasive or offer little privacy…Most of the time however, I have had good recommendations from people who have chosen this option.

B. Making the most of your trip when you are there

The second part, we will tackle now is how to make the most of it.

a. Stay put

Probably the best way to immerse yourself in the local culture is **to stay put in one place** as long you can. Being American and living in Monaco, I made a point of going back to the US regularly with the children in order for them to soak up the American culture. We experienced it in different ways: road trips with hotels and driving from one place to another, doing a big tour of the West coast in a camping car.. but what really made the difference was when we decided to rent an apartment and stay put in one place for an extended period of time. This way we made the most of the town we had chosen to live in: the kids signed up for activities and made friends, we started socializing and meeting people, we discovered new spots, beaches and parks, as well as activities and restaurants. It was a totally new experience as we trick-or-treated with local families and were invited to share Thanksgiving dinner with friends. These "immersions", in a single spot, forever changed the relationship my children have with the US. Although I know it's not possible for everyone to get away for long periods of time, it might be worthwhile to consider renting a place and staying in one spot for the duration of your whole trip. Next time, if you travel, go beyond the touristy stuff. This way you will also be able to seize the real atmosphere of the place.

If you rent a place in a local neighborhood, you will be buying food from the local grocer and necessities from nearby stores. This will allow you to get to know people that live close by. Try to look around and see how you can interact more. Normally when we travel, we get pampered up before we go, such as getting our hair cut or getting our nails done. Why not switch things around this time and get it all done locally: find the local hairdresser or barber, beautician, nail shop and get it done while you are there. Try to chat with the employee. Tell them that you are there for a short period of time and ask if they can recommend any hidden spots to visit, a nice place to eat or something nearby that is a must see. It may seem like a waste of time at first to take two hours to get your hair done, but it might make a real difference. Don't be surprised if everyone in the salon wants to recommend a certain restaurant or spot to discover. Before you leave the country, out of courtesy, remember to stop by, to relate your experience and thank them once again for their recommendations.

During one of my stays in the United States, I decided to rent a mail box and regularly went to pick up my mail or some online orders I had made. Every time, I would take the time to chat a few minutes with the lady working there. One day, she asked me if I could do her a favor: her grandfather had gone to France when he was young, and he had taken photos and bought postcards on the back of which he had written comments, but it was all in French. She was curious to know what he had written and asked me if it was possible for me to translate them for her. I brought the album home and although it did take me a little while to do all of the translating, I was happy to oblige. Seeing her smile when I brought it back, made it all worthwhile. Just goes to say, interacting with the locals can land you on some unexpected paths.

b. Eat Locally
Try to find out where local people eat, an animated place such as the market. Grab a table and simply observe the people around you. Order something typical that the waiter recommends. It's ok if you don't like it, just like my mom used to say, *"what's important is to try"*.

c. Learn something new
Try to see if you have the opportunity to **take a lesson** and learn something new:
• Take a cooking class and enjoy learning how to do a local dish
• Take a dance lesson and have fun learning a typical local dance
• Take an arts and craft class:
Some friends of mine, Michelle and her son Loup-Raphaël, for example, enjoyed creating sarongs during their last vacation and brought back their very own hand-made sarongs as gifts for their friends and family. They were not only beautiful, they had actually taken the time to learn a local craft and put their heart into creating them.

Another example: I enjoyed learning how to do pottery with a local craftsman: it was so much fun and it felt special to spend time in his workshop, watch him work and interact with the customers. It remains memorable to this day!

d. Venturing off beaten paths
Grab your backpacks and hike or walk around to **discover hidden spots**. Last time I went with my husband to the United States, we drove around and got kind of lost. We decided to park the car and enquire if there was nice spot where we could have dinner. The people we spoke to knew about a restaurant somewhere on the beach. We had quite a bit of a walk to do, but once we reached the end of the path the spot was simply amazing!!!! We ate locally fished grilled cod while watching the sun come down. And, to spice things up, this place played a game: the waiters would ask all the customers to guess at what time to the exact minute, the sun would drop behind the horizon. The winner would get a glass of champagne! It was a great idea and the ambiance in the restaurant was full of laughter and excitement. Although we didn't win and lost by one minute we all applauded the winners with sincerity. Unbeaten trails once again made this moment a winner. Since then, we have returned there so many times and we have a painting of the restaurant on our wall at home.

e. Discovering local sports

Why not **try a local sport or go watch a local match**. It doesn't matter if you don't know anything about it, just go anyway! I know this is going to seem incredible for many of you, but living in Monaco, baseball is inexistent. So, during one of our stays in Florida, I really made a point to buy tickets to visit the Tropicana Field and see a baseball match. We had an amazing time and the hotdogs that day had a totally different flavor!

But if you are going to England, why not enjoy a local cricket match, or if you come to Monaco, for example, you can watch a game of soccer or observe hang gliders jump off a cliff and land on the beach. If you are in Hawaii and have never surfed, sign up for a course and hit the waves and give it a shot. Chances are you will manage to surf a wave after only a few tries. If you are a runner, check out if there is a race organized nearby while you are in town, and if you enjoy the gym, why not sign up at a local one for the time you are there or get a day pass.

f. Check out if there is a concert in town

When I went to Corsica, I discovered a local group that sang A cappella. It was an incredible, goose bumps triggering experience. There were six men singing, each with a different tonality of voice, with no music to accompany them. You could sit and listen in admiration and awe. Believe me I bought all their records and listened to them for years even after I returned back home. While you are away, try as much as possible, to listen to the local radio, even if you don't understand a word!
During one of my travels in Namibia, we listened to the local radio and heard the bushman clicking language. They somehow click their tongue and talk at the same time. What a laugh with the kids when trying to reproduce it!

g. Buy local magazines or newspapers

If you understand the language, why not buy the **local paper** every day to see what is going on there. If you are up to date with the news you won't have too much of a problem understanding what they are talking about, and you will also be able to strike up a conversation or have questions to ask if you connect with any of the locals. If your language fluency doesn't allow you to read the paper, you can still buy magazines and flip through pages to see what the fashion is like there and you might also learn a few words!

h. Ride local

As much as possible, **use local transportation**. There is no better way to soak up the environment than by joining the crowds when riding a tram, boat, subway, bus, train or walking. If you prefer taking a cab, strike up a conversation with the driver.
Even if you do not speak very well, talk to people. **Engage in conversation**. The way I see it, you have nothing to prove and nothing to lose.

i. Go dancing

Find a local club, mingle with the crowd and simply have a good time. Just make sure you go somewhere safe!

In this last part, let's see how you can make the experience last and make it memorable.
Every time I travel, instead of writing to each and every one of my friends, I create a blog. I write it like a journal and describe what we did and visited every day. I also like to write everything that I have learned that day whether it be about local culture, history, or fauna. And then when I get back home, I bind it into a book to make a lasting souvenir of our trip, something the kids can review and enjoy later on in their life.
I usually load it up with photos. It takes a little time every day to write the page or anecdotes, that I must concede, but it's really worth the effort.

If you stayed with local people during your trip, it's a good idea to write to them and send them a few postcards from where you live.
If you have enough space in your home or if you just want to meet new people, why not propose stay-ins or daily visits where you live? You could propose to help a foreign family discover the typical spots, typical dining areas, dances, learn about historical events, and the language. There are so many things that you could do to make a tourist's day special.

A few years ago, we met an American family visiting Monaco. They were a little disappointed and evidently, not impressed. We started chatting and convinced them to come with us on a tour of our city and country. We told them all about the local gossip, brought them to breathtaking spots for photos and then directed them to a great restaurant. They had a great time and still write to us today!! It was so nice because we managed to conjure up an experience for them. If you love the place where you live, why not share your love by helping people discover it!

Change n°48
CONQUERING FEAR

48.

Are you terrified about something? Is there a fear holding you back from doing something you would really like to do? Decide today to confront it and put these fears behind you.

According to the NIMH -National Institute of Mental Health- approximately 10% of the American population suffers from some type of phobia. Knowing that we are approximately 327 million people that means that there are 32,7 million people suffering from a certain type of fear. So, if this is your case, you are not alone.

My Story

I developed a fear of driving on the highway after my best friend died, crushed by truck. She was only in her mid-twenties and at the time it was a terrible blow for me, as it seemed so unfair. One minute she was there and the next she was gone. And what made things even sadder was that she had a son, Victorien. She named him this way because he was a victory against all odds. But that's another story. I didn't think so much about the accident when it happened. It was more the sudden brutal loss that affected me and I also realized that I too could die at any moment. We all know this, but when you lose someone overnight, it really hits you. My fear of driving came later on. It sort of built up gradually until one day, as I was driving, I felt my whole body stiffen, until I could no longer move at all. I was paralyzed: I was totally overcome by fear. It was as though it totally controlled me.

It took me a long time to understand, that I was the one who needed to regain control over my body. I had once lived without fear but I had then allowed it control me. What this meant, however, was that I could live without fear again. I knew that deep down inside, it was all up to me. And so that's what I decided to do! I was going to get back up on that saddle and become fearless. Before relating my story, read on to find out more details about phobias and ways to conquer them.

Don't you think it's time for you too to overcome your wildest fear and finally… fly to Europe, enjoy a day at the zoo, pet a dog, go to a party, finally get your teeth checked, take the elevator… whatever your fear is…overcome it.

A. Defining phobia

Phobias are irrational, unreasonable, uncontrollable, intense fears triggered by a specific identified stimuli that can be an object, a living being or a determined situation.

People know that it may often appear silly, but the fear simply overcomes them and they seem to lose total control over their reactions.

1. Examples of phobias and their names

What are you scared of? Is it a fear of...

- driving on the highway
- spiders - arachnophobia
- flying - aviophobia or aerophobia
- speaking in public - glossophobia
- water - aquaphobia
- fear of the sea - thalassophobia
- fear of driving - vehophobia
- dental check-ups - or is it needles? trypanophobia
- fear of getting ill - nosophobia
- fear of open spaces or public spaces - agoraphobia
- hospitals — nosocomephobia,
- heights - acrophobia
- dust - koniphobia
- clowns - coulrophobia
- number 13 - trikaidekaphobia
- mice - musophobia
- fear of balloons - globophobia
- elevators - no official name, shall we call it elevatorophobia?
- closed-in spaces - claustrophobia
- snakes - ophidiophobia
- fear of the sight of blood - hemophobia
- dogs - cynophobia
- fear of social situations - of being humiliated while seen in public such as giving a speech
- the fear of fear - phobophobia
- the fear of darkness - nyctophobia
- the fear of everything - panophobia
- the fear of Friday the 13th - paraskevidekatriaphobia
- fear of animals - zoophobia
- fear of bananas - bananaphobia
- fear of long words - Hippopotomonstrosesquippedaliophobia. Not really sure it's true but it gave me a good laugh and just had to share.
- many of these phobias exist because, all in all, the real fear that we are experiencing is the fear of dying: Thanatophobia.

2. How do you know if you have a phobia or not?

Phobias can appear silly and most people will willingly admit it, but when a situation arises in which we are confronted with the object or situation that we fear, our reaction is often irrational and uncontrollable. When you find yourself in a circumstance where you are confronted by your worst fear, it feels like you no longer have any control over yourself and you are completely overcome by your fear. For this reason, many people decide to avoid any situation in which they could find themselves having to face what they fear the most. For example, they will drive the extra miles to avoid the highway, they won't go to Europe to avoid taking the plane, they will not get a check-up fearing an eventual shot.

3. What are the common symptoms of phobias?

How do you know if your fear isn't just a normal fear, such as a natural fight and flight response or whether it is an actual phobia? When you start planning ahead to avoid a certain situation in which you know you will have to confront your fear, you most likely have a phobia. For example, if you stop travelling to avoid taking the plane, if you start taking smaller much longer routes to avoid taking the highway, if you go all around the park to avoid cutting across because you might encounter a dog, if you take the stairs even if there are "only" 12 floors to avoid taking the elevator… there is evidence here that you are experiencing some type of phobia.

But there are actual physical and emotional symptoms as well:
- Trembling
- Increased heart rate
- Racing or Pounding heart
- Sweating
- Feeling like you are about to suffocate
- Feeling anxious
- Feeling paralyzed
- Feeling powerless, that your fear possesses you in a certain way
- Fear that you are losing it, losing all control
- Shortness of breath
- Extreme fear
- Fear of dying
- Chest pain
- Feeling dizzy
- Extreme terror
- Fainting

Symptoms can sometimes cause you to freak out or can lead to an anxiety or panic attack. But most times nothing happens and within minutes when the trigger of your fear disappears, your fear subsides.

4. What are your options?

First of all, it's important to know that many people have been treated and have overcome their phobia no matter what the cause and how long they have had it.

The next step: it could be interesting to know when this phobia started and what caused it. Many times, an event has occurred that may not even seem related to your fear, so it might be worth looking into, maybe with the help of a professional. There are different levels of phobias. When phobias are mild to moderate, self-help or the help of a friend may be sufficient. However, if the phobia is severe and if you have panic attacks it is recommended to seek professional help as it might be necessary to receive medical treatment.

5. Taking the decision to overcome it…

This is already one step in the right direction. Because it's very important to keep in mind, that in the end YOU are the one that chooses to live in fear or decides to take action. You may not control your fear right now, but you do control the way you are going to face this fear. So, take responsibility and then move to the next step: start acting upon it.

Think of it this way, whether you realize it or not, we experience the process of fear more often than we think: every time we learn something or find ourselves in a new context or in unfamiliar territory, we go through a phase of fear, as in: "I don't understand", "I am learning", "this balancing act is not easy", "what will people think of me". Uncertainty accompanies this process and some adapting will still be necessary before you are able to reach a certain comfort zone again. What is actually happening when you are in this learning phase? You are in fact failing over and over again. But all of this "failing and trying out" done repeatedly is what builds your determination over time and clarifies your intention. You have to confront your fear and decide to overcome it, take action and finally get over it. With repetition and experimentation, you will slowly rebuild your self-confidence and your fear will be a thing of the past. Quitting after one or two trials would be failing but giving it another try is one step closer to success. The way I see it, life is a never-ending school and *you* are a student.

Something to reflect upon: Many times, we imagine how things will unfold in the future, but it's important to keep an open mind: there are a million possibilities and even if you imagine the most probable ones, chances are none of them will happen. Have you noticed how sometimes life has a way of steering things? At first, it may seem as though things are going in the wrong direction. Many times, I found myself in a certain situation: I would take the time to consider what the outcomes might be and how I could react. But, in the end, none of what I imagined ever occurred and the situation turned out to be something I never envisioned. For this reason, learn to let go of the outcome, and to simply trust.

6. Accept a helping hand or read a Self-help book

The help of a friend or someone that has gone through the same challenge and is now cured, can often be of great assistance. Simply knowing that you are not alone on this path, with living proof that one *can* get over their worst fears and having someone to hold your hand and talk to, can help lead you to success. I also highly recommend reading books that help you face your specific fear or fears in general. Check the references section for ideas.

7. Rewarding

A good idea that can help is to reward yourself every time you face your fear. This associates a positive experience to your phobia. The idea is to break the vicious cycle of linking your worst fear to a negative experience. Finding a way to reward myself with my phobia of driving on the highway was quite easy. There were so many things that I wanted to do or places I wanted to go to but couldn't, because my fear stopped me from doing it. To visit a certain mall, to eat at my favorite restaurant, bring my sons to the trampoline park…it all required taking the highway. Seeing my kids happy in itself was already the biggest reward. But if you have a fear of dogs, you could reward yourself with your favorite chocolate. Carry a few squares in your bag specifically for this occasion and just as Pavlov's mice did, you will soon associate seeing a dog and getting a reward -a delicious piece of chocolate - as inseparable.

8. Break down "encounters" with the object of your fear into small acceptable and achievable confrontations.

I was lucky to have the possibility to practice taking the highway on a small portion where I live. There is an exit six minutes after entering the highway and I would do loops going onto the highway and getting back out several times in a row making it far less challenging than driving non-stop for thirty minutes. If you are scared of spiders or dogs, you could start by looking at photos or seeing tiny or small ones. Talk to yourself and learn to be realistic about the situation: it's only a tiny harmless spider, it's only a cute harmless puppy, it's only six minutes, I can press the help button in this elevator, there is always a way out, or I am at the shallow end of the pool with a friend, and there is a lifeguard.

You might contest by saying that it is not possible to do this for every type of phobia. For instance, when you are scared of flying, flights are usually a minimum of 60 minutes and there is no way out. In this case, try to focus on the moment right before the flight. Fear usually builds up progressively before you take off, sometimes even several days preceding the departure. Try to find time to relax and meditate several times a day prior to your departure. Why not practice breathing techniques that are calming and soothing? Try to reach a calm and relaxed state, while breathing deeply and slowly.

9. Therapy, with Cognitive Behavioral Therapy or CBT

CBT is psychotherapy that combines cognitive therapy with behavior therapy: the idea is to substitute faulty or maladaptive thinking patterns, emotional response, or behavior with more desirable patterns.

It often gets effective and rapid results by making you face your fear repeatedly. If you want to know more about CBT, then seek out a qualified professional therapist to explore this therapeutic modality.

10. Relaxation and breathing techniques.

A great part of overcoming your fear lies in the way you handle it. Learning how to manage it and staying calm, when you feel it coming on, is very important and can make a huge difference on the outcome. Learning to master various breathing techniques before the onset of fear, can really help you overcome the event, come out of it a lot calmer while creating the feeling that you CAN get over this. One of the worst parts of having a phobia is that we often feel totally overcome by it and we lose all sense of control.

When I was driving, my fear was such that I would become totally paralyzed. I started thinking in terms of "I am so lucky this time. No crash. Nothing happened." Later on, when I had kids and ended up driving alone with them, it really hit me that an accident could hurt or kill them or others. For this reason, I decided to avoid driving on the highway and found ways to get around it for years. However, one of the things that really helped me overcome my fear was when I was able to recognize the signs and symptoms early on in the process and respond and react to them immediately.

The day I decided to get rid of this phobia, I found that learning to concentrate on my breathing and making sure it was deep and calm was what helped me the most.

I was totally surrounded by cars. There were hundreds of cars ahead of me and hundreds behind me and I knew that I had to go on because I couldn't just stop there. There was no way out for the time being. This triggered a huge anxiety attack and in a matter of seconds, my whole body felt like one big block. I could no longer turn my head in order to switch lanes or move my feet, to press the brakes. I was frozen. My eldest son, who was in front sitting next to me, understood immediately what was happening and began talking to me in a soothing way, saying that everything was ok. He kept an eye on the traffic for me and kept telling me that all the cars around us were at a safe distance and that I had nothing to worry about. So, I kept on going at that same speed and stayed put in my lane and focused only on my breathing. Slowly, slowly, I felt my body starting to relax out of its frozen state. Gradually I started to feel my body again, until I was in total control of myself. These panic attacks reoccurred three times and then never again. Each time it got easier as I instantly put myself in "relax mode". Now, when I drive, I know how to avoid these panic attacks completely. If I do feel a surge of fear coming on, I automatically begin to breathe deeply and I quickly calm down. Usually, I will slow down a bit and my fear completely subsides within a few seconds. Learning to focus on your breathing can be truly efficient.

Note: I really felt the benefit from relaxing. However, we are all different and on the contrary, others might feel the need to yell, exercise intensely, sprint, run, practice boxing, laugh out loud, dance and sing...or maybe even cry.

11. Putting things into perspective.

Lay out flat the reality of the situation: "I am experiencing a phobia and this fear is causing my mind to exaggerate the severity of the situation and at the same time to underestimate my capacity to deal with it." I just feel it's important to make things clear and repeat it to yourself.

12. Changing the way you think

At first, I kept thinking that I could die and that if I drove the car, it just might be my last day! It's important to be aware of these thoughts regarding the object of your fear. Are there words, phrases or sentences that you tend to repeat in your mind? Or is it a mental image? Take the time to write them down and question them, and then find new positive ones to replace them. I would remind myself of all of the wonderful things that I was going to be able to do with my children, the fact that I would regain a certain form of liberty that I had lost. There is a sense of freedom in knowing that I can now go wherever I want to. I kept this idea in my mind as I drove: "I am now free to discover the world". What is your fear keeping you from doing? Deciding to be fearless starts with your thoughts, so make sure they are positive and leading you in the right direction.

13. Talking or meeting people who have overcome their fear, possibly the same one

Getting the opportunity to talk to someone who has successfully overcome a similar fear can really help boost your confidence especially if you have already decided to act upon it. They know what you are going through and will probably be more than happy to help someone who is going through what they have. They may have tips for you and their enthusiasm and pride in having overcome their worst fear will most certainly be communicative.

14. Consulting a specialist, undergoing Therapy or Medication.

If your fear feels uncontrollable, I recommend you seek out the help of a qualified healthcare professional. If your fear can put you in a dangerous situation I strongly advise you to get immediate professional help.

15. Cut yourself some slack.

Keep in mind that getting over your fear may require several trials. Hey, that's ok. Just remember that because you failed to overcome it last time, it doesn't mean that you won't succeed this time around. Sometimes, it's a question of timing, maturity, as well as acceptance.

16. What I did to overcome my fear of driving on the highway

With my fear of driving on the highway, I always found excuses not to do things. But one day I had the opportunity to go to the US alone with my two boys. But if I wanted to go, I was going to have to get over my fear of driving. This was a great source of motivation. Once the tickets were booked, I immediately signed up for driving lessons. In France, you have driving schools everywhere. I was very fortunate to get an incredible instructor who reassured me that I wasn't alone with my fear, and that he was confident I would overcome it before going to the states in three month's time. He was calm, reassuring and funny. These factors allowed me to associate driving with something positive: I knew I was going to be in good company and have a good time. I took three lessons a week and my instructor made me get on and off the highway over and over again: I would get on the highway, drive a couple of miles and get off and do this 30 times in a row until it felt actually comfortable. I knew what to expect and I was able to relax. At the end of the second week, my instructor told me I could take the road on my own for a small portion. My kids love KFC and I was never able to go because it meant taking the highway. So, my first goal was to make them happy and seeing their smiling faces when I got back home with a big bucket of chicken made me happy as well, but I also felt a big sense of pride. I kept on taking lessons until my departure but brought the sessions down to once a week. It was an investment since lessons are quite expensive, but it was well worth it.

When I arrived in the US, I chose not to rent a car immediately upon arrival since I felt tired and jetlagged after a long overseas trip. I took a cab instead and rented the car only the next day. At first, I got used to driving around town and slowly started adding highway portions. In the course of a month I actually made several long trips via the highway and was so proud of myself for my accomplishments! I took the I-275 for a distance of 46 miles, that's 54 minutes between Bradenton and Clearwater and then the I-75 for 166 miles which is about 2 ½ hours driving from Tampa Florida to Naples and then another 166 miles to drive back. I didn't really need to reward myself, because arriving at the desired destination was already a reward in itself. But every time I had some driving to do, there was a good reason for going: seeing some good friends in Naples and bringing the kids to do some indoor surfing in Clearwater are just two examples. One thing is for sure: driving, gradually and repeatedly, helped me overcome my fear.

See where YOU stand. You are more likely to overcome your fear if you take it one step at a time and feel supported in this decision to overcome it.

I was married for 17 years and although my husband was trying to be nice since he knew that driving terrorized me, his constant assistance gave me an excuse not to try, and I became totally dependent upon him to go anywhere I needed to go. Believe me, I hated it. I wasn't mad at my husband for helping; I was actually grateful every time. I was simply mad at myself for accepting this situation and being so limited.

This was my experience, but we are all different and we each handle our phobias, fears and wounds in different ways.

From the bottom of my heart,
I wish you can embrace your fear
and overcome it, forever.

Wouldn't it be fantastic if we could go through life without being scared of anything! Probably. But we must accept the fact that fear is an integral part of our existence and we have to learn to live with it and accept it. In this change we developed the idea of overcoming phobias, but what about our little fears in life that keep us from doing so many things. One of my close friends really wanted to take part in her boyfriend's triathlon training but was a lousy swimmer. She is a real athlete in other domains but because she is incapable of doing a lap without drinking up at least ten glasses of water, she would often "punish" herself and stay at home while her boyfriend and other friends would go. I asked her why she didn't take a few swimming lessons. She immediately said that she was a desperate case. But she wasn't. After the first lesson and a few simple tips she had already improved immensely, and I could see that she was feeling more confident in her ability. As I told her, it doesn't matter if it takes two, four or six months. If she continues practicing, practicing, practicing there is no reason why she couldn't join her boyfriend and the rest of the group soon.

Many times, when we tend to turn things down because we either don't know how to do it and feel lousy or we are scared to look silly in the eyes of others. Stop excluding yourself. Because *You* and only *You* are keeping yourself from what you secretly would like to experience or accomplish. Is there something you have always dreamed of? What's keeping you from doing it?

12 WEEK COMMITMENT

☆ Because every second, of every minute, of every hour, of every day counts,

☆ Because I have decided to focus on my potential to change what lies ahead of me,

☆ Because I know that **CHANGE IS POWERFUL**, rewarding and exciting,

I, _____(name), sign this contract with myself and hereby commit to doing one change every week over the next 12 weeks. (*Fill out and sign each week once the change has been completed*):

WEEK	CHANGE	SIGNATURE
WEEK 1	_____	_____
WEEK 2	_____	_____
WEEK 3	_____	_____
WEEK 4	_____	_____
WEEK 5	_____	_____
WEEK 6	_____	_____
WEEK 7	_____	_____
WEEK 8	_____	_____
WEEK 9	_____	_____
WEEK 10	_____	_____
WEEK 11	_____	_____
WEEK 12	_____	_____

I understand, that I will not do anything that will overly frustrate me, nor will I punish, or deprive myself. This binding agreement I have with myself is geared towards helping me focus on bringing positive emotions into my life (feeling proud, happy, strong, grateful, determined etc.), on doing more things that are rewarding and on committing to doing them with passion.

_____   _____

DATE   SIGNATURE

MY NOTES

_____

_____

_____

_____

_____

_____

_____

_____

_____

_____

_____

_____

_____

_____

_____

_____

CHAPTER FIVE

LEARNING TO EMBRACE PAINFUL and UNWANTED CHANGE

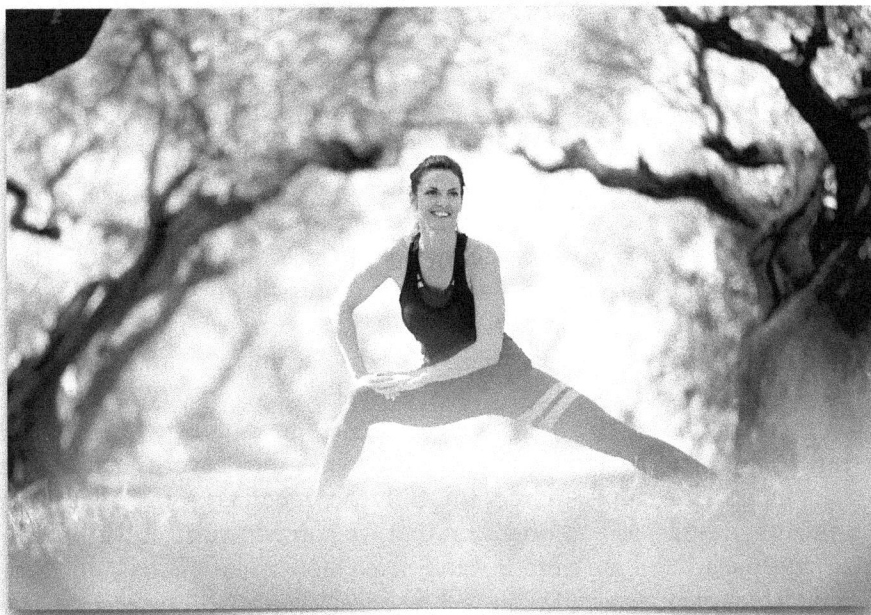

They were just thoughts
that danced through my little head…
about Aloneness.

As a child, I was often left alone. I was happy, however, on my own and I really learned to appreciate these moments with myself. Although my childhood years were not always easy, the solitude definitely brought something positive into my life: it taught me to stay in tune and connected with my inner voice.

What about you? Are you in tune with yours? Think about it…

In our busy lives we seldom have a minute to slow down: between getting ready, commuting, working, getting the groceries done, eating, taking care of the kids, the pets… it just seems as though there is always something more important to do. But meanwhile, amidst all this "busyness" lies within each and every one of us a little voice that is calling and needs to be heard. You probably know exactly what I am talking about, but it's obvious that many people aren't even aware that this voice exists.

But there most definitely *is* a voice inside each and every one of us. It's our inner voice or conscience. It's such a smart voice too, so full of wisdom! If we only took the time to listen to it, we wouldn't need laws or religions to dictate to us what to do or what to believe in. Because deep down inside we would know whether we were right or wrong, selfish or generous, loving or hating, if we were acting out of greed or jealousy… But with all our hustling and bustling, the constant noise, we tend to muffle it, by justifying "I'm too busy", or "I know you're there, but I'll get back to you later, when I have a little more time." And so, we rely on others or laws to dictate what we have to do. Meanwhile, time goes by.

I believe that for many of us, this inner voice is lost during childhood: Look at how our children are raised today and what stressful time schedules they have. When do they have the time to enjoy aloneness or simple boredom? Because, whether you realize it or not, it is during the moments of solitude and boredom that we come in contact with that inner voice. However, many people around me cannot stand being alone. The thing is, once you accept to spend some time alone with yourself, you will discover silence and quietness. You will most certainly cry, but at one point you will become calm and peaceful and amid all of this "emptiness", you will find LOVE. You will find ONLY LOVE!

Try it! Spend more time doing nothing and see how, gradually, you start to really enjoy these moments, and pretty soon you will crave them. Because it is in aloneness that you can truly strengthen and construct yourself.

And so, as I reflect upon all those years when I didn't get to attend school, and how in the end it allowed me to confront myself, for countless long hours, I am only grateful for the lesson I received: I learned to be happy in aloneness.

And what better gift than knowing that no matter what happens, whether someone dies, or someone you love deserts you, or you lose everything… you still have yourself. This gift, that was given to me fortuitously, is priceless and I will treasure it forever.

The years from 2016 to 2018 weren't easy… they really weren't, but I kept telling myself: " I know I can get past this!" That's when I think discipline and consistency kick in: I would just get up and go train NO MATTER WHAT, go to work with a smile on my face as if it was nothing. But my alone time is what really strengthened me. That's why we all have to learn to love ourselves, because the days when we are really down and have to face our problems, well, those are the days we realize that the person inside of us, is our very best friend.

Change n°49
SLEEP

Change n°50
MEDITATION, MINDFULNESS AND PRAYER

Change n°51
COMMUNICATE WITH NATURE

Change n°52
SLOW DOWN

Change n°53
DECLUTTER

Change n°54
SIMPLIFY

Change n°55
KNOW YOURSELF

Change n°56
GIVE A SMILE

Change n°57
EMPOWERING WALK

Change n°58
CHANNELLING PAIN

Change n°59
EMBRACING TRUTH

Change n°60
EMBRACE YOUR INNER CHILD

Change n°49
SLEEPING

49.

Did you know that we spend one third of our lives sleeping? Some of you are going to say "What a waste of time!"… but it actually isn't. Sleep is absolutely crucial. If you are extremely busy and presumably not sleeping enough like most people today, then you are, no doubt, either sleep deprived or in debt.

After work, you find yourself tackling a thousand more things at home and most of you end up unwinding on the couch in front of the TV. After a long day, you are entitled to some "off time", right? When the program is over, it's probably already late, and there is still a little bit of cleaning and preparing to do for the next day, which further delays your getting into bed. And when you are finally there, do you take a last look at your social network? Just a quick look and there goes a few more minutes. Often enough, I am sure you end up falling asleep knowing that you won't be getting the required amount of sleep which is, for most adults, between seven to nine hours. Since we are all different we have needs that vary according to our general state of health, lifestyle, the amount of exercise we do, and our nature.

If your goal this week is to get enough sleep, try to find out how many hours you really need for a restorative night. Be in tune with your body; listen to what it is telling you: Is it seven, eight or nine? It might even be ten!

Now, I know this will be challenging and it's hard to turn off your light much earlier than you normally do, but this is your challenge of the week and believe me, you won't regret it.

A. Why is sleep so important?

Let's start off by seeing why it's important to get enough sleep. Everybody knows that after a good night's sleep, they feel better, their eyes are bright and alert and they feel ready to tackle the new day! But those are not the only reasons why your body, your mind and your soul need sleep. How you feel when you wake up tells you a lot about the past night, but also about the day to come. After a good night's sleep chances are, you will be able to concentrate better, improve your memory, performance at work, while exercising and boost your sex life.

You will also:

- Live longer
- Feel calmer and less likely to lose your temper
- Concentrate better, improve your memory, get better results at work or better grades, if you are a student: your mind needs to rest in order to work properly
- Look rested with a relaxed face, as opposed to stressed
- Have a better chance of staying clear from diseases

- Smile more
- Feel like today is a winning day in which everything is achievable and easy
- Be in a good mood and less likely to feel depressed
- Maintain a better state of mind to make important decisions

All in all, the way you sleep can affect your whole day and how you interact with others, your appetite, your performance in sports, your efficiency at work or at school…so isn't it worth switching the light off just a little earlier? It will make your world a better place.

B. How to get more sleep

So, with your busy schedules, you might be wondering how you can manage to add more sleep?

There is only one way: you have to *make sleep a priority!* Decide that from now on you will make sure you are in bed by a certain time. Why don't you set your alarm, to let's say, one hour prior to your usual sleep time? Now you'll know that when it rings, it's time to start getting ready for bed. You could also become a little more organized by taping your favorite TV programs and watching them another day. This way, you will be able to fast forward through all the commercials and save more time.

It's also important to resist looking at your emails and social media right before going to bed. Trust me, even if you think you will spend only a few minutes, you won't.

C. Improve the quality of your sleep

Not only is it necessary to go to bed earlier, it's also paramount to find out ways to improve the quality of your sleep and I have listed below four elements that will help you and have been proven to enhance its quality. Try them all and find your way to a restorative sleep

• Have a sleep routine: create a ritual that you can repeat every night and that will prepare your mind and body to slip into a sleeping mode. It could be as simple as reading a few pages or taking a warm bath or shower. When I turn off the light, I like to take the opportunity to do five minutes of visualization. I particularly enjoy my "Give, Receive and Let it Flow" Meditation. See Change n° 11 *Love More* for some ideas. Many times, I end up just falling asleep half way through, but it's nice to know that I dozed off seeing myself in a positive way surrounded with love, achieving my goals, or in totally peaceful surroundings, depending on which meditation I chose to do that night.

- Your environment is significant as well. Make sure your room is dark, just the right temperature, which means slightly cool, and that there isn't too much noise. If need be, you might want to use earplugs.
- One thing that many people don't realize, is the importance of a light dinner. There is nothing worse than going to bed feeling full or while digesting. Also, make sure you don't drink too much liquid just before going to bed, as you might have to get up to use the bathroom in the middle of the night. Finally, avoid alcohol, as it will make you drowsy at first, but if you wake up during the night, chances are you won't be able to fall back asleep.
- Last thing: it's important to stick to a sleeping schedule which means going to bed and waking up at the same time every single day of the year! I go to bed all 365 days of the year around eleven pm and wake up between six and seven in the morning. If I have to get up any earlier, I adjust a little and make sure I am in bed a half hour earlier.

D. Could it be that you are sleep deprived? What are the signs?

As always, listen to yourself and observe certain signs, they don't lie. If your eyes feel tired and you are having a hard time getting up, chances are you might be sleep deprived. There are other signs as well, such as:

• You are moody, irritable and tend to argue or cry, anything can easily upset you
• You feel like you could sleep anytime, anywhere during the day
• It gets harder to accomplish normal every day chores
• You are less motivated to do things you normally enjoy
• You tend to drink more coffee
• You have a hard time understanding or concentrating
• You are more forgetful
• You have a lower sex drive

E. How to incorporate change

If you choose to get more sleep, you could start by applying all the points I have mentioned above on day one or break it down into increments and add a new factor every day, or every other day. You can for example do the following:

Day 1: Make sure you go to bed earlier. According to your wake-up time, calculate what is your best time to hit the sack to get your seven, eight or nine hours of sleep. Then make sure you have your lights out by that time.

Day 2 or 3: Create a routine, such as taking a nice relaxing shower, getting into bed 30 minutes prior to bed time, read quietly for 30 minutes, or meditate for 10 minutes. It will help you unwind and settle into a sleep mode. Prior to entering your bed, make sure that you have turned off all your electronic devices.

Day 3 or 4: Eat your dinner earlier. Research suggests that you eat two hours prior to going to bed. So, if you are turning the lights out at 10:30 pm, make sure you don't eat anything after 8:30 pm. If it's not possible, then just make sure you eat something light and that you leave the table feeling just right. There is a pleasant realm where you are no longer hungry, but you don't feel full. That's what you're aiming for.

Two or three days later: you can drink an herbal tea or take a look at essential oils and incorporate them into your sleep routine.

After a long day, it's totally understandable, to feel the need to have some time for ourselves to unwind and relax. For some, going to bed earlier feels like a punishment: you didn't get the time to do something such as watch TV, read a book and so you naturally tend to delay the time of your nightcap. But this is a misconception. If you sleep more, you will be able to do more and do it with a smile on your face. Chances are you don't need to add two to three extra hours of sleep; you possibly only need an extra half hour or an hour to be at your best. So, seriously think about it, and see how a slight shift in your night routine can change your entire life for the better.

Change n°50
MEDITATION, MINDFULNESS AND PRAYER

50.

Our thoughts and words have direct consequences on our lives. At times they may appear insignificant, but they can actually have drastic repercussions. There is no need to praise meditation as it has been widely touted and most of us are already well aware of the many benefits. But let me ask you a question: do *you* meditate? Are *you* mindful throughout the day? Do you pray? Do you actually take the time to do these things? I know how it is: it's just like exercising and eating a balanced diet, you are aware of their benefits but how many of you actually do it? If you always wanted to meditate, feel curious of the benefits and outcomes, why not decide this week to establish a meditating routine? Make an effort to pray more often, spend some time with your GOD, whoever he might be for you, and be more mindful throughout the day. Make a real commitment!

If you decide to take up meditation, prayer or mindfulness, it has to be as important as eating or sleeping. And, come to think of it, in a way these techniques provide essential food for your soul; so, make the extra effort to find the time!
To help you get started, here are a few questions and answers that might interest you.

A. What is meditation? What is mindfulness? What is prayer?
a. Defining "meditation"
The dictionary defines meditation as: a continuous and profound contemplation or musing on a subject or series of subjects of a deep or abstruse nature; or contemplation of spiritual matters. I prefer:

Meditation is that space of silence in between two thoughts.

b. Defining "mindfulness"
The dictionary defines mindfulness as: the trait of staying aware of (paying close attention to) your responsibilities. I prefer:

Mindfulness is a state in which you are fully aware of the moment and at the same time are capable of observing yourself "being fully aware of the moment", you see the scene from up close and in its entirety.

c. Defining "praying"

For the dictionary praying is: addressing a deity, a prophet, a saint or an object of worship. I prefer:

> ***Praying is not asking or begging.***
> ***Praying is when you open your heart***
> ***and accept with absolute faith***
> ***whatever it is you are going through,***
> ***no matter what the outcome might be.***

For certain people, praying is simply the act of reciting a prayer or asking for something. However, when praying you should be connecting your entire being, "mind, body, and spirit", to a higher purpose; you should be in total osmosis with who you are, and your inner self. Once you enter this state, you can ask, be receptive and capable of receiving.

Over the years, I have practiced meditation, mindfulness and prayer but have come to the conclusion, that they all serve the same purpose: they allow you to step back and have a moment of communion with yourself. In such a state, one is more receptive to what is happening inside and around them. Thus, one becomes more capable of responding to "LIFE" the right way.

For this reason, I have merged all three of them together in one change. I understand that they are all different and it's up to each and every one of you to choose what works best for your needs.

I honestly believe that although we need alone time to get to know ourselves, if we desire inner growth, the best school ever is being amongst others. Alone time is necessary to find your inner-calmness, reconnect with yourself and feel centered. It becomes like a reference point you try to return to during the rest of the day. With time, you slowly learn to be in a constant state of self-observation as well as observing others. Finding out who you really are, how you and others react and interact is one of the best ways to gain inner wisdom and peace of mind.

To meditate, pray or be mindful, the absolute requires no school, no technique. They are innate, and they simply need to be done. Just like you don't necessarily have to be a Christian, Muslim or Hindu to pray. All you need is faith. And you don't necessarily need a place to worship such as a church or a mosque: your body is your temple and you simply need to commune with yourself. Meditating, praying or being mindful can be done anytime and anywhere: just do it, do it right now, at this very moment, wherever you are. Be fully PRESENT.

Start by seeing, observing, listening without a word. Do it without judgment or emitting any criticism. Do it with an open loving heart. I even feel like saying, lovingly. When you pay attention and let all of your senses awaken, you reach a beautiful state of inner quietness and peace.

Note: Stop finding excuses and start meditating. Countless times I have spoken to friends and colleagues and they always hold the same speech: "I don't have the time" or "I have tried and I can't stop my mind from blabbering" or "I would love to meditate but I need someone to guide me." Just as you surely would benefit from hiring a personal trainer to exercise properly, you don't however need one to learn how to walk or go out for a little jog. Without a doubt, you will most likely benefit from a qualified yoga instructor. But if you don't have the time, the money, the knowledge, you can also start by simply sitting down quietly, breathing calmly and observing what happens.

B. Why do it?

With the lives we lead today, both our minds and bodies need a break. Time often seems to be an issue. Although it may seem contradictory at first, meditating will actually allow us to save time by calming us down and increasing our faculty to concentrate. While rushing through our days without taking the time to exhale and breathe, we tend to do things quickly, impulsively, while not allowing ourselves to see the complete picture. Indeed, to make the proper decision, it is really important to see things objectively, in their entirety. How can we do this when we are always on the go, in a hurry or busy? When we do things too quickly, we make hasty decisions. Allowing our body and mind a little time to slow down and relax while meditating, praying or being mindful, allows us to collect the information gathered, sort it out and see the situation we are in, in its entirety. Then, we can see things as they really are and make more sensible decisions.

But meditation also…

- Brings peace of mind and allows you to reach a state in which you feel utterly happy
- Makes you feel like a better person on the inside and, with time, you see yourself becoming a better one on the outside as well, as you slowly start integrating the notion of acceptance, patience and love
- Allows you to understand the irrelevance of many issues that normally preoccupy you. Getting upset for certain things just doesn't make sense anymore.
- Changes your vibrations, what you emit, allowing you to attract moments, events and people that vibrate more like you
- Heals. Meditating brings peace and you reach a state where you understand that "Love" is all that matters. This feeling of peace and love heals you within.
- Will have you spreading more love thus contributing to making this world a better place
- Allows you to be more aware of your thoughts and actions. If you pay attention to what you say and think, to the way you do things and how you interact with others, you will soon see that you feel more in control of your life as well. Taking the time to slow down allows you to collect yourself, take a step back and analyze the situation. Isn't it time you became the captain of your own ship?
- Rids you of your inner tension, leaving you less anxious about what lies ahead. When you are calmer, life is easier and you are more capable of handling others, you become more productive at work and have loving thoughts for the people around you.
- Allows you to sleep better. Meditation can really help if you have subject to insomnia or not sleeping enough. We often can't sleep because we are thinking about our problems. By meditating regularly, you take the time to address these issues at a certain moment during the day, which will allow you to sleep better at night. A good idea would be to add a moment of visualization in which you envision yourself going to sleep and having a wonderful sleep and then waking up feeling energetic, radiant and ready to face the day!

- Will have you focus your attention on the task at hand, become more present and centered
- Will find you feeling more grateful! When you meditate, make an effort to spend a few minutes being grateful about what you have. Go over your day, or your life in general and give thanks for all the good things you have. Be grateful for the big things such as your health, your friends, your family, and your job. But be grateful as well for the little things, such as someone's kind words or support, the drawing your child gave you, or having a little bit of time off to meditate…Taking the time to be grateful for everything you have, will remind you how lucky you really are and become more appreciative of what you have.
- Will Increase your vitality, leaving you completely energized. Meditation has a way of energizing you and making you ready to tackle what lies ahead!

Other benefits….
- Gain control of your temper
- Feel serene and laid back
- Inner peace & silence
- Diminished need to overeat, smoke or drink
- Attunement with your intuition
- Awareness of your emotions and how certain events and factors affect you
- Improved patience with your spouse, children and co-workers

When times are tough, sometimes there is only one thing left to do: *go with the flow* and let life handle your problem. If you feel like you are struggling all the time and there seems to be no solution, take the time to meditate or pray. Decide to trust LIFE completely: life has its ways of taking care of things. Then get up and move on with your life… with faith that things will soon improve.

It's important to understand that inevitably sometimes you will not be able to calm down and things won't feel like they are flowing. You will be nervous, fidgety with thoughts constantly pouring in: accept it, relax, as it is all part of the process.

C. How to practice?
a. Finding the time
The hardest part is to actually sit down and do it. But, believe me, once you start reaping the benefits, you will be feeling so good that you won't need any motivation to continue.
You can also set an alarm for fifteen to twenty minutes, in case your time is limited or you can let yourself go and stop when you feel it's the right time.
Many times, people complain about the numerous thoughts that keep buzzing in their mind. Let me tell you something: if you wait for your thoughts to calm down, you will never start meditating. IT'S NORMAL to have your brain churning thoughts incessantly and pop from one idea to another. Learn to pay attention to recurring thoughts, since it's most probably something that needs to be addressed. Quickly write down one or two words as a reminder on a piece of paper and once you are done meditating, get up and get that task done, if possible. That way it will be one thing less to think about during your next meditation session

b. How to meditate

As I said before, if you wish to meditate and don't know where to begin, I suggest you do not overcomplicate the whole process: start off by making some time for it. Various types of meditation can be done with your eyes closed or open, sitting or lying down, but can also be done while walking or being active.

Find your personal meditation style, see what works best for you or explore different ones, according to the time of day and mood. And remember: what works for you now, might not work later and it's ok to change. However, in order to meditate successfully, normally people find it easier to stick to the same time and place. The key is to keep trying; it's all a question of trial and error.

Once you start your meditation simply relax and let your mind settle, and then observe your thoughts, your emotions. Are you feeling angry, stressed, excited or happy?

Now is the time to really get to know yourself.

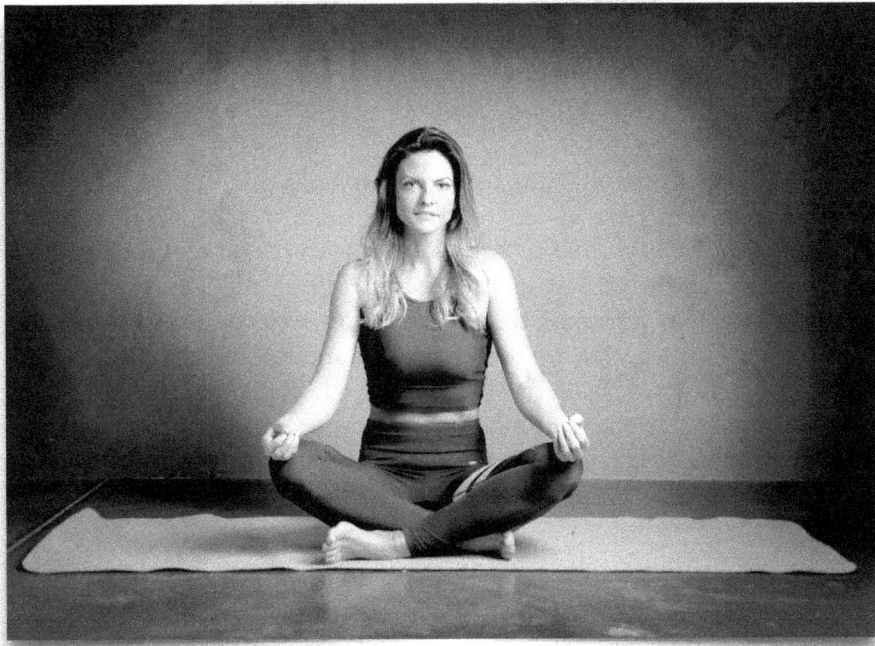

c. How to be more mindful

Being mindful means being more present at every single moment. It requires you to slow down and give your full attention to everything that is going on within and around you. When you first try being mindful, you will quickly see that it is impossible to remain this way the entire day. For this reason, it might be better to choose certain moments throughout the day, such as when you are driving to work, eating, going for a walk, or putting your children to bed.

The key here is to do what you usually do, relax and be aware of what is going on around you, but also how you feel about it. Try to notice how certain things affect you and in which way: what annoys you, what leaves you indifferent, what makes you lose patience or on the contrary the things that make you feel good inside. As days go by, you will notice an increased ability of mindfulness throughout the day. You will also quickly notice that it is absolutely necessary to slow down in order to be more mindful. Slowing down and fully experiencing what you are doing, will, however, become truly satisfying and bring you more inner peace.

Mindfulness requires you to focus more on one thing at a time. For example, if you eat while working, are you focusing on your work or on the food? Probably both, which means you are not able to truly focus. Maybe you are working a little more and simply nourishing yourself without noticing it, without paying really any attention to what you are eating.

This is why so many people end up eating again only one or two hours after a meal: because even though they have already eaten, the brain was concentrating on something else and consequently, eclipsed the rest. If you want to become more mindful, keep your attention focused on to the task at hand. See yourself as the sun with all its sun beams. When you do something, you must direct all your rays to the ONE thing you are doing and then light it up. This way you are totally present and mindful.

Throughout the day, try to name the emotions you are going through. Pay attention to your thoughts and then tag them: *That was anger, or jealousy. That was joy or compassion.*

Try to be honest with yourself: it's only between you and yourself. Being able to identify your emotions will help you in your quest of becoming more mindful. I often find that it helps me come to terms with the chatter in my mind. Once I admit that I am jealous, angry, or hurt I know what emotion I need to work on or replace and it allows me to move on with the rest of my life.

d. How to pray

As I said before, praying isn't just asking or reciting a prayer. Prayer is a sacred act in which you come in communion with your GOD. Just as with meditation and mindfulness, you need to relax. Breathe deeply and feel your body becoming more peaceful and serene. Eyes closed bring to mind what is troubling you. At that moment, you can do two things:

Clearly and precisely, "say out loud in your mind" what it is that you are feeling: you have to literally hear yourself saying a clear and precise sentence that expresses your emotion. Then breathe and surrender. Tell your God that you trust him completely, that you have total faith in the fact that he is helping you to resolve your problem. Most of the time when you are in a challenging situation, it's either that you fear change with the loss it implies, or that you don't like the situation the way it is, and you would like it to change.

At some point, we all experience tormenting thoughts. Before tackling any problem however, one should first get rid of all the negative emotions. And the best way is to ask your God or your inner guide to help you remove and replace these feelings with their opposite emotions. So, every time a problem arises, name the emotion you are feeling, and observe it as it monopolizes your entire mind. Learn to replace it with thoughts of love, compassion, forgiveness and by affirming *out loud in your mind* "I completely trust God" or " I unconditionally trust the Universe".

It might take a day or two, but your heart will have loving intentions again. It is then time to come back and pray for help to finally resolve your problem. I think it's always a good idea to show that we make an effort towards improving a situation before asking for help.

I love this prayer by Saint Francis of Assisi that helps you in this respect:

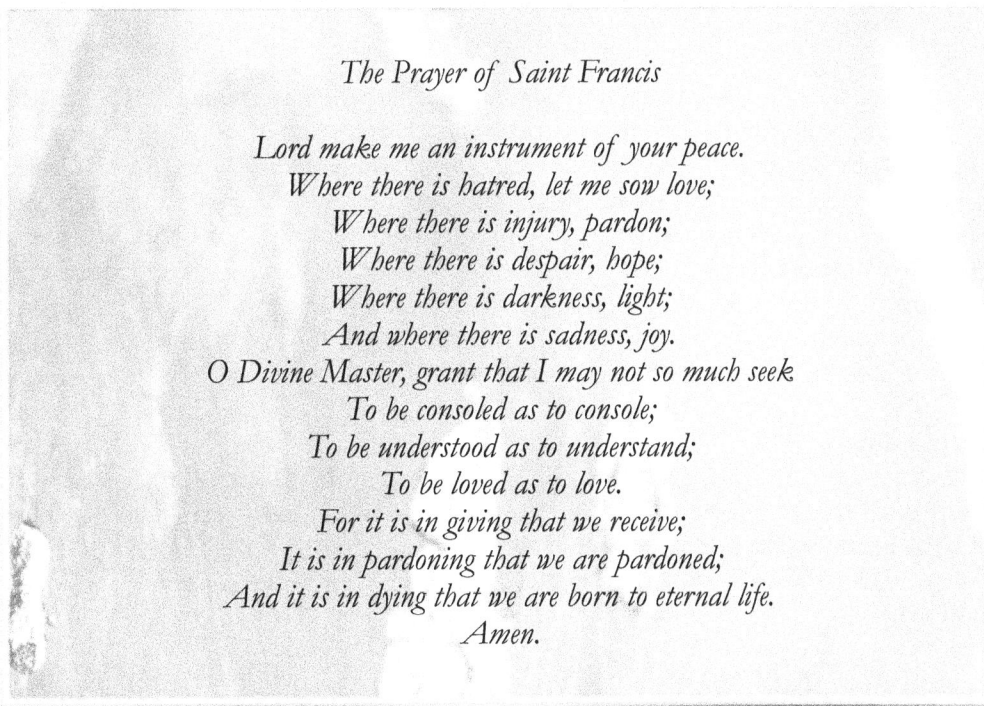

The Prayer of Saint Francis

Lord make me an instrument of your peace.
Where there is hatred, let me sow love;
Where there is injury, pardon;
Where there is despair, hope;
Where there is darkness, light;
And where there is sadness, joy.
O Divine Master, grant that I may not so much seek
To be consoled as to console;
To be understood as to understand;
To be loved as to love.
For it is in giving that we receive;
It is in pardoning that we are pardoned;
And it is in dying that we are born to eternal life.
Amen.

I always tell my children that when they are in a "difficult situation" there is always some form of action that can be done to avoid worsening it: saying they are sorry or letting the other person express themselves while remaining nice and calm are just two examples.

Another option is to choose to say absolutely nothing. What exactly are you feeling? What emotion has overcome you? Are you feeling pain? Are you suffering? Don't answer with words. Instead let yourself *feel* the answer. Acknowledge it and embrace it totally. Accept your pain, your hatred, your jealousy. It's time to be honest with yourself. Breathe deeply and ask your inner Guide to help you accept and replace this negative emotion and find the right solution to your problem.

When you find yourself in a difficult situation, a thousand thoughts start churning in your head. That's when fear or doubt kick in and take your mind under control. It can literally feel like "Hell" up there. Learn to become aware of these emotions and take immediate action: as soon as an idea, that expresses fear, doubt or negativity pops up, you must address it on the spot and keep at it incessantly until it loses all of its impact. See it, name it and then, just as a friend would, tell yourself some kind and reassuring words.

Keep in mind that each and every one of your thoughts, words or actions has an effect on your body, mind as well as environment. Indeed, when you feel stress, anger, resentment or keep emotions bottled up, your body is clearly affected. When facing these types of emotions, it is obliged to leave its state of homeostasis to adapt and adjust accordingly. But your body can only accept up to a certain point. When pushed out of its comfort zone too far or for too long, it ends up reacting - you no longer breathe the same way, the energy doesn't flow freely anymore, your organs and various body parts become stressed and contracted - and that's when you start receiving certain signals such as various aches and pains, feeling tired or having skin problems.

So, isn't it time you grabbed the reigns and took control of your mind? It takes a bit of practice but, sooner than you think, you could be spending your days channeling and harboring mostly positive and loving thoughts. Once you do, you will be, on a more regular basis, in a state of inner peace which can only, in turn, have a positive impact on your exterior environment - how and when you interact with people around you.
Think of the benefits that a simple mind-shift can have, as it can go far beyond anything you have ever imagined. In this entire process, meditating, being more mindful and praying become essential tools as they allow you to push the pause button, put things back into perspective and reach a state of inner calmness.

Accepting illness
The minute you are diagnosed with cancer, all of those thoughts going on inside your mind become very difficult to handle. Indeed, you can quite easily find yourself totally overcome by fear. And it's understandable. For this reason, I really wish to share a few of the things that truly helped me to accept the situation along the way, and experience it in a more peaceful manner.

Accepting treatment and medication

Every time I was administered or had to take some form of medication, I always did it willingly, not only with acceptance but also in a state of gratitude. "This medication is a gift here to heal me." I would always take a moment, eyes closed, to give thanks for the treatment I was about to receive.

Not too long ago, a person I know who was undergoing chemotherapy, told me that she had a hard time accepting the fact that they were injecting "poison" into her. Her words were very violent but that's how she really felt. Although I can understand her point of view, I believe it's essential to tackle the situation in a different way, by being open and receptive in receiving your treatment. If you believe it's poison, your body will inevitably tense up as you take it and be unwilling to receive its benefits. Thus, the importance of practicing acceptance and giving thanks. Every time I would receive an injection or undergo radiotherapy, I would close my eyes and imagine beautiful pink or rainbow-colored hearts entering my body. I would envision thousands of tiny little colored ones flowing into me and spreading throughout my body. It was the way I found of transforming these difficult moments into happier ones.

You are not being punished

Never once did I see my cancer or tumor as a form of punishment. Never once did I ask myself: "What have I done to "deserve" this?". The way I see it, cancer was simply the way my body chose to express itself. Something was not right. I had turned a blind eye and avoided a situation and I was not living "my truth". Had I tackled it earlier, I most certainly would not have had this cancer. From the beginning it was clear that it was a message, sent not to harm me but to "save" me, and that it was now time to start dealing with it.

Healing Meditation

Meditating when you have cancer is an essential part of the treatment. It's a moment that allows you to bring more peace and love into your world. Since I had breast cancer, I imagined a bright light, the "light of love", flowing in and out of my breast. As I inhaled, I consciously breathed in love, and upon exhalation, I let all the love go back out into the world. The idea is to let it flow freely back and forth, by receiving the gift of love, but also spreading it out into the universe, without ever clinging onto it. Indeed, this flow of love must always remain in constant motion.

Note: I already developed this idea in a previous change, but I would like to remind you of this important aspect. Many times, I read that one needs to inhale good things, such as love or a healing light and exhale everything that is negative or bad. I have a real problem with this, since it is my belief, that our surrounding world is a beautiful place and not a trash bin into which we can dump our negative emotions. You might ask: what does one do with all that negativity they have built up inside? My answer is quite simple: There is no need to get rid of it. All you have to do is replace it. Change fear into faith, transform thoughts of sickness into thoughts of health, hate into love. That way you can receive love, but also spread it back out into the world. With today's growing concern about our environment, it's important to make a conscious effort to preserve it. What better way than spreading more love back into our world.

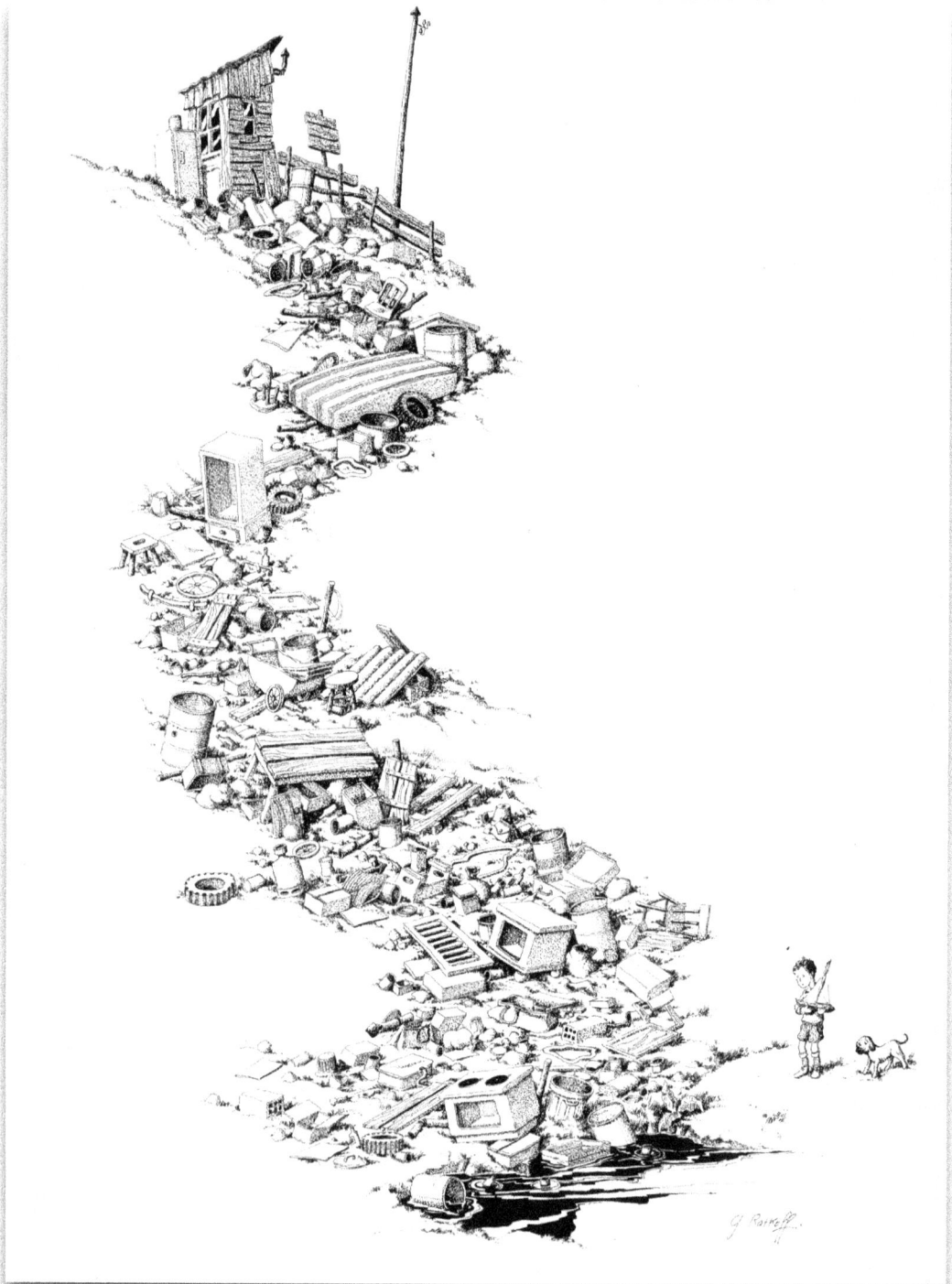

The world is polluted enough as it is.
Let's avoid dumping negative thoughts into it as well, and focus on spreading more love.
Love and a thousand hugs to my father for this beautiful drawing.
Illustration by Georges Ratkoff

Change n°51
COMMUNICATE
WITH NATURE

51.

With the increasing amount of people living in cities and with the hectic lives we lead, we tend to lose ourselves in our list of daily chores. We forget what was, once, an essential part of our lives: nature! At one point in time, we were in constant inter-communication; it was a question of survival, our senses needed to be in total communion with all the elements surrounding us.

Although cities can be beautiful, they are synonymous with chaos, pollution, noise and crowds. Nature, however, brings a vision of beauty, vast open green fields, fresh air to breathe and the sound of birds and rustling leaves. The city fills our lives with needs and occupations that always turn us outwards, whereas nature requires nothing and allows us to get back in touch with who we really are on the inside.

Whether we acknowledge it or not, we are all like sponges, receptive and responding to the world around us. Think of a gong. When you hit it, the sound propagates to its surroundings and everything starts to vibrate in unison. Well, the same holds true for people and environment:
• People have the capacity to transfer their moods – whether good or bad - to those around them
• Environment also has this faculty: when we have the opportunity to be in a peaceful setting, such as nature, a church, or a quiet room, we absorb the vibrations emanating from that specific place

So, if you are in a moment of stress or are feeling down turn to nature and draw on its resources: put on your walking shoes and head outdoors to the countryside, nearby woods, a beach, the park or the mountains and reconnect… chances are, when you get back home, you will feel recharged and uplifted again.

A. Benefits of Communicating with Nature
There are numerous benefits to getting away and spending some time in nature. Here are the many advantages:
• It reduces stress and allows you to sleep better
• Soaking up some sun allows you to spend some time with an important someone, Mr. Vitamin D
• Taking the time to reconnect with nature allows you to clear your mind, bringing clarity and improving concentration
• It makes you happy and brings a sense of fulfillment

- Going for a nature walk is a great form of exercise! Let's face it, if you have to choose between a treadmill or a walk in the woods with the everlasting change of scenery, the smell of pine trees, the pleasure of seeing little squirrels hoping around... what would you choose? And have you ever tried walking-off your problems? Walking has a powerful effect on your mood. After only a short brisk stroll, observe yourself and see how your mood and your self-esteem improve, how energized you become. A great idea is to finish this off with a cool, or better yet, cold invigorating shower.
- Getting away, even for a few hours, makes for a real break
- An outing with the family is a great opportunity to spend some quality time together. Make it fun by adding a picnic or a few games.
- Being outdoors boosts creativity. Kids especially love to create things and it helps develop their imagination.
- Spending time in nature makes you more aware of your environment and of how precious it is. You will learn to respect it and will want to make a conscious effort to preserve it, when you are outdoors, but also back home, such as not wasting water or using more "eco-friendly" products.
- Have you ever heard about grounding or earthing? The idea is to walk barefoot on the ground in order to receive the negative charge emanating from the Earth. In today's world, full of computers, WiFi, cell phones and what not, we are surrounded by devices that emit positive ions. Grounding allows you take the time to reconnect with mother nature's negative ions. Note that swimming in the ocean or a lake also recharges your body with these negative ions.
- And what about meeting new people: Have you ever noticed how, many people who live out in the countryside, in the woods or in the mountains are often very simple, laid back, generous and spontaneous? Make the most of this moment by taking the time to chat with them and embrace their simplicity.

B. Outdoor activities to choose from

To get you motivated, here is a list of outdoor activities you can look into:

- Swimming in the sea or lake
- Gardening
- Walking
- Hiking
- Rock climbing
- Beach strolling
- Yoga or exercise in nature.
- Cloud gazing
- Sleeping in a tree house
- Going for a botanical walk and learning about plants and trees
- Ballooning
- Mountain biking
- Horseback riding
- Camping
- Windsurfing
- Outdoor adventure camp
- Zip-lining
- Meditating outdoors
- Paddling
- Kayaking / canoeing
- Surfing
- Snowshoeing
- Walking barefooted
- Visiting a Japanese garden
- Canyonning
- Treetop adventure course (or high ropes course / Accrobranching)
- Learning to use a compass in nature
- Fishing
- Outdoor exercising
- Team treasure hunts

C. Getting back in touch with our best teacher, Mother Nature

When communicating with nature try to listen to its messages and learn from them. If you observe your surroundings, see how you can subtly find answers within nature itself. Just like the poem "The Road Not Taken" by Robert Frost, you will see some signs and they will get you thinking about the events you are going through at the moment.

> ### Two roads diverged in the woods...
> ### I took the one less traveled,
> ### and that has made all the difference.

a. "Tell me, Tell me" listening to nature's messages: A game I invented and used to play as a child. So, open up all your senses and be receptive. Listen to the relaxing sounds, see the colors or how nature has its way, smell the grass, the wood, the pines, hug a tree trunk and look at nature's messages.

I saw this tree once that managed to grow off a tree trunk, at the edge of a lake. What were the odds? How did it grow there? I couldn't help but feel amazed by it. There are thousands of trees all around it, all cooped up together; but this little fellow chose to do its own thing…and it was beautiful. And so, I asked myself: what is this tree trying to tell me? Is there something I can learn from this vision? That tree was perfect, right where it was. It blended to perfection with its surroundings, although it chose a totally different path from others. After a few moments of reflection, I came up with this lesson:

> ### You don't have to be like everyone else to fit in.
> ### Be unique!

I saw this message, but maybe if *YOU* look at it, you will see something else and receive a different one. That's ok. What we see is in accordance with what we are living and going through in this present time.

Maybe when you look at this picture, you will think: *"Miracles can happen!"* or *"Even if I am alone, I can grow. I will be ok. Life has its way"*.

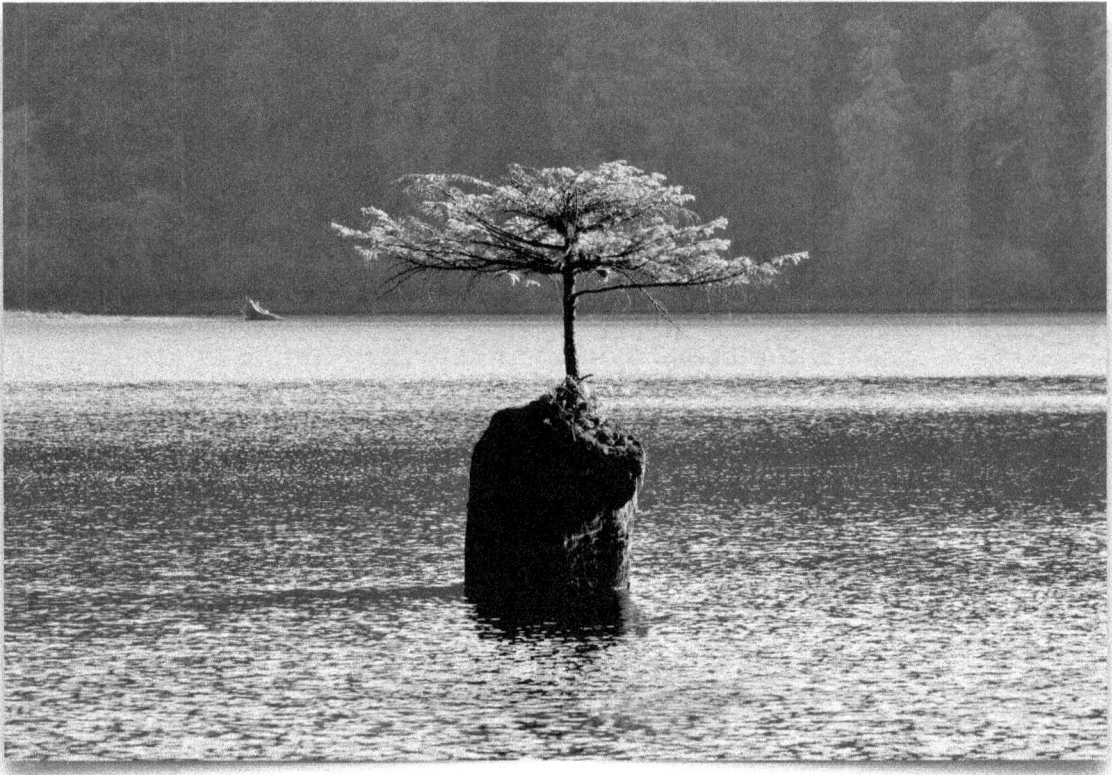

What do YOU see in this picture?
I see_____

WORK SPACE

D. Communicating with the clouds

Another "exercise" you can do is to look at the clouds and dissolve them. Lie down on the ground and find a small isolated cloud and focus your attention on it. Imagine it represents something that's bothering you in your life right now, such as a problem, a mistake you made, an obsessive, recurring thought that you are having or on the contrary, your wildest desire. Stare at this cloud and make it disappear, and as it dissipates tell yourself mentally that your problem is dissipating too. If it's a desire you are focusing on, then imagine that this cloud is your wish and as it is spreading apart, your wish is picking up more space and spreading out to the universe. While this is happening, tell the universe that you trust it to take good care of it and believe that it is now actively trying to make it come true.

E. Sharing a moment in silence

Another idea is to share a walk with someone special. The goal here is to soak up the energy and the beauty of your surroundings, side by side with another person, perhaps your partner, a friend, your child or your pet. Try, as much as possible, not to talk, unless you want to point something out. At first, it may seem a little awkward. It will feel almost intimate. You will be together, but each one in your aloneness. It's nice to know that you can share a moment with someone and not be obligated to talk. Maybe at one point you will share a glance, a smile or a kiss. You will see that a connection will grow between the two of you, creating a special new bond.

In a world that pressures us with money and gadgets, where is the happiness? Think about it: the things that make us really happy, carry no price tag: succeeding in doing something, passing an exam, falling in love, making someone else happy….

Let's take sex for example. Why do people enjoy it so much? When having sex, one lives in the moment. We are not lost in our thoughts or worrying about the future. It's a moment when we focus on giving, receiving…sharing and simply letting go.

As much as possible, when you're out in Nature, try to embrace it totally. At first, it will take a little bit of commitment on your behalf to do it regularly and to integrate the idea that you have to WANT to connect with your surroundings, to really reap the benefits.

So, embrace nature and keep the following in mind:

Buddha found wisdom sitting under a tree, not by reading books or worshipping a master.

We ARE nature.
You are nature.
We are all a part of nature…so go find yourself!

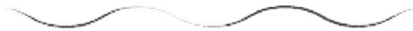

Change n°52
SLOW DOWN

52.

If you look at your day objectively, how much of it is spent doing one thing at a time? In today's connected world we are more likely to be multitasking, than focusing 100% on our present occupation. Think of it: how many of us eat while watching TV, drive while talking on the phone, read while listening to music or are lost in their thoughts while supposedly listening to others?

The other day I was told that a cop stopped a car and was in total shock to see the woman driver who was simultaneously driving, breastfeeding her child, smoking and talking over the phone!!!! Talk about multitasking!!!!

But let's admit it: in order to get through one of our days, we really have to be an efficient juggler.

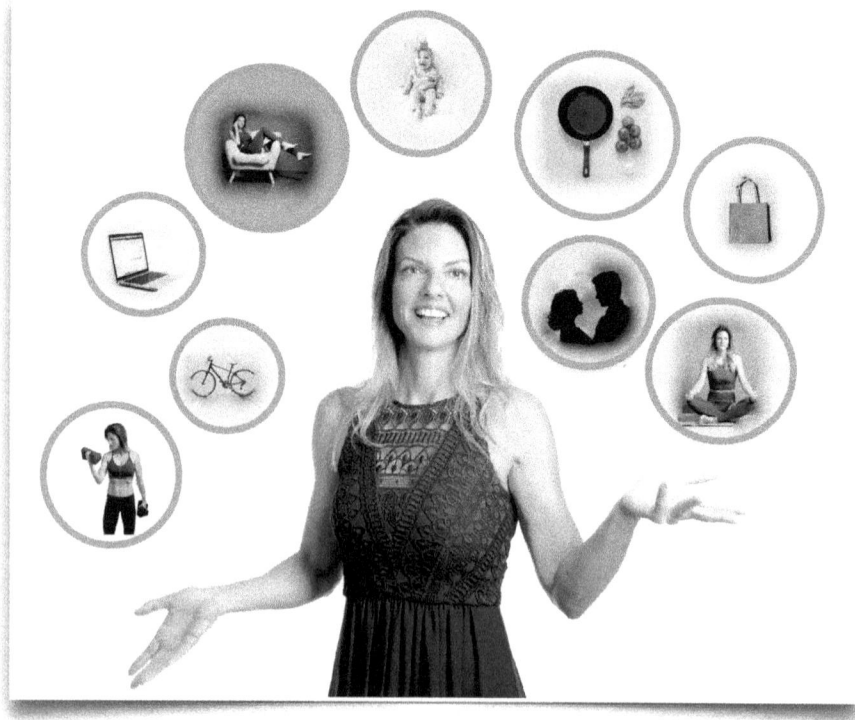

It's almost impossible to have it all done without undergoing any stress. But what's the point of doing it all, without being able to savor any of the moments? Even when we are alone, we are pressured by all the things we have to do, like cleaning, phone calls to make, going to the gym and all that social networking that didn't even exist 20 years ago!!! The problem is that we have totally lost connection with all of our natural rhythms and tend to hang in there thanks to our nerves or another cup of coffee. But we *do* need some time off, we *do* need to slow down. Our vehicle needs to stop and get its tank refueled or it will eventually run out of gas.

So, before you rush off to your next obligation, ask yourself: Is it really urgent or can it wait? Do I really have to do my entire "to do list" or are there some things that I can delegate or put off until later? Am I feeling guilty about relaxing? Does everything really have to be perfect? Could it be that I am scared of confronting myself, my aloneness…my emptiness? What do I fear of discovering?

Why don't you decide this week to focus on slowing down a bit. Who knows, once you try it, you might want to be that way for good. Make a conscious effort to be 100% in the present moment: wake up and instead of rushing out of bed, take the time to reconnect with that special someone who is lying beside you with a hug, a kiss or more. Savor your breakfast while sitting down and maybe enjoy the view from your window, be present when driving, try to do one thing at a time at work and give your full attention when spending time with your kids or friends.

A. Advantages of Slowing Down

There are many advantages to slowing down. To name a few:
• It improves your sense of well being
• You will be less stressed, thus more able to calm your anxieties
• Your body will be more relaxed, free from all the tension it gets when you are overly stressed. You might want to cultivate the habit of stretching and breathing every hour
• You will be more patient with co-workers, your partner, children and friends and most likely won't feel the urge to yell as much. Which brings us to the next point…
• It reduces the number of times you get angry
• It will raise your self-esteem. When we have too many things to do and just can't get them all done, we tend to get the feeling that we are a failure. So, do less and do it well!
• You will feel happier: you have the time to enjoy each moment
• When you slow down, you have the time to see yourself, realize that you have a part to play and that you belong here…you *ARE* needed
• It may seem somewhat of a paradox, but by slowing down you will actually get more done. When taking the time to do things in a more relaxed way, ultimately you become better organized. For example, you won't be wasting time coming back for forgotten items, or let certain things slip from your memory causing more work in the long run. The day will slowly unfold and you will do everything in a concentrated, calm manner.
• You will be less distracted. If you do things calmly, you will be more concentrated and won't be as affected by what is going on around you. It will increase your capacity to focus on the task at hand. This is definitely a time saver and a guaranty that things will be done properly.

B. What will happen if I slow down?

I know what your thinking: "If I slow down, then my laundry will pile up, my house will be a mess, I will be able to do less of the things that matter to me, such as seeing my friends or going to the gym, and my work colleagues will see me as someone slow and inefficient." STOP!

OK, your house might become a little messier but then there ARE things you can do about that, it's called DELEGATING. You might not be able to do everything you wanted…but wasn't the moment sipping that Latte or reading a book sooooo relaxing?

If you take the time to slow down, then you will be able to thoroughly enjoy the moments that really count. When was the last time you:
- Spent some time with your kids giving them your full attention, meaning no phone, no other occupation?
- Read a book on your couch, in a park or at your favorite coffee shop, even though you know you have a ton of chores that need to be tended to?
- Visited relatives and took the time to really be there for them: play games, chat, or have a bite to eat?
- Talked with your neighbors or chatted with the people who work at your local supermarket?
- Took the time to take care of yourself: taking a nice long bath, getting a massage?
- Allowed yourself to take a nap, star gaze or lie down on the grass at the park for 10 minutes? I honestly don't remember doing this one in a very long time: that's on this week's Bucket list!
- Turned the TV off and went for a walk?
- Took your time really savoring each bite and enjoying your meal? Check out Change n° 22: *Eating Mindfully*.
- Drove slower and accepted not to be stressed by anything that could happen along the way?
- Talked slower: took the time to think about what it is you really want to say?
- Stopped interrupting and listened more? I really have to work on this one!!!
- Didn't bring your entire home with you when you went away on vacation? By this I mean you didn't bring any work or your entire social network with you.
- Went to a concert and spent your time enjoying it, without filming or networking?
- Did one thing at a time?

C. Suggestions on how to slow down
- **Do less.** When we have too much to do, but not enough time on our hands, the best thing to do it is to kick a few things off your list. You don't have to get rid of it for good. You could, for example, decide not to watch TV two nights a week in order to do something else, such as spending some quality time with the family. Why not take some time to talk and listen to the kids, shoot a few hoops with your partner, go for a longer walk with the dog and recreate a bond with those who share the same roof.

- **Go hide.** Every once in a while, try to find a place where you can be alone for five minutes and use this time to reconnect with your inner self. If you are at home, it could be your room, your bathroom or even a closet. Go lock yourself up, shut your eyes, breathe slowly and deeply, and savor the silence, the peace and quiet. Every once and a while we need to escape the life we live in, in order to be with ourselves again. Only a few minutes suffice to bring your stress level down, to recharge your batteries and have you ready to face the world again.

- If you have more time, you might prefer to look into meditation. Read Change n° 50: *Meditation, Mindfulness and Prayer.*

- **Decide to drive slowly.** Plan your car trips ahead of time. Every time you stop at a red light, remind yourself to stop internally as well and breathe deeply. Why not create a tape to remind you to relax and ride safely.

- **Leave early.** In order to slow down, it might be a good idea to leave five minutes earlier than usual so that when you arrive at destination, you will have five whole minutes, to lie back in the car before getting out. You can shut your eyes and relax, read a book, sip on coffee you brought with you, or listen to one of your Personal Empowering Tapes that help you feel stronger and more self-confident. See Change n°05: Create your very own P.E.T. - Positive Empowering Tapes.

- **Delegate.** If you have children at home, it's time to have them contributing to household chores in order to relieve you from all of these tasks you have. Take the time to teach them how to do the laundry, how to empty the dishwasher, take out the garbage, or walk the dog. Also, learn to accept when others offer to help. We often say "No", but people are often happy to be of assistance. Put your pride aside and accept a helping hand. When things get quieter, you can return the favor.

- **Learn to say "NO" to others and to yourself. Learn to see where your real priorities are.** When my friends will read this, they will probably laugh! It's true, it's really a problem for me to say "no". I tend to automatically say "yes" and then realize later what my "yes" implies. But I am getting better and better at it. I have found that you can say you are busy or really can't assist someone because your schedule won't allow it… there is no need to be rude or defensive, you can refuse and say "no" in a kind way. If you are trying to slow down, then you are going to have to do less. Tell your friends and family that your schedule is already hectic or that you are tired. At first, they will insist, but over time they will end up respecting your choices.

- One point where I really progressed was to actually **say "no" to myself.** I always had these self-imposed obligations and a whole list of them too. Are you like that? My house just had to be clean, the ironing had to be done, my papers had to be in order before I would even consider doing anything for myself. At one point however, I had to really decide where my priorities were and I realized that, although I love to have my home spotless, cleaning was not absolutely necessary. It wasn't always easy, but I have learned to put my priorities like writing my book, meditating, exercising first, even if it means having my ironing load pile up or finding dust balls here and there around the house. Once, my son reproachingly told me that the kitchen needed cleaning. I told him that if it was a problem for him, then he could do it. Believe me, that put an end to the discussion… and he never mentioned it again

- **Focus. Focus. Focus**. Slowing down doesn't necessarily mean doing less. What actually happens when you slow down, is that you are in a better mindset to concentrate. When you are quieter on the inside, you are more capable of giving your full attention to what you are doing on the outside. The goal is to bring that state of inner calmness into what you are doing. So, before you start to work, take one minute to breathe deeply and connect with your inner self. Once you feel peaceful, decide what you are going to start with and try to stay concentrated on this one task. It's not always possible, I know, with our hectic jobs, the phones ringing, the constant interruptions… but every time an opportunity arises, seize it and reconnect with your inner self. Once you are able to do it a few times a day, slowly, slowly you will be able to do it more often, and for longer periods of time.

To conclude, slowing down is the best way to notice all that is going on around us, enabling us to be more present, to be in the moment. At times we need to be a "Do-*er*" and get things done. But there is joy and gratification in *being* rather than *doing*, so *BE* more by *DO*ing less.

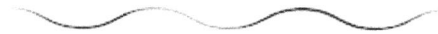

Change n°53
DECLUTTER

53.

I don't know if you are like me, but when I have a problem, my mind becomes preoccupied and keeps going over and over the whole situation. I find that I can no longer read or concentrate on anything. For this reason, cleaning up and putting things in order has helped me calm down and put things back into perspective.

If you are going through a challenging moment and want to bring more peace into your life, taking the time to clear up your entire home, car and garden can be just the thing you need to get back on track. Slowly, slowly as you start clearing up each drawer, as you tidy up each and every closet, it will feel as though the clouds in your mind are dissipating as well. I kind of like to make the analogy with hiking. As you hike through your life and herd along that heavy backpack, it gets harder and harder to move forward. Once in a while, it's nice to stop and put that load down, dump it all onto the ground and see what it is exactly you are tugging along with you each day. It's nice to go through your stuff and chuck the things that no longer interest you or are no longer valid. When it's all done, there is that moment of relief when you see how much lighter the load has become, which allows you to get back to your hike, feeling ready to tackle a new journey.

> ### If you want a clear mind, start off by cleaning up your room!

A. What is de-cluttering?
Definition of clutter: *fill a space in a disorderly way.*
In other words, *to « de » clutter means to empty that space of its "disorder".* When your drawers and closets are bulging and every spot you have in the house is saturated, it's time to declutter and create some more space.

B. Start applying to your everyday life
You want to go through every single one of your drawers and closets to see what needs to be given or thrown away. The best way to do it is to tackle one thing at a time: start with all the clothes, then all your books, papers, various objects and finally all those sentimental things that you just simply love.
It's not as easy as one could first imagine: clearing your clutter means letting go of things that belong to you and even though they are just objects, they withhold memories and have a sentimental value.
But as you declutter, think about applying the lesson to your everyday life: Should I cling onto these memories and keep on living in the past? Is this issue really worth the trouble? What if I decided to simply let it go?

C. Why do we hold on to things?

There are many different reasons why we feel the need to keep all our stuff:

a. We think that one day **we might need this object** and regret throwing it away.

Advice: Give it to someone who can really use it. Knowing that it is making another person happy usually puts an end to any regret you might have.

b. We feel guilt about throwing away: : Indeed, many people in the world have nothing and here you are, throwing away items that someone else may need.

Solution: *You could choose to host a give-away yard sale or donate to the Red Cross or another similar organization.*

What to do when these objects were **gifts**. Once again, donate so that the gift has a purpose and has a new opportunity to be useful.

Advice: *Take the time to remember all the gifts you gave away to friends and family. Do you expect them to keep these items forever or would it be ok if they got rid of them to clear up a little bit of space? It's time to move on with your life and you can't do that if you are herding along tons of things. It's time to change, free yourself, and lighten up your load.*

Solution: *Why not take a picture of these special items, gifts or memories? You could save the pictures or even frame them to see these gifts every day.*

c. You wore a piece of clothing just once, or never: it's happened to all of us. We buy something and it's there, we look at it, like it, but we never wear it. The only solution is to get rid of it, once and for all. You will NEVER wear it, do you hear me? NEVER !

Your possessions are like Linus's security blanket. Having them around, **brings you a sense of security**. Many people refuse to bring change into their lives for fear that they might feel uncomfortable, and out of their comfort zone. Once you have cleared your home environment, you will gain wings and much more willingness to discover new things and tackle new opportunities.

Solution: *Select and save some of the items you cherish the most. You don't want to have an empty cold home. The goal here is to clear things out, move forward with your life, and not create an impersonal "hotel like" atmosphere. Make your home warm and welcoming. If you possess special items, display them so that your home feels like "a home" and reflects who you are.*

d. It is just too overwhelming! Oh yes! I know the feeling. It is simply too much and you don't know where to begin. The best thing to do, is set aside several days such as a weekend or a few days of your next vacation, to do just that.

Solution: Tackle one drawer at a time or one category at a time, whatever suits you best, and get it done. Once you start seeing how blissful it feels to have your interior uncluttered and in order, you will never want to go back.

e. Another reason why we hang on to our stuff comes from our **fear of change.** For example, why hang on to all of your books?

Solution: *Bring them to the local library and donate them, knowing that you will be able to come and read them in the future. You and I both know that there is a high possibility you will never do that but it's nice to know that you can.*

Knowing that there is no room for fear where love is concerned, release the grip you have on things by letting go of certain belongings. All things must flow: back and forth, you receive and then you give. Because in the end, when you think about it, nothing is ever really yours.

f. Finally, **why bother cleaning up**? You may feel that in one week you will be back to square one, in other words, a messy house.

When decluttering you must make the inner decision that you are doing this for good. It's just like when you quit smoking or want to lose weight, you start with the goal of never smoking again or never regaining the weight. Once you have cleared out everything you no longer want, the next step is to put away those things you wish to keep. In order to do this, find a specific spot for similar items, place together papers, kitchen appliances, towels, each in only one spot. Organize in a logical way.

Solution: Go over all those little things that really annoy you on a day to day basis such as "where are my keys?", "where did I put that letter?", " I hate putting away laundry", "my kid's toys are everywhere "

Address each and every one and try to find a solution.

Have a specific spot for your keys, such as a hook, a drawer and use them systematically when you walk past the door.

Have a file that is readily available in which you can place all incoming mail, if you are not going to take care of it right away. This way, when you have a little bit of time, you can sit down and take care of all these letters in one go.

For the laundry, you could designate turns in the house. I think it's better to have one person doing the laundry all week and another loading up the dishwasher and swap the following week instead of having them do something different each day.

Your kids' toys are all over the place? They empty their room and clutter the living room. Kids like to be around you. Why not have a specific spot for toys in the living room or in the hall between the bedroom and living room? Also, teach your kids to pick up their toys and put them away as soon as they have finished using them.

D. How to declutter?

In order to make it simple, you really need to set aside a certain amount of time or several days to declutter your entire home. Do it all in one go. I really do not think doing one closet a day is the way to go about it, but then we are all different and you have to find what works for you. Keep in mind, however, that you want your place "clutter free" fast, to feel the emptiness, the cleanliness… and feel the full effect of freedom.

a. Organize your decluttering

Why not organize your clean up theme by theme instead of room by room? If you do the living room first and file all the papers you have there and then move on to your desk where you have to do some more filing, it just doesn't make sense. Gather all the documents you have in the house on one table and go from there. It's a good idea to have one binder or box in which you place all the papers that need to be taken care of. After everything is cleared up, create a habit of each week setting aside some specific time for paperwork:15 minutes should be amply enough.

b. Scheduled cleaning up

It might be a good idea to set aside a specific time every week to get the cleaning done, according to your time schedule. For example, you could decide that every Friday night is laundry night. Have the kids and husband know they have to get their bed sheets and dirty clothes in the laundry basket by a certain time or they won't be washed. Tuesday nights, when the kids have practice, you could bring along your paperwork. Find a place close by and get two things done in one go.

E. Clutter affects your mind

a. Clear your work space to help clear your mind

Whether you are aware of it or not, having a cluttered environment affects how you feel. Working or getting things done in a clean room, office or kitchen brings pleasure to your mind: it feels sharp and can concentrate on what needs to be done. Seeing your room or space all tidied up allows your brain to relax and ease into work, unstressed. When I was writing my book, just one glance at my desk and I knew it would be impossible to work there: too many papers, too many books, or sticky notes. I would often grab my bag, my computer and a few documents and escape to a nearby coffee shop. Even though it was a busy place, I knew I would be able to work hard for two hours: no mess or things to clean up, and I had nothing else to do but focus on my writing.

That's when I realized how clutter actually affected my brain and the way I worked.

b. Stop procrastinating

There is yet another type of clutter that needs to be addressed and that's all those "mind cluttering thoughts" that cause you to procrastinate. You know what I am talking about: all those things, phone calls, promises you made that have to be done but you keep putting off until later etc. If these thoughts are upsetting you, it will be hard to focus on anything else properly. Take two minutes to think about it. Is there maybe something that you can do, such as write a quick message to ask for a little delay or give a call to say you haven't forgotten what you have promised to do and commit then and there, when you will do it. If something is really troubling me, I find it better to tackle it immediately or else those thoughts will simply come back incessantly.

c. Learn to enjoy the process

For many decluttering and cleaning up feels like a chore and a burden. Why not try to find ways to make it fun? Decide in your mind that while you are tidying up, this is "me time": You could take the time to think a few things through and straighten things up in your mind as well. You also could observe your mind and your thoughts: what's troubling you right now?

Or why not put some music on loud and sing and dance while cleaning up your mess?

You could also ask a friend to help you. Once you have finished your place, you could tackle your friend's home.

Make things look pretty, in order, and have them smell good. You could sort out your clothes according to color, have all the same coat hangers or place a few decorative flower or fruit shaped soap bars inside your drawers to enjoy the smell every time you open them.

Make people happy by donating or giving away. Try not to chuck things away. Sometimes it's a lot easier to just give away the bags but why not see if specific items could make a certain person happy? Get a box and put little labels on what you wish to give to whom. I had this dress that a friend of mine loved. I knew it would make her really happy to have it. As I wasn't wearing it anymore, I boxed it up in a little package and the next time we sat down for a chat, I gave it to her. I will never forget her beaming smile when she opened it!

If you want to bring some change into your life, decluttering should be one of the first things to address. When things are where they should be, you can focus on what really matters. How can I sit down and write my book when I see all the messy dishes in the sink, when the floor needs vacuuming and I know I have some mail to take care of?
So, start by decluttering your home and when everything is in order, notice how you suddenly feel ready to embrace new challenges.
Remember:

Less is more.
Say less, listen more.
Own less things, and you'll experience more freedom.

Change n°54
SIMPLIFY

54.

After a long day or whole week at work, we all crave for a little time to unwind and relax. Some of us might choose to go out and have a drink or enjoy a nice restaurant with some friends, others might prefer to be entertained by going to the movies, theatre or ball games. But what if this week we decided that we wouldn't spend a dime on *after work* activities? Yes, you heard me: a whole week without spending anything superfluous. At first, it may seem a bit challenging to undertake. You might even wonder if it is at all possible. Will you be bored? Won't it be lame? What will your friends think?

A. Why simplify?

The first thing that might come to mind is your friends: You're ok with trying out something new, but what about your friends? They will never accept it. But let's get things straight, partaking in free activities doesn't necessarily mean that you have to stay isolated in your own home or cultivate your vegetables in your back yard. In fact, it's all about being creative and taking the time to think it through, in order to get it organized.

Why don't you decide this week to go out into the world with open eyes and open arms? See all the FREE opportunities that are readily available to you and seize them. You will be amazed to see just how much fun this goal can turn into. There are so many things that we take for granted that have always been there. It seems as though there is always something better to do. For example, when was the last time your curled up in a blanket with a cup hot coco in the company of a true friend and simply enjoyed a chat or watched a great movie instead of going out? Embracing simplicity means finding joy in the simple things in life such as cloud gazing, watching people go by, really taking the time to listen to a friend or a relative.

Think "simple". Tell me honestly, if you had to choose between going on a date in a crowded, noisy restaurant or watching the sunset while sipping a glass of wine with the same person on a beach or lying on the grass at a nearby park, what would you pick? HHHmmm! I know I wouldn't have to think twice! Why not even do it alone and take a bit of time to be with yourself?

The thing with simplifying is, that it usually means we are going to have to slow down. And you know what that means….
That's when we start seeing things the way they really are.
That's when we begin to face what we feel deep down inside.
That's when the truth about our existence comes up to the surface.
Did you ever find yourself in the situation whereby you have 10 minutes to relax, perhaps at the end of a yoga lesson and, instead of relaxing, your mind starts wandering off to that "to do" list of yours?

This week, make it a goal and go all the way: instead of cramming your life with "moments" and activities, why not do the opposite and fill it with simplicity. Start tonight, invite a special friend over and spend a relaxing time together, just the two of you. Have your friend come over with some fruit and cheese and tell her it's "simplicity dinner", meaning that you won't be cooking tonight. Prepare a tray with raw vegetables, olives, crackers, ham and turkey slices and simply enjoy. Being just the two of you will make this moment so much more profound and can only deepen your relationship.

B. Simple activities to choose from

To help you I have listed below some ideas that you can do this week that are totally free. Try to do at least one each day!

- Go to the library or a bookstore. Take some time off to read more in general, whether for yourself or for others. Why not share a special moment and read a book to your child or to a relative that is alone?
- Call a friend or relative you haven't called in a while and catch up.
- Get up early to watch the sunrise or after work, stop and see the sunset. Enjoy! Why not program a sunset or sunrise meditation or a yoga sunrise or sundown workout.
- Simplify your meals by eating "simple" foods: as an example, grab a real fruit instead of a processed or packaged one!
- Enjoy the great outdoors: get out and take the time to breathe
- Have a special night with your special someone, just the two of you to talk, listen and reconnect.
- Send a "romantic" date to your other half for the coming evening and make it special.
- Go for a long walk
- Tick off all of those things that you *have* to do. Get them finally done and over with! Clear up your desk, file all your papers, get your accounts up to date, get all your mail done.
- Take special care of yourself and take the time while doing it
- Go camping out in the wild or in your back yard! The kids will love it!
- Spend an evening with the family laughing: program to watch funny videos or sketches.
- Take the evening off to write your goals down or do a vision board
- Spoil your pet with attention, cuddles, games or go for a long walk.
- Simplifying means having less around the house: so why not go through your closets to see what can be given away.
- Rediscover your creativeness by writing, sewing, cooking, painting, singing…
- Reconnect with your partner by reading a book together about relationship, love or any other topic and then discuss it: Make this a moment of sharing and find out what both of you really think.
- Spend an evening with a friend and listen to all of your old favorite songs
- Go out to take some nature pictures or why not try to make some artistic ones with animals or objects or by trying out portraits
- Spend an evening with the family looking at all your photo albums or visioning them on a screen
- Go swim laps

- Create a time capsule with the children in which you write a letter and program to read it in five or ten years
- Do a clothes swap with your friends where you swap the clothes you no longer wear.
- Have a Karaoke night. Sing your heart out!
- Go visit a free museum
- Go to bed early
- Have a family reunion where everyone has his say
- Go hiking
- Dress up night. Have fun with the kids and let them wear your clothes. Swap with your other half and dress up as a woman or man!
- Make your very own movie from scratch with your family or some friends. Invent a story with a plot and an easy text to learn. You'll need to have one person designated to be the cameraman. Action! Have fun editing it and then visioning it together.
- Have a no TV night! Reconnect with the family. Play board games or enjoy a game of basketball/frisbee or baseball.
- Put some music on loud and dance your heart out!
- Take the time to make a delicious meal together with the rest of the family, set a beautiful table and enjoy it!
- Daydream
- Do nothing

Go from a life where processed foods, TV, social networking, crowded superficial clubs are replaced by a life of togetherness and simplicity and see how your life gets a deeper sense of meaning!

Change n°55
KNOW YOURSELF

55.

As a child, have you ever had a diary or later on, wanted to write your life story?
Why not start filling out a diary or gathering up the willpower to write down all your memories? At first it might sound daunting, especially writing your memoirs, but it's actually a great exercise.

I don't know if any of you have read the book *Wild* in which Cheryl Strayed decides to walk the west coast of the United-States all alone carrying a huge backpack. As she walks, she goes over many details of her childhood and adult life and her progression by foot becomes a progression that allows her to understand who she is. The walk turns out to be real therapy. No matter what her thoughts or feelings were, she insisted on pushing forward. Her past memories kept popping up in her mind but as she walked, she had nothing better to do than to give them her undivided attention. After a 1000-mile hike, her wounds were totally healed and she felt ready to embrace a new life to its fullest.

Writing your journal could be an amazing tool to help you understand why you are the person you are today, and why certain things are not the way you think they ought to be. By analyzing yourself and being 100 % honest in the process, you might just take the lid off some of the issues that needed to be addressed.

Diary or a life story?
A diary is a lot easier than writing a biography in the sense that you can start today: write whatever you want and the number of lines you wish.

A life story will necessitate some reflection before you start writing as well as laying out a plot. What exactly do you want to write about: your entire story? Do you wish to focus on one or several major events and then move on from there? Remember, there are no rules. So, you are totally free to write what you want and leave out the details that are irrelevant or that you do not wish to talk about.

1. My experience writing a diary
For years, I held a journal in which I simply wrote everything I did. I chose intentionally, however, not to criticize people or write things that could hurt anybody's feelings. Every time I wrote something down, I kept in mind that someone, someday could read these pages, my husband, my children, my in laws and I absolutely did not want my loved ones feelings hurt by something I wrote. I just wanted to be able to read these diaries again in the future and remember all the things I did or that we shared together. I did however express anger, discouragement, tiredness and those kinds of emotions that were natural daily emotions that a young woman and mother could feel, but I never wrote hurtful words towards anyone.

Having my best friend die in a sudden car crash when I was in my late twenties made me realize that everything could be over today, in a instant or tomorrow, and I didn't want to leave writings behind that expressed things that might not be understood by others or might eventually hurt them. But this is personal and some of you might even ask what's the point of writing at all. I see my diaries as photo albums: you are free to flip through them and they bring back memories of good and bad times. You don't necessarily need to write a legend under each photo as each one comes with many different memories. When other people read my diaries, they will have a totally different and more neutral read, which won't be the case for me. At several occasions, I took the time to look through some of my writings and really enjoyed strolling back into the past to relive the days when I gave birth, the moments when my sons made their first steps, and the times when I travelled to different parts of the world. Although I stuck to the essential, each line would systematically ricochet to other memories.

2. My experience writing a blog

Later, as the kids got bigger and the homeschooling became a handful, I stopped keeping the journal and created a blog, which I wrote only when we were away on vacation. At the end of each trip, I would get it printed into a book. Just as I did with my diary, I chose not to write personal issues. I stuck to writing about our journey, the experiences and things that we learned about the country, and the customs. There are, however, some moments of stress, irony and life lessons that I did chose to share.

I am glad I wrote these "BlogBooks" and now I have a cupboard full of them that the kids can flip through and might want to read some day. These" BlogBooks" took a lot of time to create. While on vacation, I would often wake up very early in the morning, write about what we did the day before, and choose which photos to add. I really enjoyed the process and always kept in mind that one day, my children might cherish reading them.

3. My experience writing a book

The book that I wrote and you hold in your hands this very moment, was in a sense therapeutic since I have had to go over and question many issues in my life to write about them. But just as I have done with my diaries, I have chosen not to write anything against anyone who might have hurt me in the past. I kind of feel like saying: "What's the point?" The purpose of my book is to move forward and heal, not to seek revenge in any way whatsoever. Quite the contrary. I have learned to accept and forgive. I just wanted to explain how I did it in order to help others move forward in a positive way.

"What goes around comes around"

We often hear people saying that the wheels spins but I don't really believe this, at least not in the way most people do. I have already developed this point in the book, but it needs to be addressed here to prove a point. I don't believe that people who are mean, will one day pay for their mistakes and I don't choose to be good today to receive something good in exchange. I try, as much as possible, to be nice and kind, because it makes me feel good about myself to be this way. I know deep down inside, that no matter how good I am, life will not spare me and that I will get my load of burdens, heartbreaks, sicknesses and problems, because that's just the way life is. When something bad happens to me, I do not sit and wonder: "What did I do to deserve this?".

No. I will more likely sit and ask myself: "OK. What is the lesson that I can learn from this challenge? How can I come out of this bigger, stronger and wiser?" I know a lot of people believe that they are responsible for everything that happens in their lives, while others take no responsibility at all. Some people also believe in reincarnation, that they must "pay" for the things they have done in previous lives. And then you have those who believe that there is life after death while others are convinced there is nothing. There are many, many theories. I am not saying any of them are wrong, I just choose to say that I don't know for sure and, for this reason, I want to make this life super special and try to do the best I can. I wanted to explain why I have chosen not to say certain things: I feel, deep down inside me, that it's the right thing to do. But some of you may, on the contrary, really need to express such painful moments. And readers might gain a lot from reading your experiences and how you handled them. We are all different and have different needs. So, listen to yourself and see what it is that you want to do and then start writing.

What to write about?

The only rule here is that there is no rule. It's your diary, your story, so you can write exactly what you wish to write about. For instance, you could choose to write only about one specific topic in your diary:

1. **The Day to day Diary**: just take the time to write about your day, what you did, who you saw, how you feel. In this type of diary, you are totally free to write about everything and anything.

2. **The Feelings Diary:** You might be at a certain point in your life where you feel the need to find yourself. In this case a "Feelings Diary" might be what you need. Every day, take the time to reflect upon your inner emotions. Try to be honest: see the good, but also the bad in you. Admit your faults. Question yourself. Pour it all out on paper; it can really be therapeutic. Go into the past and dig out everything you can remember: bring out the tough times when you really struggled. Remember how you coped with challenges. Did you just accept them, or did you grow from these experiences? Take the time to go over the good moments as well. It's also very important to go over all of those positive emotions you experienced in the past. And what about the future? Do you spend your time imagining the worst for yourself; always thinking that the situation obviously won't go the way you would like it to, because, "*it never has in the past, so why would it in the future*", right? You probably think that if you imagine it enough, you will be fully prepared for the disappointment when it actually happens, and this way it won't hurt as much. But you are in fact living in constant FEAR. Take the time to FEEL these fears, but also to realize what you are doing to yourself and then write it all down on paper. See the recurring patterns going on in your life. Being aware of them is already moving you one step forward towards healing.

3. **The Memories Diary:** take a stroll down memory lane. You can do this freely and write down one memory after another, without following any particular order. Or, you could do some research, such as going through your photos and begin at a certain age and work your way up to today.

It might be nice to add photos and drawings to back up your writings. Why not plan a trip into the past as well? You could, for instance, go back to where you used to live as a child, to describe your old school, playground, and neighborhood.

4. The Question Diary: In this one, you decide to ask yourself a different question every day about yourself, your past, your beliefs, your dreams, you name it. Just pick a question and answer it. Why not prepare an array of questions ahead of time, so that you can simply pick and choose one when you have some time to write. Some are easy and might take a minute or two, whereas others might take more time or necessitate a bit of research. So, depending on the time you have at hand, you will know which question to choose. You could also write the questions in the diary ahead of time and plan ahead to do some research to have it all ready by a certain date. This one is fun and will sometimes require some detective work.

5. Goal Oriented Diary: In this diary, the idea is to keep track of your goals and write down a few lines each day to see how you are doing, stay motivated, and see what needs to be changed to make sure you reach your goals. Goal setting will inevitably come with ups and downs and it's important to accept it as normal. A goal-oriented diary will help you stay on track and motivate you to keep pushing forward. I have set myself many challenges: Some were quite easy, such as drinking more water, while others, were really challenging such as:
- getting more muscle definition on my arms. This particular goal took me several years to achieve, but I kept regularly putting that goal back on my list.
- Doing chin-ups.
- Quitting coffee.
- Getting in the habit of taking cold showers.
- Leaving the table feeling just right, having eaten just the right amount of food. I also struggled with this goal for a number of years. Today, I don't even have to think about it, I am totally in tune with my body and it has become second nature.

Every day, write down what you did to get one step closer to your goal, what your challenges were, or what made you deviate. If you are visualizing or listening to your motivational tapes, write it down and describe how you felt after the session.
If you suffer from fear of failure, write all of your fears down and try to understand what is causing them. Add a few affirmations or some motivational quotes at the end to create an extra boost. You could also add some photos of your goals thus adding your visual sense to the picture. Remember: the more you incorporate your different senses into the whole process, the more it feels real and the closer you are to making it a reality.

At one point I had envisioned myself going on the Oprah show to talk about my book to hopefully help as many people as possible to change and reach their goals as well. I visualized it and even sprayed her favorite perfume onto my diary, my vision board, in my home… every time I would smell the fragrance it would remind me of this amazing goal I was moving towards and it would empower me to keep pushing forward.

6. Gratitude diary: More and more books and articles talk about being grateful. What's the big deal behind all of this "being grateful" business? Many people tend to wake up complaining, go to work complaining and come back home still complaining. Maybe now would be the good time to look at everything you have, instead of focusing on what is not going right or what you don't have. Cherishing the present will help you appreciate even more the good things that come into your life. Keeping a Gratitude Diary means writing down:

- all the good things that have happened to you throughout the day
- the beautiful things, a special moment you experienced such as a kiss, a hug, or something touching that you saw
- the little things, such as having the time to sip your favorite coffee in that little café you love, or the fact that someone did something kind or helpful for you
- the big things: a promotion, a proposal, good news
- the quotes: if you read something that inspired you and made you see life in a more positive way, write it down
- the name of the books and movies that inspired you positively. Try reading more autobiographies about exemplary and successful people or watch success stories on TV. Let these people inspire you to succeed as well.

All of these things can help you become more positive, more appreciative and grateful for the life you have right now. So, if you are inclined to dwell in negativity or are stuck in a rut right now, this might be a good option for you.

7. Life Lessons diary: I truly believe that every day and everywhere there are messages for us to receive. It's all just a question of opening one's eyes and looking at life around us as it unfolds.
This can be done:

- By observing other people: by doing so, we learn about character and how each person reacts in different ways and how these reactions are so dependent on so many different factors such as our mood, our previous experiences, whether we are under stress or tired. It might be interesting to take the time and ask ourselves how we would have reacted in a similar situation? What lesson did you learn from what happened?
- By observing ourselves: by doing so, we see our mistakes, our flaws, but also our successes and our good qualities. It's important to acknowledge the fact that you were jealous at a certain point or that you went too far and lost your temper. Why? What triggered these reactions? But it's just as important to recognize that you were kind or efficient in other instances. Get to know yourself in each situation.
- By observing nature: for this point you might want to check out Change n°51: *Communicate with Nature*. Nature has messages and it could be fun and interesting to write about the ones you can interpret each day. Take a photo and add it to your text for a visual impression.

8. The quote or "line of the day" diary: this one speaks for itself and only necessitates finding one inspirational quote each day. I, for my part, love quotes and I have sticky post-its all over that I love and that keep me motivated. A good idea is to create your own quotes according to what you learned or quote some funny things that people or your children might have said in order to remember them.

My kids have told me so many amusing things!

Just to quote a few amusing ones they came up with:

When we went to see the musical "Dirty Dancing" my eleven year-old son asked me: "Why is it called "dirty dancing"? Are they going to dance with garbage bags?"

My niece, Elea, before going to bed would ask if we could "turn the black light on". She thought that when you flicked the light switch, you had two options: a light that would make colors appear or a light that would turn everything black.

My son once told me that he had to correct his dramatical errors (instead of grammatical).

Another time, when my son was five, I attempted to explain to him the meaning of the word "contagious". I told him that when you catch a cold or the flu, the fact that you can catch it from someone else makes it contagious. I then asked him to use the word in a sentence to see if he had properly grasped the meaning. He looked at me and said: "That's an easy one: a ball is contagious because you can catch it."

Quotes don't necessarily have to come from famous authors... sometimes life lessons come from the people you least expect.

9. Photo or Drawing Diary: If you are an artist or love taking photos, this diary could be just what you are looking for. I have seen many travel diaries in which people draw or take photos of the places they visit. Why not do the same thing for your every-day life? Turn this one into something similar to a report. Take photos or draw the people, the places, the food, the objects, the nature around you and capture a moment. Add a legend, a quote to each selected memory or even a whole paragraph. It's all up to you. Who says you have to travel to keep a photo or drawing Diary?

10. Who, what, where, when, why diary: In this one, you answer these five questions every day. Who did you see? What did you do or what happened today? Where did you go? When did it take place or when was the last time you experienced or did this? And eventually ask yourself various "why" questions?

11. Reflection of the Day Diary: in this one you will want to write short essays about different topics whether political, social or personal. When I chose this title for the diary, I had in mind those letters women used to write in the 19th century that were a mine full of information about how people lived, dressed, but also what their concerns were. For example, you could choose to write a satire about today's society or simply write what your beliefs are regarding various topics and concerns. You could read the paper or watch the news and choose a topic and eventually write what you think could be done to solve these issues.

12. A theme based Diary: If you have a subject that interests you in particular, why not write a diary about it. Perhaps you are passionate about sports such as yoga, swimming, triathlon, surfing or perhaps travelling, fashion, food, gardening, science, the news, current affairs or politics. Whatever the topic you choose, take the time each day to research and write about it. Print out any documents that relate to this subject and read about people who have succeeded in this domain. In this diary, you can write down everything you have learned or that is related to the subject at hand. Become a pro. Let's say you are interested in surfing. You could write down how you have progressed, collect photos of yourself or beautiful surfing shots, research how to improve your different techniques or view surfing videos on the net. And why not read biographies about the best surfers in the world? Become a living encyclopedia about your passion. Make this diary super special by adding colors and making it fun and pleasurable to look at.

When I was young, I had a diary in which I wrote all my favorite songs. We didn't have printers or internet at the time, so I used to listen to the songs on the radio and write down the lyrics as fast as I could. Every time the song would air, I would rush with my pen and paper and fill out the missing blanks. When I had the entire song, I would copy it into my special Songs Diary. Today, with internet and computers, things are so much easier: search, click and print! But you can still enjoy learning the lyrics of your favorite songs and maybe add photos of the artists or interesting information about them.

13. A Dream Diary: You could write down all your dreams and try to interpret them. There are many books and websites that can help you grasp the meaning of your dreams. Usually, you look up a specific word, such as "tooth", "earthquake", "rainbow" and you get an interpretation. I usually examine what is going on in my life and try to see how my dream applies to current events.

I once dreamt that I was going to visit someone in a hospital. To my surprise when I opened the door of the hospital room, the person who was lying in the hospital bed was myself. Not quite understanding how this was possible, I then had doubts about who *I* was. If "she" was "me", then who was I? I went over to the mirror to look at my reflection. What a shock it was when I realized that the face I saw was an older version of myself, all covered with wrinkles. It hit me that the older version of myself, was how my younger self was feeling inside: she was feeling old, tired and sad. I grabbed a glass and filled it with water and as I offered it to my younger self, I smiled and looked at her with love, knowing that what she was in desperate need of, was self-love.

Writing your Life Story

To write your life story, there are three options:
• The easiest way to do this one is to buy a diary workbook that has everything already laid out for you and that simply requires you to fill out the spaces. All you do is answer the questions on each page. There is no need to begin with page one. You can easily flip through the pages and start wherever you wish. There will be an array of questions and the whole thing is pretty straightforward. If you really wish to write a book about your life, it might be interesting to begin by filling out this type of diary beforehand, to get you started and discover what you wish to talk about.

- You can write a book from scratch. You will need to write a plot and the general structure of the book beforehand. There are a number of books to help you write your life story. I suggest that you read one or two of these books before starting, as they will be very useful in helping you organize your thoughts and map out the steps. Remember to always have a pen and paper at hand, so you may write down any ideas as soon as they pop up. I have found that while writing this book, I would get a flash of an idea anytime, anywhere. You can also add them to your "notes" application on the phone or tape it on your Dictaphone.
- You can get someone else to write the book for you. Yes, you can actually hire a professional writer to do it for you. But don't think that it will be any easier. You have to tell the writer your story, talk about anecdotes, reveal emotions, describe what you endured or lived… and believe me, it's not an easy exercise and will require that you get your ideas together. If you are not much of a writer but would love to write your life story this might be the best option for you. However, this might come out as being rather expensive. It's just an idea, but you could go on campus and ask students or professors that are studying or teaching "creative writing" if they would be interested in participating in this project. You could probably get away with a much better rate.

You could also sign up and attend a course to learn how to write. If you feel passionate about writing, this might be a great way to start.

Additional points:

It's important to take pleasure in writing your diary: this is a time to be creative, alone with yourself, and ask questions. You are totally free, so make the most of it.

On days when you lack inspiration, remember that it's important to be disciplined. As much as possible, try to write every day, even if you only write a few lines or a single paragraph. You could make it a rule to write at least one line a day. Regularity will keep the journal going. Try to see this journal as your journey. Each word is like a footstep that is taking you somewhere, with your final two footsteps being the words "The End."

Don't forget to date your writings. It may seem irrelevant now, but in a few years, you will be happy to know when you wrote it.

If you are not happy with your writing style, I recommend reading more and perhaps creating a word bank. Every time you find a new word or an expression that you think might be useful, write it down into a specific notebook. Every once in a while, review and read the words one by one, to help freshen your memory. Don't try to copy someone else's style. Be yourself. Remember you are unique and you have something to contribute, that is unique as well.

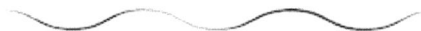

Change n°56
GIVE A SMILE

56.

Although you don't have the power to change the world, you CAN, however, have an impact on the people around you… with your smile. Why don't you decide today to make a difference? Get up and begin smiling at the world. Offer a smile every opportunity you get…and you know what? Chances are you will get one right back.

**Smile and then observe the magic happening:
as you light up so will the world around you,
it's contagious**

Keep this in mind and remember that the opposite holds true as well.

You see, a smile is a bit like a yawn: ever notice how a yawn can get all the people around you yawning and drowsy? Well the same holds true for a smile. Smiling can trigger an unconscious automatic response and will most likely make your interlocutor smile right back at you.

You don't believe me? Try this little test. Go on internet and type in successively the words: "sad face", "crying face", "surprised face", "angry/or yelling face". Observe how you are feeling, what expressions your face makes. You could even film the sequence to really visualize the impact other people's emotions have on you. Now, type in "smiling, happy faces", "funny faces" and "laughing out loud faces". What different expressions did your face communicate this time? Are you now convinced? I call it the ripple effect. Once your smile is triggered, your mood is boosted and the people around you not only see it, they also feel your vibes.

So, starting now, when you grab your keys and walk out the front door, remember to take your smile with you. Something to reflect upon… Once you cross the threshold who would you rather encounter, one hundred smartly dressed people or one hundred smiling faces? Which group do you think would have a greater impact on the course of your day and on your mood in general?

If you want more peace and serenity in your life, or if you are feeling down, start by smiling a little more. You don't need to have good news in order to smile…there are many different reasons to do so. Open up and look around you: observe nature…and smile at its beauty. Look at your children or your loved ones, and smile for gratitude. Remember a funny memory…and smile with laughter. Look at everyday life events happening right now around you, and smile for being able to be there to see it.

1. Why smile?

It may seem obvious, but did you know:
- Smiling, even if you are not happy, will lift your spirits and make you feel better
- When you smile, your face lights up and you appear more beautiful
- Smiling is a gift and it's free!
- Smiling is contagious: just do it and see how you make other people happy!
- Smiling makes you appear more self-confident. People will see a person who feels good about themselves
- Do you want to meet new people? Smiling makes you far more approachable
- Don't forget, when on the phone, the person at the other end can actually "hear" you smile
- A good handshake and a true smile with a direct eye contact portrays competency!
- One smile induces the same positive effect as eating 2000 bars of chocolate! And a smile is calorie free!
- A simple smile *can* change things: so, smile and see how your entire day can shift for the better

2. How to do it?

Read below to find out ways to make your smile really come through:
- First, take good care of your teeth. I am not saying that you cannot smile if your teeth aren't picture perfect. However, a smile with the leftovers of today's breakfast visibly stuck between your two front teeth won't have the same effect as a beaming clean smile! Although, you might trigger a good laugh, which is actually better than a simple smile! Just remember to brush and floss your teeth, see your dentist regularly and why not start whitening them up with baking soda? You'll never know the impact your smile has until you use it and observe its powers!
- Start paying attention to others. Open up to the people around you on the bus, in your neighborhood, at the supermarket. Notice random smiles and how you automatically give them back. If you don't, then seize these opportunities and start practicing! When interacting with strangers - such as when you walk into a store, when you are served at a restaurant or holding a door - offer a smile and make someone's day!
- Do the confidence pose or try the confidence walk. For the confidence pose, just stand in front of the mirror in a "soldier pose" and while standing tall, shoulders back, tummy in, look at yourself straight in the eyes and then add a big fat smile on your face! For the confidence walk, check out Change n° 04: The "Confidence Walk". Do the same walk and make sure to add a smile on your face. Try out different types of smiles depending on what you encounter! (read below for a list of these different types of smiles).
- Take the time to figure out what makes YOU smile. Is it spending time with a certain friend? Is it eating in a certain restaurant or visiting a special place? Is it watching a certain TV show? Make a list of 10 things that make you happy and smile and try to knock out the whole list this week.
- Make it a goal this week: day one, make one person smile or smile at one person. Day two, make two people smile or give two of your smiles. Day three… you got the point.

- If you find it difficult to go out and start smiling at people, you can always begin by smiling in your own home, with your family or even when you are all alone. Why not try the "Smile Meditation"? It's very easy: just sit as you would when meditating, close your eyes and smile…and keep smiling whether you are meditating for five, ten or 15 minutes. Every few minutes make your smile broader and then even broader to finish with an "ear to ear smile". Observe how your mood changes.

Of course, at first when you decide to smile more it will seem a bit awkward and feel unnatural. But that's ok, even if you feel like you're forcing it a little bit. You will quickly see that it still works.

Remember to smile with your eyes as well. Add genuineness and empathy into your expression and make it truly sincere.

You have no idea what power you have in your hands: your smile and your attitude can totally change the course of your day and everyone else's as well. For this reason:

Every time you smile see it as a gift:
wrap it with love and give it with the desire
of making the other person happy.

3. What is your smile saying & expressing?

When you think of it, how many different smiles can you express during a single day? It got me thinking and I came up with the following list:
- The polite smile
- The shy smile
- The sexy smile
- The commercial smile
- The fake smile
- The laughing out loud smile
- The surprised smile, when an unexpected good thing happens
- The victory smile
- The moment of complicity smile
- The thoughtful smile
- The happy smile
- The up to no good smile, you know, when your kids are up to something!
- The proud smile
- The breathtaking smile
- The "I am in love" smile

And there are so many more smiles to choose from, depending on the occasion! I am sure you can find one to suit your mood right now!

At one point in my life, I felt so much pain inside that I couldn't stand or sit up straight anymore, since I could literally feel deep pain within my heart. It was as if I had this weight pressing down upon it and it just wouldn't leave. Every second, every minute of each day felt painful and never ending. I knew I was going through major depression, but I refused to consult a doctor, because I knew he would prescribe anti-depressants. For me, it was out of the question to start going down this path. Although it seemed that this pain was insurmountable, I knew deep down inside that it was just a question of time. And so, I isolated myself, I meditated, prayed, slept and I cried a lot too… but every day I forced myself to go out and face the world: I would do my confidence walk, I would listen to my P.E.T.s and I would open up to others and smile.

It took time, a long time, but eventually, one day, I smiled and laughed spontaneously and it hit me: this depression was losing control over me and I was on my way up again.

Many times, you will find that you are simply not in the mood to smile, you are going through tough times and it's just too much. Do it anyway. Let your inner turmoil aside for a few seconds and focus on what is going on outside. Smile. Keep faith on what lies ahead. You can get past this pain and your heart will smile wholeheartedly again.

A heart doesn't just love, it can actually smile.
So, whenever you can,
place a smile on it.

Change n°57
EMPOWERING WALK

57.

When in emotional pain, the hardest part is to get your attention away from what is hurting you. When you are going through a breakup, have lost a loved one, or are going through deep depression, all you feel is complete sadness, a sense of total emptiness and you tend to obsess over the situation. It's as if nothing could fill the void, nothing really matters anymore and you lose all interest in what life has to offer. You also have this sense of helplessness, whereby you feel that nobody can do anything for you and nothing can help. In these moments of despair, you often feel crushed and powerless and you wonder if you are ever going to make it through…. The emotional pain is such that you don't see how you are going to be able to be yourself again.

A. Things will be OK again, eventually

It's important to know, in these moments, that things WILL eventually be "OK". You must never lose faith. That's when experience comes in handy: if you have suffered in the past, and have gone through very hard times before, you *know* that you will "survive" this.

I find it strange that people always tend to prefer playing the role of the victim, constantly complaining and dwelling about what has happened to them in the past, when they should in fact be proud of the challenges they have overcome. Indeed, although they have suffered, if they are still here today, never once were they defeated. Why not decide to change the way you see things: you are no longer that victim. Okay, you have been in the boxing ring a few times but you were never knocked out. You ran a few marathons but relentlessly managed to cross the finish line every single time. Sometimes, it sure felt as though you were drowning but you have always succeeded in reaching the shore. That's because you are a fighter, a survivor and a winner. So, start imagining all of those podiums you stoop upon, the medals and trophies you earned and now visually place each and every one of them on a shelf in front of you. Yes, you have quite a few victories to be proud of.

So, remember, and repeat to yourself as many times as necessary: whatever you are going through right now, you had numerous victories in the past. *You* are victorious and *will* get past this.

Keep faith that sometime in the future, whether it be near or a little further away, things are going to be all right again. Trust time and always remember that an ending is only the end of a chapter in your life. You have a whole life-book to write and there are many more chapters to live that promise to be full of adventure, love, ups and downs, laughter and lessons to learn. The key to getting back on track is to take "baby steps" every single day. At first, doing so, even for one minute, may seem like too much already. It doesn't matter, keep believing and trying every single day. Only *you* can force yourself to regain control of your life.

Although it may seem as though you are in total darkness, there is a light somewhere. Search for it. At first it may seem quite dim but once you found it, you are assured in knowing that it will lead you on the way out.

B. A personal realization that might help: the difference between letting go of pain and embracing it.

I don't know if what you are about to read will make any sense to you, but I would like to share a personal experience that was an eye opener and that, undoubtedly helped me move forward with my pain.

I had always heard that when you find yourself in a difficult situation, such as when you are suffering or feeling very sad, the best thing to do is to just let go, stop struggling, and completely release what is worrying or hurting you. One day, I decided to give it a try.

It was at a time I was left completely heartbroken. Although I tried, no matter what I did, I just couldn't seem to get over the grief and pain and move forward with my life. I had tried to imagine seeing the person who was connected to my emotional pain, as floating away, while I felt total acceptance. I visualized this several times a day… but deep down inside, I still felt that I just couldn't let him go, or to be quite honest, that I didn't *want* to let him go. I clung on to him desperately, with the hopes that he might come back. Time went by and my efforts to let him go came to no avail. This puzzled and annoyed me, until one day, it hit me. The idea dawned on me that letting go doesn't mean you have to make "what is hurting you" go away, but it means that you have to ACCEPT and *EMBRACE it!*

This was a great discovery for me and it really helped me move forward with my life. I no longer had to let this person go. What I was supposed to do was accept the fact that I didn't want to let him go and accept the fact that I was in pain. So, that's what I did: I accepted the pain and that it was killing me. I accepted the fact that I was desperately clinging onto him and would do so by admitting to myself: "I am clinging onto him. It's ok. I am in pain and am suffering, it's normal to cling onto him. I love him. It's ok to still love him."

Instead of "letting go", which felt like I was forcing myself to do what I didn't want, while fighting against my inner feelings, I just embraced the fact that I didn't want to let go. I embraced the fact that I was in great pain. I embraced the fact that I felt like crying. In a way, letting go, embracing, accepting all mean the same thing, but the slight nuance really helped me in my healing process and this is why I wish to share it with you today. And so, from then on, every time I felt myself clinging onto him, I just mentally repeated these soothing words: "I am clinging onto him. It's ok. It's normal." And every time I thought about how much I loved him, I told myself: "Everything is okay: I love him. I am going to be ok." And every time I felt the tears coming, I would tell myself: "You are in pain BB, it's normal to feel like crying. Don't fight it, don't force yourself to stop those tears from falling. You are going to be ok. Just accept it. Embrace it."

Handling the situation this way made a huge difference on how I felt: Knowing that I didn't have to force myself to do anything I didn't want to, really helped me to finally let it all go.

C. A few things you can do that might help

There are many little things that you can do, such as:

- Call a friend every day and talk or listen, even if you really don't feel like it
- Make sure that every day you watch a funny movie or TV series, even if you don't want to
- Push yourself to do things for others. Sometimes focusing on other people instead of your sadness, can give you a little boost or keep your mind off *you*
- Sing out loud in your shower, in your room, in your car. Put on your favorite music and pour your emotions into it.
- Allow yourself to cry your heart out, but for a limited time only. Literally put the timer on for 5 or 10 minutes and let it all go. But when the alarm goes off, get up and get a move on. This advice was given to me by my sister. It's important to evacuate all those emotions but don't let yourself drown in them. Tell yourself "I am going to cry for 10 minutes, and then I am going to take a cold shower, call a friend, watch a funny movie, or go for a walk.
- Do some gardening or cleaning up
- Go see a professional therapist who can help you. Call and make an appointment
- Reconnect with nature: get out and spend some time in a peaceful place such as a river, a lake, the ocean…

D. My experience embracing pain

a. Walking the pain away

A few years ago, I read this book, about a woman going through a terrible depression. She didn't know how to cope with it. She ended up losing her job and stayed at home just feeling sorry for herself.

A friend of hers came to pick her up and drove her out of the city to this small cottage by the ocean. Before leaving her there, she said: "You are most welcome to stay here as long as necessary and you can spend your whole day feeling sorry for yourself, if that's all you are up to. However, you have one obligation: every single day, you have to get up and get out for a long walk on the beach. No excuses, whether you are tired, it's raining or storming, you must get out and walk." And that's what she did.

She also had to ride her bike to the little town nearby to get some food every week, since she didn't have a car. The young woman kept her promise and slowly, slowly these walks invigorated her and became an essential part of her day: She walked all through the winter season through rain, thunderstorms or heavy winds… By the time spring came, faith had come back and she started to believe that life still offered possibilities. I just wish I could remember the title of this book, so I could reference it and read it again!

b. Pouring your pain into cooking, gardening or whatever you love to do

When you think of it, you can pretty much pour your pain into any activity you want: by engaging in sport, reading, playing chess, gardening, or creating things. For example, if you love cooking you can find great joy in growing your very own vegetables or herb garden. You will get to spend a little bit of alone time tending, picking, chopping, simmering; the entire process can be truly healing.

c. Accept the fact, that it is going to take time

Years ago, I lost my best friend in a car crash. It's always a shock when someone disappears in a sudden, brutal way… but it was even harder for me to accept her death, because we were both in our twenties and she was the mother of a little boy. I just couldn't understand why something so unfair could happen to her and her son. She hadn't even had the time to accomplish any of her lifetime goals yet and she shared such a special bond with her son. I wondered how he was going to cope with it all. I remember feeling devastated and not wanting to see anyone or do anything. Although I always exercised with passion, I didn't feel the courage to get out of the house or even take a shower, for that matter. As the days passed by, however, I told myself that I had to go out for a run. And so, I would get dressed and head outdoors. The first few times, I only had the courage to jog a few minutes before turning back home, realizing that this wasn't going to be possible. But I persisted and did it every single day. And with time, I managed to increase the length of my jogs.

When going through difficult times, it's important to cut yourself some slack and just simply accept the fact that you are in pain, and that you will need time to get over it.
But the most important thing to remember is that it *will* pass. So, if you are going through great pain right now, hang in there.

E. Turn your walk into an empowering tool

a. How to use your walk to empower yourself

I found that one of the best ways to get back on track was to go walking. The way I saw it, walking was moving forward. It didn't really matter where I was going: I had to get up and go for a walk. Every time I would pass the front door, I would step out determined to empower my mind. For this reason, I call it my "empowering walk" and it has helped me numerous times: not only when I have lost someone, but also on those days when I felt down or stressed out, when I had low self-esteem or felt totally discouraged. It's pretty basic and easy to do: You simply have to put your walking shoes on and walk out the door. No need to have a destination: let your feet lead the way. Stay in the now and don't project yourself into the future.
This walk is to be done alone, preferably in total silence. If it's not possible or you would prefer being with someone, just make sure you both remain silent and respect each other's moment of solitude.
It can be done anywhere, but I find walking in nature far more effective and easier to stay connected with how you feel, than walking through the turmoil and noise of the big city. However, this is not always an option, so don't let it stop you from trying.
No need to search for performance: that is not the goal.

- At first, simply walk in silence, and try to bring your focus on your breath. Feel the air as it enters your nostrils. Be aware of yourself while breathing calmly.
- Once you have reached a certain state of inner peace, stay centered within yourself and connected to how you feel. Mentally repeat the words "quiet", "peace"," calm" or any other word that you find has a soothing effect on you.

If you find that there is simply no way to stay centered, practice point a) and b) below, "Listen to a pre-recorded tape" or "Reach your 5 senses Walk". It might help you keep your mind of your inner turmoil.

Focus on your bodily sensations: how do your feet feel when they touch the ground? Do you feel any discomfort from walking? How is your posture? Are you standing nice and tall with your shoulders back and your chest wide open?

- When you feel centered, spend a few moments observing your thoughts. Are you obsessing over one specific topic? Is your mind bouncing from one idea to the next without really focusing on anything in particular?
- To stop the over analyzing, over thinking, procrastinating, I suggest two methods, that have really helped me:

b. Listen to a pre-recorded tape

To be in tune with yourself, I find that it's important to be in total stillness. However, sometimes my mind just won't stop chatting. Does that happen to you too? When this occurs, I find it helps to listen to one of my tapes: I need to have a voice that is louder than the one inside my head. At times, I enjoy listening to nature sounds or soothing music, but at other times, I feel the need to put on a motivational tape.

What I normally do is create my own tapes in which I talk encouragingly to myself. I have made several of these tapes to attain specific goals depending on what I was going through in life. I have countless recordings, varying in length from 1 to 4 minutes, in various topics. I think it's important that you write them yourself. We all need to work on something specific, so it just makes more sense to create your own.

To make things easier for you however, I have tailored a series of different tapes according to what you might be going through. On my website, you will find a wide selection.

c. Reach your FIVE senses walk

Another walk, that I call "the _FIVE_ senses walk", has helped me open up and give my full attention to what is happening around me.

Just read below and start your new journey using your five 5 senses:

For five minutes simply concentrate on your breathing. Feel the air coming through your nostrils, breathe in and out deeply, expanding your rib cage while standing nice and tall. Then, ask yourself the following questions:

- **What do I see?** Look around you and observe everything: people, nature that surrounds you, the sky. Pay attention and continue breathing. Enjoy this for one minute.
- **What do I hear?** Open your ears and listen to all the sounds around you: the loud ones, the discreet ones, people talking, birds chirping, cars driving, the sound of the branches and leaves under your feet. Reconnect with your surroundings for one minute and breathe.

What do I smell? Breathe in and out deeply and smell. What can you distinguish? Perfumes? The salty air, the smell of food, the smell of trees or flowers? What does it remind you of? Be totally in the present moment and have fun trying to guess what the smells are and where they come from. Experience it for one minute.

What do I taste? This one is optional. If you brush your teeth before going out for a walk or keep a tic-tac in your pocket, you could even add the sense of taste to your walk. I place a tic-tac in my mouth and just simply enjoy the minty sensation I get!

How do I feel? This one is twofold. You can either do one or both, as in one after the other.

- **How does your body feel?** First, straighten up and tuck your tummy in. Do you feel any pain anywhere? Breathe through it. Do you feel tired? Inhale the fresh air, inhale the sunshine, inhale the power of the wind blowing and if it's raining, let the cold drops hit your face and wake you up. Let the elements of nature come inside you. Relish this for one minute.

- **What mood are you in?** How are you feeling? Happy, sad, angry, stressed...? Straighten up, smile and breathe deeply. Try to find one word that expresses how you feel right now and then let everything go. Relax, breathe and repeat in your mind for one minute "I let go".

The last minute, open up all your senses at the same time. Be totally connected with everything that surrounds you: the smells, the sounds, the sights, how you feel.
This walk takes approximately 11 minutes and is truly invigorating. You can repeat the whole process again for a total of 22 minutes or simply get into the habit of starting off your walks this way and remaining in the moment the rest of your walk.
At the end, take a few minutes to close your eyes and be in peace. You can sit on a bench, stand in the middle of the woods, lie down on the beach or the ground, sit in a meditating pose and just think "PEACE." Embrace the moment completely.

Now off you go! Wishing you a beautiful walk and hoping you reach your destination, the only destination that really matters: your enduring inner peace.

> **Wishing you a beautiful walk
> and hoping you reach your destination,
> the only destination that really matters:
> your enduring inner peace.**

Change n°58
CHANNELING EMOTIONAL PAIN

58.

Every time life rains on me, in order to hang in there, I constantly remind myself, that I am part of nature and just like a plant, a reed or perhaps a flower, I know deep down inside that it's time to grow. As life goes by, I like to keep this image in mind, and as I look back at all the difficulties I had to face, I can't help but notice:

- how with each and every one of these stumbling blocks, although I may have fallen, my roots became thicker and reached deeper into the ground,
- how my stem became more resilient yet more flexible. I am stronger but also more capable of seeing my mistakes. I learned that at every given moment *I* can choose how I react,
- how my branches and leaves have taken up more space, in other words I gained in confidence.

When the sun shines, these are the happy days, I open up to life and bloom. And when it rains, on sad days, I am still growing, but in another direction… underground, deep down within myself.

> *Just like you need sunshine and rain to see a rainbow,*
> *you also need laughter and tears*
> *to see the true colors of life.*

A. Different kinds of emotional pains, defining yours

For as long as man has lived on earth, there has been pain, and there are so many different kinds:

- The Pain of losing a loved one, a parent, a child, a friend, a much-loved pet
- The Pain of heartbreak whether at 16, after 20 years of marriage or from a passionate one-month experience
- The Pain from failing after having given it your all
- The Pain that comes from not knowing who you are or where you come from.
- The Pain from being separated from your loved ones, feeling so alone and homesick
- The Pain from disappointing yourself, feeling like a total failure
- The Pain you get from feeling helpless when someone you love is suffering and you would like to do so much more than just be present
- The Pain that comes from injustice, when you are unfairly accused of something and have to suffer the consequences although you are innocent
- The Pain from having to choose between two different things that both mean the world to you

B. How do you manage your emotional pain?

When going through a challenging moment, you have different options in regards to pain:

- You can choose to refuse it, denying its existence. I call it the "boomerang strategy" because sooner or later, it will come right back at you. How do you know if you are ignoring it? Well, if you are overdoing intense exercise, doing too much shopping, partying, turning to a belief system in an excessive way, using substances or relying on anti-depressors, doing anything in an exaggerated and addictive way. These are examples of running away from your pain. Initially or at some point, you might feel the necessity to go through this phase to help you accept what is happening to you.

- You could also accept the pain by giving up and settling for it. This one leaves you with a bad taste in your mouth, as if you didn't have a choice and that your only option was to settle for less.

- Finally, you can acknowledge your pain completely, face it and look it into the eyes. This means you must explore your pain, understand it, see it as a message that life is sending you, telling you that things are not "OK". It's in fact quite similar to physical pain. When you start feeling ill or any kind of ache, your body is trying to warn you that somewhere inside of you, something is not quite right.

So, keep this idea of a message hidden within your pain and repeat to yourself:

> **Life is giving me a lesson.**
> **It's time for me to grow.**

C. It's Time to Face Your emotional Pain

To help improve your state, take the time to do the following:

a. **Accept the pain**, don't try to fight it off or ignore your emotions. It's time to face how you feel deep down inside and most probably allow yourself a good cry. As long as you are not disturbing anyone, you can even yell, or scream it off.

b. **Ask questions**. Don't let your pain overpower you. You must learn to use it. We could compare this situation to the technique used in martial arts, whereby you use the opponent's strength to defeat him. As your opponent attacks you, you move aside, leaving him no choice but to come flying forward and end up crumbling onto the ground. Use this same technique for your pain. As it tries to crush you, step aside for a few moments and stop to reflect: What is the real cause of this pain? For example: Is it really about the loss, or are you lonely and scared? Is it because you failed? Did you really work hard enough or are you just making excuses? You are alone with yourself now, so no need to lie. It's time to be totally honest. It's really important to know what the true emotion hiding behind your pain is. Chances are, if you are sincere with yourself, the reason isn't the one you are crying about right now. Next ask yourself: What am I to learn this time? What is the lesson behind this pain? What is this pain trying to tell me? Take the time to write down your answers.

c. It's time to act on the pain. Ask yourself "What can I use this pain for?" The goal is to have a positive approach regarding your pain. Yes, I say a positive approach. Always try to see things in a constructive way. Ask yourself how you can use it to become stronger.

For example, if you have just lost a loved one, ask yourself why you loved this person so much, what were their qualities? Why not decide to honor this person with a gift of being a little more like them. Were they generous with their time with others? Did they laugh a lot, or know how to listen when you were down? Remember what you loved about this person and start doing it in return.

Did you just get dumped? What was the real reason for the breakup? Were you too possessive and jealous? Why? Do you lack self-confidence? What could you do to boost your self-confidence? Maybe muscle up or lose a little weight, take acting lessons. But then maybe it wasn't you. It might have been the other person depreciating you or purposefully making you jealous. Why did you allow it?

The goal here is to ask yourself what the true cause of your suffering is, and to try to find a way to never end up in this kind of situation again.

d. Rediscover your passion or what you are passionate about.

Look at your life objectively. What do you love doing? If you can't think of anything, look back and see what you loved doing as a child? What were you good at? See if there is something that soothes you or helps you feel good, such as nature, being around others, singing, composing etc.

It is not generally perceived this way, but pain is a FORCE. You have to do something with it instead of allowing it to consummate you. Some have understood this and have chosen to express it in writing, others by drawing or singing… they pour their emotions into something and come out of it taller, stronger.

Promise yourself, starting now, that you will take this pain and use it to create something, so that in the end, a beautiful "gift", I like to say "fioretti", which means a "little flowers" in Italian, bloom from these painful times.

Every artist in the history of time has poured their suffering into their songs, paintings or writings.

Because my relationship with my husband was not going well and it looked as if it wasn't going to improve, I was obliged to put my homeschooled children, back into regular school in September. It was a challenging moment for both of them. My youngest son, Diego, told me as he came back home from school one day, that he always felt sad. He had this sadness inside him that just wouldn't leave him. Then he told me that the only time he was happy was when he was singing. So, I decided to sign him up for a musical and it was the best thing we did! It got him singing all day and really boosted his self-confidence!

Just a few months prior to putting my children back to school, I had started writing this book and was very enthusiastic about moving forward with this whole project. Little did I know, however, the number of obstacles I was going to face and that my life would soon be spiraling out of control. Indeed, in a matter of days my husband and I were facing divorce and I was diagnosed with cancer.

All these dramatic events initiated a whole series of medical and legal appointments in the upcoming months. To make things worse, in the middle of all this mess, I met someone… and fell in love. It's as if I was on a roller coaster ride… events, over which I had absolutely no control, just kept happening to me. By the time spring arrived, I turned 50, just completed radiotherapy, my husband and I had filed for divorce and I was left crushed and heartbroken. Here I was, penniless, job hunting, still feeling cancerous and my heart torn into little pieces. Not easy to face job interviews with confidence… I felt NAKED! If I would have been out on the streets naked, it wouldn't have made much of a difference. I am not much of a crier, but during this period, boy did I cry. I cried my heart out.

I have to say, however, that although I felt like I was drowning in my tears, I never lost faith and kept telling myself: "I know this is going to pass. It's just a question of time. I will get through all this. Things are going to be OK again." This thought stuck with me and when August arrived I told myself "Hey, you are still here. You made a minor improvement, but it's still an improvement. Imagine November! Yes, in November you will be feeling so much better, hang in there." And when November finally arrived, I told myself "Look! You made it, and you are feeling a little bit better. Just imagine January!"

These long months felt like forever. I never suffered this way before. Every hour was endured and felt never-ending while my nights remained sleepless. Although I was moving forward, I was only capable of facing one minute or even one second at a time: that was all I could handle. The idea of having to go through an entire day was unbearable, so dealing with it one minute at a time was the way I found to "survive". For some of you the word "survive" might seem exaggerated, but I was really in survival mode: every second of the day was a challenge.

I don't believe anybody in my entourage was aware of this…

I did go through a clinging phase, where I hung on to whatever I could… but eventually the time came, when as if my head was still underwater, something clicked, time stopped, and I took a moment to ask myself why was all this happening to me, or in any case "what could I learn from it all?". And it hit me that all my experiences could help me write a better book. Maybe my cancer, my divorce and my heartbreak were the missing chapters I needed to experience, in order to write a better one. Maybe, if I wanted this book to help people, it was necessary to be face-to-face with all of this. How could I help others, if I hadn't experienced what they had or what they might be going through. Being empathetic is one thing…but living the real deal is another!

It convinced me, all the more, that I had to move forward with the writing. And although at one point, it was literally impossible to write even a single line, because it felt like my head was about to burst, the thought never left me, that all I was going through, was a necessary part of the whole process. I went through my "extreme phase": swimming in the frozen sea every day in January, February and March, running sometimes 25km a day and on average over 100 km a week. It may not seem a lot for certain people, but keep in mind, I was also fighting cancer. So, I had my running away phase too. But when the crying subsided, I started returning to my desk and tried to write again. Sometimes I would sit for hours with my head buzzing and without being able to concentrate at all. But as time went by, I managed to concentrate for longer periods of time and somehow, jumped over each hurdle one at a time.

- Lack of time hurdle: when I complained that I didn't have enough time to write
- Interruption hurdle: when my husband and kids interrupted me incessantly for trivial matters while I was desperately trying to write. *You are all forgiven!*
- Cancer hurdle: when fear enters your mind and you lose that mindset. And then there are also all those time-consuming doctor appointments,
- Divorce hurdle: the arguments and the stress of not knowing where I was going to be in a few months and how I was going to survive financially
- Finding a job hurdle: more time needed, while having to question my self-worth AGAIN!
- Heartbreak hurdle: this was the toughest one for me to handle. I guess in these difficult times I really needed support and knowing that my relationship was going to end, it had a devastating effect on me.

Once I managed to jump over all these obstacles, I knew that nothing, anymore, could stop me. I was going to focus on ONE thing: finishing my book. In the end, all of this had strengthened my will to get it done!

One morning, I set the goal to finish writing my book, with a due date. I stuck the cover, as I imagined it, on the wall in front of my desk, and on the cover page of my cell phone. From that moment on, I decided to perceive these hardships with a positive approach: it became obvious that they were necessary events. This book, in fact, was helping me by keeping me busy, encouraging me to move forward, and focusing my mind constantly on the future.

e. Letting go of resistance

When you are confronting pain, there comes a time when you have to surrender to it. There is no need to fight or resist it. The way I see it, situations are all just a question of perspective. For me, at one point it was as if the world had shut its doors on me. I was a caterpillar lost in its own suffering and probably feeling sorry for myself. Why a caterpillar? Because when the end is near, it buries itself…and for me it seemed like I had reached an ending. But this is the exact moment when you must stop clinging, when you have to stop resisting and learn to let go…to surrender. Sometimes there is nothing you can do but admit your own powerlessness. And, slowly, slowly, the doors open again and you realize it's not the end after all. As I write these words, I am not totally healed. I was going to write "I am waiting for my wings"…my butterfly wings. I realize, however, that this is incorrect, these wings are not something you can simply expect. So, let me rephrase that: "As I write these words, my wings are under construction and I am the one building them!"

When it comes to surrender, I love a certain poem inspired by the Fables of Aesop, entitled *The Oak and the Reed*. On the one hand we have the oak, who is big and strong and on the other, a simple reed, apparently quite week, in comparison. One day, they both face a terrible storm: the oak tree resists with all its might but in the end is uprooted. The reed, however, makes no effort at all and it simply bends over forward. The moral of the story is that you have far more to fear, when facing a problem, if you decide to stubbornly resist it. Sometimes it's best to simply accept the situation.

f. Turning a negative into a positive

Easier said then done, right? How can I have a positive insight when I am sick, jobless or heartbroken? How on Earth can I find something positive, when inside my mind things are all going buck wild? Whether you acknowledge it or not, you can always find a positive aspect in everything or at least create one? Let me give you an example:

When I turned 52, dark times seemed to be behind me, and I was starting to feel like I had my life under control again. Unfortunately, my biological clock wasn't on the same wavelength, and chose to hit the menopause button on start. For those of you who don't know, one of the downsides of menopause is that you are subject to having "hot flashes." You get them numerous times throughout the day. Your entire body literally and without warning starts heating up as though you were in a pressure cooker and within 30 seconds you are left feeling as though you just did a two-minute sprint: your heart is beating faster and you are all covered up with sweat. I would literally get puddles on my stomach, back and chest, every time. Your clothes and underclothes turn damp and as the sweating occurs regularly, you end up feeling sticky and smelly! Basically, it makes you feel uncomfortable. I didn't want to dread them and tried to accept the fact that it was a natural process and did my best to embrace it, but my first two months were a bit of a struggle.

Then, one morning, as I was in the middle of a healing meditation in which I was letting love and light surround me completely, something happened. As I lay there feeling loved and imagining this bright light shining and penetrating me, I also felt a hot flash coming. The heat made my meditation more real and intense. I embraced the heat and decided that from then on, every time I would get one I would take the opportunity to take a 30 second break: I would embrace it and imagine that it was healing and spreading love throughout my body. From then on, I saw myself looking forward to the hot flashes, really wanting them to come so that I could use the heat, direct it to healing myself completely, body and soul.

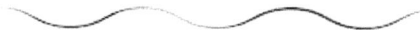

Change n°59
EMBRACING TRUTH

59.

This week choose to be 100% honest with yourself and with others. Admit that you have made a mistake when you are wrong, learn to say "I'm sorry."

A. Being honest with yourself and others

Did you ever notice, when in a certain situation you are aware that you are wrong, but instead of admitting it, you automatically turn to denial? You know, when deep down inside, your inner gut knows you are mistaken, but instead of acknowledging it, you quickly come up with some sort of lame excuse, or a seemingly plausible explanation.

And I wonder, why is it so hard to admit that we are wrong or that we made a mistake? It's a question worth pondering upon... Pride? Probably. The way we were raised? Most certainly. Our own mindset? Without question.

As toddlers we accept to make mistakes: it's part of the process of learning and growing up. But slowly, slowly with others making fun of us, our parents becoming more demanding, and our wish to make them proud, with our "comparing-competing school systems" that chooses to base education on results rather than making learning a more enjoyable process... as we grow up all these elements contribute to the belief, that making errors is something unacceptable... even humiliating.

B. For many, making mistakes is unacceptable. What if we changed that and started accepting our errors?

Why don't you decide to acknowledge your errors: accept them totally. I know what you are going to say:
"No one else does it... why should I?" And it's true. When does anybody ever come up to you and say "You are right! You're totally right. I am sorry. Thank you for pointing that out to me!"?

a. The mistakes we make

Every day, we meet a lot of people. We are surrounded by family and friends, and let's face it, we all make mistakes as a result of:
- misinterpretations
- being a beginner and learning a new skill
- doing something without paying attention, from lack of concentration, because we didn't really listen or properly follow the instructions or because we are tired
- setting goals too high
- our clumsiness
- we didn't study or learn our lesson

b. Allowing for trial and error

There has been this theory, called the "10.000 hour theory", whereby it is said that to master any art, you will need 10.000 hours. Although it has since been contested - indeed, a predetermined number of hours is no guarantee that you will master your art completely - it is interesting to note that to master a certain skill we mostly rely on trial and error and not whether we are initially gifted. In other words, to be good at something you need to practice, practice, practice. You remember your mother's words "If at first you don't succeed, try, try again!" What this means is that during these long hours of practice there will be a lot of mistakes, there will be moments of doubt and discouragement, but you will also be blessed with progression and eventually, success.

Another interesting point that has been developed, is the fact that there are two different types of mindsets: the fixed and the expanded mindset. People who have a fixed mindset are concerned about how they will be judged, whereas those with an expanded mindset are concerned with improving. For those of you who have a fixed mindset, becoming aware of this fact, allows you to make a conscious effort to change: you start understanding that it is far more important to improve yourself than what others might be thinking of you. When in a learning position don't be too hard on yourself and accept failure as part of the ongoing process. Forget those that are watching you, or if you can't, then tell yourself that in the nearby future, these same people will eventually see you achieve the results you were once trying to attain.

c. Acknowledging your mistakes

All this is to say, that mistakes are all right. It's fine to fail, mess up, be clumsy, or tired. These things happen and shouldn't discourage you from trying something new or even put you ill at ease. Next time you "trip", accept it. Say out loud in your mind: "I missed", "I made a mistake", "I am wrong" but don't forget to add "but it's OK, I am learning", "it's OK, next time I will know better", "It's OK. Why did I make this mistake exactly? Oh Yes! Now that I know why, I know what to work on, to avoid finding myself in that situation again."

C. It's O.K. to make mistakes

So, this is the first phase: stepping back and admitting your errors. Lead your life as you normally would but notice how you make mistakes and how you handle them. Is it difficult to admit your own errors to yourself? Is it hard for you to handle making a mistake in front of other people? Do you acknowledge them openly, if someone points them out to you, or do you deny them and find excuses?

See where you stand and then decide to go the next step: **Acceptance.**

> *Once you understand that making mistakes is "normal",*
> *the next step is to expect them to happen,*
> *accept them and learn how to handle them.*

As I am writing this chapter, I just started a new job as a secretary for an important company. There are a lot of different open cases to understand and master, as well as many different things that have to be done, in a specific way. Every task is required to be handled promptly and efficiently. No need to tell you that being under pressure, I made quite a few mistakes, most of which I would never have made, had it been in another context. It's highly frustrating, and all the more so, when you are trying to make a good impression. The fear of losing my job also did me a disfavor. Some people tend to succeed better under pressure: this is not the case for me. In fact, I tend to make even more mistakes.

After a while, however, I saw that it wasn't possible for things to go on this way… If I kept this attitude, I was sure to fail. That's when my close friend, Rachel, told me: "Let it go! Just relax. Do your best and learn as much as possible. What's the worst thing that could happen? Yes, you *could* get fired, right? Well, who knows what the future has in store for you. One thing is for sure however: you will, eventually, find another job. It might even be better than this one. Who knows. So, just relax."

It was exactly what I needed to hear. And although I wasn't able to apply it at all times and still stressed on occasion, I did try, as often as possible, to keep things in perspective. I told myself that there would be more mistakes and that if it didn't work out, things were still going to be ok.

It's hard to make mistakes, isn't it?
It's hard to fail. Wouldn't it be nice if you were always good at everything you did?

I can't help but think of the famous tennis player John McEnroe and how he handled his mistakes: yelling and throwing his racket. He made no effort whatsoever to control his anger or temper. For him, losing was simply unacceptable. If you look online, his outbursts are memorable. Luckily, we don't all handle our mistakes and failures the same way he did. But whether we show it or not, it is stressful, annoying, aggravating when it does happen.

D. Taking action

As much as possible, accept the fact that you have made a mistake:
At first, as we said before, admit them, start of by being honest.
Then, take action. Start with the little things, such as when your spouse or a friend corrects you. Readily admit your mistake with a short quick sentence. No need to elaborate about it. You could, for example, say: "You're right it is…." or "How did I get that wrong? Indeed, it's…".

You could also take advantage of the fact that you made a mistake to compliment the other person: "You have got an awesome memory" or "You are absolutely right" or "you're always so good with…".

This is actually a good way of turning the situation around. Instead of focusing on your error, pinpoint the other person's abilities and see how your interlocutor's pride presents itself. Accepting your mistakes and, in the process, making someone else happy: now that's what I call a win/win situation.

Slowly, over time you will be able to accept these little mistakes quite naturally. And then, just maybe, you will find it might be a good time to acknowledge some bigger ones... maybe from the past.
We all have these "lost apologies" bottled up inside us. When the opportunity arises, why not take advantage of it, admit that you made a mistake, whether it is a big one, or simply the way you handled the situation.

I have an amusing, and also, in a way, sweet memory of something that happened to me as a child. I was in 3rd grade and I had a crush on this boy in my class... his name was Olivier. The teacher had planned a dance for the end of the year performance, and we were supposed to be in couples. Olivier had no desire to dance with me; he made that quite clear, but in the end, I don't know how it happened, we ended up paired together. He did everything to make me pay for it: He didn't smile, ignored me, and purposefully missed taking my hand when he was supposed to. Although the show was a big success and it may seem futile, as I was only nine years old, I was deeply hurt by this boy's attitude.
The years went by... and one day when I was 15, out of pure coincidence, Olivier and I ended up meeting and chatted for a while. As he got up to leave, I remember, he looked at me and said: "I'm sorry for how I behaved in 3rd grade, I sure was stupid back then." I never saw him again, but his kind words stayed with me forever. I was truly touched, that he acknowledged the fact that what he did was hurtful and chose to openly say he was sorry about it...even if it was six years later. As the saying goes, "Better later than never."

Another story, but this time, it was *my* mistake...

I had just finished high school and I was living with my great aunt and great uncle in the south of France. They were always kind to me - and I take the opportunity, although they have long left this world, to say *thank you* for everything they have done for me.
I was a little quick-tempered and a bit rebellious about certain issues at the time, namely my family. My Great Aunt Tony, short for Antonine, was adamant about the fact, that it was *my* duty to keep in touch with my parents. I felt that it was unfair, since neither my mother, nor my father made an effort to call or write. One day, I got really upset and decided to pack my things and leave. For a few days, I slept in a friend's car or on the beach and then moved in with a friend. But as the days went by, I felt terrible leaving them this way, without even saying goodbye, especially after everything they had done for me. And then one day, although I was terrified, I built up the courage to call. It was my Aunt that answered the phone, and do you know what she said? I was expecting a reprimand, a long tirade about how ungrateful I was... but in fact, to my biggest surprise I got quite the opposite: "My darling. Thank you for calling. When are you coming home?" And when I came back home, although she was such a petite in frame, she took me on her lap and hugged me with genuine love. She died in her sleep a few days later...

I can't help but wonder what I would have felt, had I not called to say I was sorry. That thought dawned on me and lingered there for a long time. This story, however, taught me three things:

N° 1: it taught me to admit that I was wrong and learn from my mistakes.

N° 2: it taught me to be forgiving. I was so thankful for my Aunt's forgiveness and all through my life it has served me as a lesson. It was obvious that she was an example to follow: at many different occasions, I remembered her act of kindness and chose to be like her, and to forgive others as well. We all make mistakes, and most of the time we all deserve to be forgiven. I was genuinely sorry for what I did, and receiving her forgiveness was truly a gift of love.

N°3: it taught me to be proactive and do something in return to thank the person for their forgiveness. When my Aunt died, I was devastated, but I remembered her last words… the ones she said when I was sitting on her lap. She told me that my parents would never make the first step. I had to be the smart one. I had to be the one to keep in touch with them. And so, I promised her that I would do my best to keep in contact with them. It didn't happen overnight. It actually took years, but eventually the doors opened and I was able to connect with them. I don't know if she is looking down on me now, but I do know that she is proud of me for having kept my promise.

Although saying you are sorry or admitting your mistakes may seem challenging in the beginning, it can turn out to be a blessing afterwards. Some of you might ask: "and what if your Aunt hadn't forgiven you?" What if the person in front of you shuts the door? Well remember that it's a good thing to get it off your chest and to have asked for forgiveness. Maybe they will not forgive you, but at least YOU know you have done the RIGHT thing. There will be times when people refuse to forgive you. You can't force anyone and you wouldn't want to anyway. Who wants to be forgiven if it isn't done with sincerity?

Let me open a parenthesis here: May this be a life lesson and may it remind you, to be forgiving in the future if someone ever asks *you* for forgiveness. Now that you know how much it hurts to move on without it, remember that your decision might make a difference in someone else's life.

When I divorced, there came a point when I absolutely needed my ex-husband to acknowledge his mistakes. I needed to hear it from him, that he understood why I had left. I really felt that if I wanted to move forward with my life, he *had* to say "I'm sorry." But we kept having the same discussion over and over again, until one day it hit me that I would never hear those two words I so wished to hear. What I really came to realize, was that we were two different individuals, and even though we lived together for over 17 years, we had not experienced the relationship in the same way. As I reflected upon this, I asked myself: "Who am I to decide for my ex-husband? Who am I to tell him what he has to say or do?" My focus should be on changing myself and not on trying to make him say what I wanted to hear. I understood that it was time for me to accept my fair share of the responsibility.

My husband was truly suffering at that time, because of my decision to divorce him. Although I may have had, according to me, good reasons for leaving, I couldn't deny the fact that he was in deep pain and felt devastated. I realized that after 17 years of marriage, many of which were wonderful, I owed him an apology as well. For that reason and even though I knew I would never hear it from him, I understood that it was going to have to come from me.

What has this experience taught me? Never to expect others to admit their mistakes or to say they are sorry, as you may be waiting for years. We are all human beings with eyes, ears and feelings and although we might seemingly live through the same things, we all see different colors, hear different melodies and experience each situation in a unique way. And so, you ask me: How is that going to help you to move forward? I'm just saying it might be worth a try to take the time to put yourself in the other person's shoes and really feel what they are going through. I'm not saying it's going to be easy: it's a process and it requires some digesting. It's called empathy.

Whether you are up to doing it or not, it's your decision, but that's what I chose to do: I really took the time to understand my ex-husband, to feel his loss and pain and it helped me put things back into perspective, calm my anger, and stop putting the blame on him. I had my reasons for leaving, but it was now clear that it wasn't all about me.

I know of a Sanctuary not too far from where I live, called Sanctuary Notre Dame de Laghet, and the Saint there is known for her numerous miracles. I went up there and took a slip of paper and asked for forgiveness for both my husband and I, to be able to move forward with love and respect. I then drove home and asked my ex-husband to join me for a cup of coffee and I told him what I should have said long before: "I'm sorry."

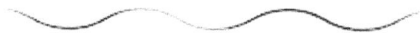

Change n°60
EMBRACE
YOUR INNER CHILD

60.

The other day I was sitting at my favorite coffee shop and savoring my double black ristretto. Somehow at Planet's Café in Monaco, they seem to make the perfect coffee that sets me off for a perfect day. How many hours have I spent there researching and writing for this book? I can picture the waiters' faces and smiles even from my desk at home. It's funny how you can see people every day, enjoy their presence but have no idea who they really are, what their interests are, whether they are single or in a relationship, what they are like after work... I take the time here to thank the whole team: it's priceless to arrive somewhere and know that you will always feel welcome. All I have to do is smile, say hello and a few moments later, I know, that one of them will come over with my cup of coffee.

To get back to what I wanted to write about... I was sitting at the coffee shop and watching people as they walked by: mostly men and women going to work, mothers with their strollers taking their little ones out for a walk, or retired folks going to the local supermarket. It's summer right now so the kids aren't at school and since it's early morning, many of them are headed towards the beach. Some just tag along, some are crying and others are laughing... each one living in the moment. Not one of them is preoccupied about their future, about what to prepare for lunch, about obligations that must be met. And as I observe one of them laughing out loud and looking at his mom with glittering eyes, I can't help but think: where did that spontaneity disappear? Where did that careless laughter go? Do my eyes still express love and laughter at the same time? When was the last time I really burst into tears or laughter?

And it all made me think: where did that child, I once was, go? Is she still there?
Why not take the time this week to go and find HIM or HER again?
Now doing this doesn't mean you have to act silly, we are not talking about being childish. We are just looking to connect with who you once were, how you reacted to certain situations and remember what you enjoyed doing. Who knows, maybe, you can take the time to do them again.

A. How can you reconnect with your inner child?

Here is a list of things that you can do, to help you bring back the spontaneity, the creativity and the vitality you once had as a child. Give it a try!

BRINGING BACK or RELIVING YOUR CHILDHOOD MEMORIES

a. With Food:

- Have a dinner with only junk food or your favorite childhood food! Do you remember when you were child and used to say: "When I grow up, I will eat only what I want!" Make a plan and do it. If you have kids, let them join in the fun. However, make sure you are eating exactly what *You* like. Preparing a special tray for each person with the foods they love is probably the best solution, since we don't all have the same cravings.

- Buy your favorite cereal even if it's Fruit Loops! and have it for breakfast!

- Have a picnic with exactly the same delicious foods your mother used to prepare and take a stroll down memory lane: Fried chicken and potato salad were one of my favorites. Even a better idea, why not call your mom and tell her you miss her and her wonderful cooking and would love to share a picnic with her again!

- Buy food you used to love as a child that maybe you don't allow yourself to eat anymore. Now, take the time to savor it. Do you still enjoy it today? Maybe not and that's ok. Remember how much you used to love it and how happy it used to make you when your parents would buy it.

- Play the guessing game: let someone blindfold you and then taste different foods while you try to guess them. The one making you test the foods had better be nice because it's their turn next!

b. Rediscovering your childhood activities:

One of the best ways to feel like a child is to partake in playful activities that you really enjoyed doing as a child. Why not do them again or share this moment with your own kids. You could:

- Go on a swing at the park and go as high as you can!
- Decide to spend an afternoon completely carefree with no obligations, no responsibilities.
- Roll or tumble down a hill.
- Make a snow angel or a snowman.
- Go roller skating
- Build a sandcastle
- Climb a tree and sit up there for a while; enjoy viewing life from another perspective.
- If it's raining, put your boots on and go on outside without an umbrella, walk through puddles and enjoy getting all wet. Then go back home and why not have a cup of hot coco with marshmallows on top?

- Have a nap after lunch. Just lie down and let yourself go for a few minutes. Chances are you will snooze off.
- Play pretend: imagine you are a great chef and cook something delicious, imagine you are a famous artist and while you are painting let your imagination run wild, walk in the street and imagine you are someone famous or beautiful!
- Hop, skip and jump, use a hoola-hoop, play hop scotch or use a jump rope!
- Have a sleepover. Why not enjoy a sleep over at a friend's house, or have one of your special friends sleep over. Catch up, watch a great movie and why not a enjoy a pillow fight!
- Wash the car and just have fun doing it!
- Play hide and seek!
- Go to a trampoline park!
- Go to a toy store and do every single isle! Remember the games and toys you used to love playing with.
- Have a board game night

c. With books and DVD's:
- Go to the library and find the books you used to love as a child: Alice in Wonderland, The Secret Garden, Cinderella and read them again. See how you understand these stories today, how your perspective has changed now that you are an adult.
- Read comic strips
- Watch the movies you used to love as a child. I really enjoyed watching again the "I love Lucy" and "Gilligan's island" episodes with my kids and they loved it. But you might also want to watch the classics such as "The wizard of Oz" or "The Sound of Music".
- Why not flip through your childhood photo albums and stroll down memory lane? You could share this moment with your parents.

BEING MORE CREATIVE

- Get your pens and pencils out and draw! If you never were a good drawer, buy an adult coloring book. There are a lot of meditation drawing books as well.
- What creative activity did you enjoy as a child: see if there is place nearby that allows you to try it again. When I was a child, I really enjoyed pottery and when I had the opportunity to redo it a few years ago, I was so happy! But it could be anything: quilting, sewing, macramé, creating bouquets, finding your way in the woods with a map and a compass, fixing car engines or building things.
- Get creative with paint! When was the last time you did finger painting? Why not cover your wall with paper and do a huge painting! If you are not a good drawer, simply put in lots of colors, polka dots, hand and footprints! Why not share this moment with the kids? Observe them to see how they respond and imitate them, just for fun.
- Look online how to create a fort: and then get out in the woods with a couple of friends and build one. Bring a snack and drinks along and when it's done, enjoy it inside the shelter you created.

BE MORE SPONTANEOUS

Children react in the moment according to how they feel. Try to be more spontaneous by:
- Sharing more love: tell the ones you love "I love you", give and ask for more hugs. When you need or feel love, express it!
- Learn to rediscover your emotions: let yourself go and laugh wholeheartedly when the opportunity arises. Don't fake it or force it, simply laugh. And when you are sad: cry! Let those tears come out. Learn to express your inner emotions again. And how about stomping your feet and clenching your fists if you are mad and saying "NO!"
- Sing more often! Who cares if someone is listening. On my wall I have this huge sign that says: Sing and dance as if no one can see or hear you! Loosen up and enjoy!
- We always contain ourselves for fear of hurting others: why not say what you think for a change? Try to find a kind way of saying it, but say it nevertheless. We are not talking about blurting out every single word of truth like in the movie "Liar Liar", but just gathering up enough courage to say what you think once in a while.
- Remember when your three year old hit the "why" phase and required an explanation for everything? Why don't you similarly ask question people when you don't understand something : For example, when someone says: "Things must be done this way". Ask them why? Or someone makes a statement and you don't quite see what they are getting at, and some explaining is required... Instead of doing as you usually do and pretending that you understood them, ask the person to repeat or give you more details. There is no shame in asking and most people are happy to oblige.
- If you are cooking, gardening or fixing the car, accept to get dirty or messy. Just concentrate on the task at hand and do the cleaning up after.
- Live in awe and amazement of everything that surrounds you. Take a few seconds to look and see all those things you take for granted, or are simply used to seeing and don't notice anymore: nature, people, kindness. Enjoy the simple things.

HOW TO RECONNECT WITH YOUR INNER CHILD

a.Meditate and renew contact

I particularly enjoyed reconnecting with the child I once was. Have you ever tried to come in contact with yourself as a child before? It's quite simple: remember a setting you once lived in such as your old room or a place you loved to go to. Imagine yourself sitting down with that child you once were and take it's hand in a comforting way. Smile at each other. If you had a tough childhood and things are pretty good all in all for you today, reassure that child you once were by telling it that you are ok today: you have a job, a partner, friends… If you are going through tough times, tell it what you are going through and that you are thankful it listens to you.

If you have a question that needs to be solved, or you are in a situation in which you really don't know what to do, ask your inner child a clear question and wait to see what the answer is. You will be surprised at how simple the solution might be. However, maybe you will not get an answer. That's ok as well. Just give that inner child another hug and thank it for spending some time with you.

I found the experience deeply moving and it brought tears to my eyes. There were so many times when I was little where I felt lost and all alone: it was a great experience to go back and reassure that child I once was, and to show her: "Hey look at me, there was and is nothing to worry about: I am doing just fine!"

b. Write a letter

If you are not much of a meditator, why not write a letter to your inner child? First acknowledge the difficulties it went through as child and tell it that you have managed to surpass those problems.

Take the time to reassure this child and to tell it that everything is ok today. If there are still some things you are struggling with today, explain that you need to move on with your life. Invite the inner child to move on with you so you can do this together.

I like to write and mail letters even if it's only symbolical. The idea that the letter is actually travelling to get somewhere even if it's back to me, makes me feel like it's moving forward, it's being processed. When it reaches you again, you don't necessarily have to open it. You can simply put in a drawer with all your other letters.

c. Draw a picture of your childhood

If you are not much into writing, why not try to draw or paint your childhood. How do you picture it? What colors would you choose to best describe it?

Would your page be full of details or half empty? What technique would you choose, something childlike, as finger painting or more adult like? Thick or thin markers or a paintbrush? Realistic or abstract?

Let your painting or drawing rest a while and get back to it with fresh eyes. Do you see anything? Does anything strike the eye? How do you interpret it now?

If you don't see anything you might want to ask a close friend to check it out and tell you what they see in this picture that you might not notice yourself.

d. Draw a list of the good and the bad

Why don't you draw a list of all the good and bad things that happened to you as a child? Look back and take the time to go over your entire childhood and place in two columns all the events you went through: your successes, your failures, the things that made you happy or sad, the events that brought great changes into your life, in what way they were positive or negative….

e. Play with Aesop

To finish, try to remember how you felt most of the time as a child. Find an image that best suits this feeling. For instance, during my childhood I mostly felt like a mouse: tiny and insignificant. I was there but I wasn't noticed. Many times, I was a silent, passive observer.

Maybe you felt like a fox because you always felt the need to be cunning in order to get attention or to get through the different challenges that were imposed upon you.

Or did you feel more like an elephant, either overweight or feeling that your presence was always a burden for others? You might have always felt unwanted or too much.

I give examples of animals, but you could very well be a thing or an object such as a car or a frame.

Some kids, who have very rigid parents, are not allowed to express themselves and might feel they were the image their parents wanted them to be. They never had the chance to show who they really were and what they aspired to become. In this case, they might feel like a picture. As children, they were "picture perfect".

You could also be a book or a film. In that case, what type of book or film were you? Adventure, classic, drama, comedy, or action? You are the main character: how would you describe yourself? What book or movie that already exists would you compare your life to? If there aren't any, what movies and books inspired you, and why? What is it that moved you, that made you love it? Why not read or watch it again. Is there something in it that you have always wanted to do? Maybe there is a message for you, just waiting to be read.

Next, take the time to find the image of who you are today. I definitely do not see myself as a mouse anymore. I actually see myself as different animals, all at once: a roaring lion is one of them. The way I see it, the lion is laid back, but deep down inside it's got that incredible roar. I want to roar at life and say: "Watch me, here I come!". But I also see myself like a little monkey, always busy and curious: I love life and see all of its opportunities and everything it has to offer. I want to embrace everything I possibly can and make the most of it.

**What about you,
who are you today?**

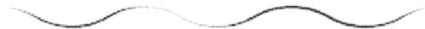

I AM READY...

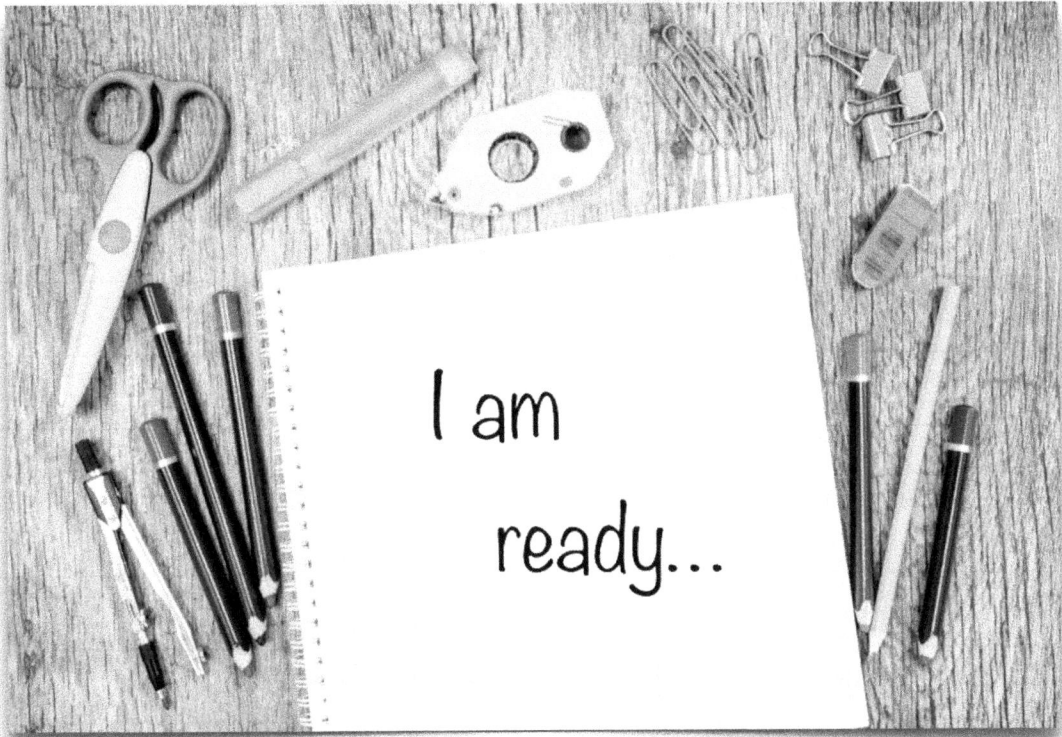

What are you ready for? Take the time to go over something that is troubling you and decide to put an end to it, once and for all, no "*ifs*" or "*buts*" attached. It's time to move forward with your life and accept what is and *Change*.

Let go of what is holding you back. Stop clinging onto it. Set yourself free. If it's painful, accept it without letting resentment or anger fill your heart. The time has come to let it all go. Imagine yourself blowing on a dandelion and let the wind spread your loving and accepting thoughts to the outside world, and toward whatever or whomever is hurting you. You have now planted the seeds of *Change*.

Eventually, there will come a point when you feel "Ready" to move on. When you get there, grab a piece of paper and write down what you are ready for. Place the piece of paper under your mattress and get on with your life. Who knows what exciting new change will start growing your way…

MY NOTES

WORK SPACE

_____

_____

_____

_____

_____

_____

_____

_____

_____

_____

_____

_____

_____

_____

_____

_____

_____

FINAL WORD

We often let ourselves settle into a comfortable routine and get upset when something pops up, unaccountably disturbing our peaceful lifestyle. And then paradoxically, we also tend to complain about the fact that our days repeat themselves in a "work-eat-sleep-repeat" pattern. But, what if we intentionally brought elements of change into our lives? What if we rediscovered the joys of learning and decided to improve ourselves by trying to master new things such as a language or a new skill? And what would happen if we switched our routine around and discovered unusual places, noticed different colors and tasted surprising new flavors? What if we brought little changes to the way we look, live, eat, exercise and work?

Change is Powerful and can have a truly positive impact on your life. So, step out of your comfort zone, learn to be more open to change, and see just how your life can turn into a fulfilling and exciting adventure.

Embracing Change
can mean rediscovering the pleasures of learning,
but also seeking and adapting to new situations of your own free will

Embracing Change
can mean packing your bags and moving off to the big city for that new job,
finally doing what it takes to lose weight and lead a healthy lifestyle,
or choose to live differently or go around the world!

Embracing Change
can mean putting your foot down and leaving a dysfunctional relationship
and finding the strength to start anew!

But Embracing Change
also means accepting painful events such as death,
heartbreak or sickness;
they are a part of life as well and tell us it's time to grow.

So, let these thoughts simmer in your mind
and ask yourself what would happen to *YOU*,
if *YOU* started to embrace
the **Power of Change**…

Many years ago, when I was 28, I had a job interview to work for a prestigious bank in Monte-Carlo. I was excited about this opportunity and was ecstatic when I saw that the interview was going well. When the discussion came to a close, the Director turned to me and said that there was just one more thing: I needed to give a handwritten letter for my handwriting to be analyzed by a graphologist. He told me to scribble down a few lines, anything I wanted, and send it to the bank.

When I arrived home, I was a little puzzled and sat in front of my blank piece of paper, not really sure what to write. I really wanted this job. I took a few minutes to breathe and think about it. I could feel that I was stressed about writing the "wrong thing" and not landing the job. At that moment, a Chinese Proverb I had once read popped up in my mind.

You may have already heard it: "A blessing in disguise". It went like this…

There once lived a peasant who raised horses. He lived on his farm with his beloved son.

One day, one of the peasant's best stallions managed to escape.
When the neighbors heard the news, they all came to comfort the peasant and his son.
To their biggest surprise, the peasant wasn't upset at all.
This is what he told them:
"Unfortunate? Fortunate? Who knows.
Those things happen; they are a part of life.
One must accept them."
The neighbors left but were a little intrigued by the peasant's reply.

The stallion came back eventually, accompanied by a beautiful young mare.
This time the neighbors expressed their joy when they came to see it
and they congratulated the peasant for his luck.
Once again, the man didn't react as expected.
He simply said:
"Fortunate? Unfortunate? Who knows.
Those things can happen.
Whether they are fortunate or unfortunate however I do not know."
The neighbors left thinking that he was a strange little peasant indeed.

That week as the son was trying to break the new mare,
an accident happened: she slipped, fell and landed on the son's leg.
From then on, he would have a limp when he walked.
The neighbors couldn't help feeling sad for the peasant's misfortune,
as he only had one son. Indeed, the injury made it difficult for the young man
to work and the peasant wasn't getting any younger.
The neighbors expressed their concern for both of them.

But the peasant went on as he usually did,
seemingly unaffected and this is what he told them:
"Unfortunate? Fortunate? Who knows.
Accidents are a part of life.
One must accept them.
Whether this event is unfortunate or fortunate, however, I do not know."
The neighbors left, concluding that this peasant didn't have it all together.

The son was never able to walk normally again but,
when a few years later the country was invaded
and all the healthy valid young men were sent off to fight for their country;
the peasant's limping son was spared.

You already know the peasant's wise words:
"Fortunate? Unfortunate? Who knows...."

This story teaches us that only time will tell the whole story.

And so, I thought about this job and told myself to relax: it didn't really matter whether I got it or not. If I did, great, but if I didn't, well something else lay ahead for me.

I looked at my empty sheet of paper and wrote down the story about the old farmer and hand delivered it. As I opened the doors to exit the bank, I was serene, and as I stepped out onto the streets, I smiled, knowing that, no matter the outcome, I would accept it and it would be ok. Little did I know then, that many, many years later I would be sitting here writing a book to encourage people, no matter the outcome, to embrace…

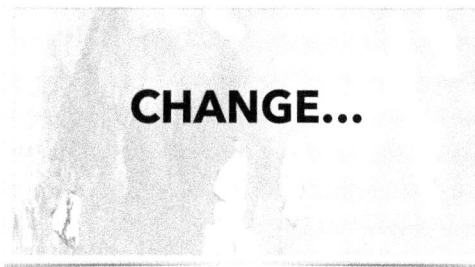

CHANGE...

REFERENCES

Change n° 02 Stand Tall

Remember to do your research! Here are just a few suggestions you might want to look into:

Posture, Get it Straight by Janice Novac. There is the book and the DVD.

The A.P.I. (American Posture Institute) for those of you who would be interested in taking an online course about posture.

Change n° 04 The "Confidence Walk"

Charisme Myth by Olivia Fox Cabane. It will change how you perceive others and you start understanding how you have a hand on what others thinks of you.

Check out the *"Who is"/ "Who Was"* series

Change n°05 Believe in Yourself - Create your very own P.E.T.

Think on These Things by Krishnamurti about observing your habits.

Feel the Fear and do it Anyway by Susan Jeffers

Change n° 07 Be Inspired

La Pensée au Coeur du Corps by Philippe Lamache (Book in French. Translation *"Mind Over Matter"*).

Change n° 09 7 Rings to Learn 7 Different Things

Ultimate Sticker Puzzles: License Plates Across the States: Travel Puzzles and Games Paperback

Change n° 13 Hydrate

Remember to do your research! Here are just a few suggestions you might want to look into:

- www.waterbenefitshealth.com
- Check out the International Bottled water Association – IBWA : www.bottledwater.org, to get to know and understand the different types of bottled water (spring, purified, mineral, sparkling etc.), to know how long and how to store bottled water and much more.

Change n° 14 Daily Dose of Goodness

Remember to do your research! Here are just a few suggestions you might want to look into:

- *Juice* (Recipes for juicing, cleansing and living well) by Carly de Castro, Hedi Gores and Hayden Slaters
- *108 Chakra soupes* by Helen Margaret Giovanello. Please note that this book is in french.
- *A Fresh Start* by Susan Smith Jones (more than 250 recipes!)

Change n° 15 The Big 5 Challenge

Remember to do your research! Here are just a few suggestions you might want to look into:

- *Juice* (Recipes for juicing, cleansing and living well) by Carly de Castro, Heidi Gores and Hayden Slaters
- *108 Chakra soupes* by Helen Margaret Giovanello (the book is in french)
- *A Fresh Start* by Susan Smith Jones (more than 250 recipes!)

Change n° 17 Try Something New

Remember to do your research! Here are just a few references to find seasonable fruit and vegetables you might want to look into:

- www.eatseasonably.co.uk: You can find a poster or a tea towel with all the vegetables and fruit classified according to the different seasons.
- www.fruitsandveggiesmorematters.org: You will find a list of vegetables classified by color that will also inform you about the benefits of the fruit or vegetable you are interested in.
- www.Disabled-world.com: Color wheel of fruits and vegetables: you will find a list of all the fruit and vegetables according to color, what their contents are and in what way they are beneficial for you.
- *The Healing Power of Nature Foods* by Susan Smith Jones

Change n° 20 Self-Observation

The Kingdom of Happiness by Krishnamurti
The Greatest Love of All sung by Whitney Houston

Change n° 21 Rules Between Meals

The Slow Down Diet by Mark David. This is truly my reference book about finding peace with your plate.

Change n°23: Read! Read! Read!

Remember to do your research! Here are just a few suggestions you might want to look into:

- *The Illustrated Cook's Book of Ingredients* – Select, prepare and cook with more than 2500 global ingredients. Published by DK Publishing.
- *The Visual Food Lover's Guide* – Includes essential information on how to buy, prepare and store over 1000 types of food created and produced by QA International and published by John Wiley and Sons
- *The 150 healthiest foods on Earth* by Jonny Bowden
- Nutritional Values for common foods and Products at www.nutritionvalue.org/
- The Food composition databases: http://ndb.nal.usda.gov/ndb/search/list

Change n° 26 Get out and Walk

Remember to do your research! Here are just a few suggestions you might want to look into:

- *What country is most active* by Withings September 4th, 2014

Change n°28: Hot and Cold

Remember to do your research! Here are just a few suggestions you might want to look into:

- *Curarsi con Acqua e Limone* by Simona Oberhammer (If you speak Italian)
- *Se Soigner Grace à l'Eau et au Citron* by Simona Oberhammer (If you speak French)
- *How to Eat, Move and Be Healthy* by Paul Check about cold showers. Check out his post about cold showers as well.
- Cold shower therapy: Joel Runyon at TEDxLUC (a 10:47 mn video) A must see on Youtube! « How I crushed « The 30-day cold shower challenge » and the Great life secret it unveiled » on www.thefeelgoodlifestyle.com

Change n° 29: Physical Assessment Checklist

Check out webmd.com for information about Probiotics and Prebiotics.

Change n° 31: Train Right

Remember to do your research! Here are just a few suggestions you might want to look into:

- I particularly enjoy watching Athlean X VIP for great tips. Don't let his muscles scare you: his explanations are for everyone and what's more, he analyzes every exercise so you really understand what you are doing and why. Make a point of watching one of his videos daily and you will really become knowledgeable!
- Douglas Brooks DVDs and books : He is the reference in the field
- Frederic DELAVIER check out all of his books as they allow you to visualize exactly what muscle you are working out

Change n°32: You are your very Best Friend

The Giver by Lois Lowry

Change n°33: Do the BB "BEST²"Workout Ever

N.A.S.M. - National Academy of Sports Medicine - provides certification programs for entry-level and advanced practitioners in the sports medicine, performance enhancement and health and fitness industries. The NASM-CPT certification is accredited by the National Commission for Certifying Agencies (NCCA).
A.C.S.M. Whether in the field of sports medicine or amid experienced exercise professional, ACSM is considered one of the most highly sought after certifications in the industry — a credential that is known as the gold standard around the world.

Change n°36: An Exercise Challenge

Remember to do your research! Here are just a few suggestions you might want to look into:

- *Posture, Get it Straight* by Janice Novak (or How to Look Ten Years Younger, Ten Pounds Thinner and Feel Better than ever!) Sounds too good to be true? Try it!
- Check out on youtube "We did 100 push-ups every day for 30 days" https://youtu.be/TlQ8txalLYg or https://www.youtube.com/user/buzzfeedblue

Change n° 37: Get ready to change jobs

Remember to do your research! Here are just a few suggestions:

• When browsing through job descriptions, the language can be quite technical and difficult to decipher. Check out www.thebalancecareers.com to get a clear comprehension of what a job description means.
• Check out www.balance.com to find a list of verbs to use and avoid when writing a resume.
• You will also find on this website a list of the words to use in regards to the type of job you are applying to. Check out "list skills by type".

Change 38: Back to School

Remember to do your research! Here are just a few suggestions:
• Check out : The IDEA World Nutrition and Behavior Change Summit.

Change n° 39: Talk and Listen

Remember to do your research! Here are just a few suggestions you might want to look into:

• Check out the following two handbooks to help you increase your vocabulary:
    - Word Power Made Easy by Norman Lewis (The complete Handbook for building a Superior Vocabulary)
    - Word Smart by Adam Robinson (How to Build a More Educated Vocabulary, with more than 1400 words that you need to know)

• *The Charisma Myth* in which Fox Cabane explains in detail exactly how to talk to gain added charisma.
• *The Conversation Handbook* by Troy Fawkes. He recommends that you make a list of all the topics you are interested in and improve the way you talk about them.
• To discover and improve your visualization techniques, I recommend *Creative Visualization* by Shakti Gawain
• To cut out swear words for good check out :
    - "101 Great Cuss / Swear words alternatives"
    - "Holy Rackafratz! 101 more funny swear/cuss word alternatives."

Chapter n° 44: Completing Things

Remember to do your research! Here are just a few suggestions you might want to look into:

• *10 Days to Faster Reading: Zip Through Books, Magazines and Newspapers* – Understand and remember everything you read by the Princeton Language Institute and Abby Marks Beale.
• To improve your vocabulary: *"Word Power made easy"* *The complete handbook for building a superior vocabulary.* Each chapter gives you a list of words. They explain, in detail, each and every one of them and in which context you should use them. There are plenty of exercises and review exercises. A must read! You can also check out: *« WORD SMART more than 1400 words you need to know to communicate effectively, to speak and write persuasively, to improve reading comprehension, to score higher on the SAT, GRE and other standardized tests.»*

- To improve your memory and mental math skills why not try Dr Kawashima's *Train Your Brain*" and "*Train your Brain More.*" My kids still talk to me about these books today!
- I also recommend the Singapore Method in maths.
- I love the "Who Was" and "Who is" Penguin series, to improve your knowledge of history. for example, that published a great number of books – between 70 and 100 pages each - about famous people or important historic events.
- To become more knowledgeable about wine, there is a manga called *Drops of God* by Kami no Shizuku that is really interesting that tells you the story of two very different young men who wish to inherit a wine empire. While reading the story, there are tons of details about wine, the regions where they grow, how the wine is prepared etc. Simply amazing: a fun and great way to learn.

Change n°48: Conquering Fear

Remember to do your research! Here are just a few suggestions you might want to look into:
- *Facing the Fear (and doing it anyway)* by Susan Jeffers can turn out to be an amazing tool to help you come to terms with what is troubling you.
- The Anxiety and Phobia Workbook by Edmund J. Bourne.
- Check out Fearof.net – the ultimate list of phobias and fears: to get to know more about your phobias.

Change n°53: Declutter

Remember to do your research! Here are just a few suggestions on how to declutter might want to look into:
- Marie Kondo books *The Life Changing Magic of Tidying*, that sold over 2.6 million copies !!, Although I do not quite agree with all of her principles (she basically tells you to throw everything away), I did find some important information inside regarding home decluttering and cleaning. You might want to check out her other book, *Spark Joy,* which is the illustrated version of the book that will show you how to fold and file and what your closets and drawers could actually look like. I also enjoyed a manga written by Kondo that tells the story of a woman who transforms her home, work and love life using Marie Kondo's principles.
- *Clear your Clutter* by Karen Kingston, another good read that I highly recommend. For her, clearing your clutter goes all the way: not only does she advocate getting rid of all the stuff you have piled up at home, she also explains why you do it and makes you aware of other domains in your life that need some serious cleaning up. We are talking of all the different aspects of life.

Change n°55: Know yourself

Remember to do your research! Here are just a few suggestions:
Wild by Cheryl Strayed

Writing Prompts: The Ultimate Self Exploration Journal. 'Who Am I?' and 199 Other Transformational Questions and Creative Writing Prompts for Self Reflection and Personal Enlightenment Paperback – June 22, 2018 by Gerald Confienza

Self Discovery Journal: 200 Questions to Find Who You Are and What You Want in All Areas of Life (Self Discovery Journal, Self Discovery Questions) Paperback – January 15, 2018 by Gerald Confienza

Find Your Passion: The Ultimate No BS Workbook. 186 Questions, Prompts, and Exercises to Find Your Passion, Work on Purpose, and Leave a Lasting Legacy by Gerald Confienza

Start Where You Are: A Journal for Self-Exploration August 11, 2015 by Meera Lee Patel

Change n°58: Channeling Pain

Remember to do your research! Here are just a few suggestions you might want to look into:

• I love the poem *The Oak and the Reed* by the Fables of Aesop, reviewed by Jefferys Taylor

Change n°59: Embrace Truth

Remember to do your research! Here are just a few suggestions you might want to look into: the

• 10.000 hour theory, by Malcolm Gladwell, whereby it is said that to master any art, you will need 10.000 hours.
• *Mindset* by Carol S. Dweck, another excellent read that I found highly interesting and that gives great insight on this topic. She goes about explaining the two types of mindsets: the fixed and the growth mindset.

Change 60: Embrace Your Inner Child

Remember to do your research! Here are just a few suggestions you might want to look into:

• Mary Pierce books

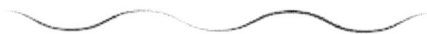

ACKNOWLEDGMENTS

The book is now finished and will soon be in print. Four years, in other words 1460 days have gone by almost to the day and as I flip through the pages I can't help but realize how much my life has changed in this lapse of time. Indeed, when I started I was married with my children homeschooled. Progressively, however, I divorced, was diagnosed with cancer, had to put the children back to school, move out and get a job. I also fell in love and was left heartbroken… Life has its ways of changing things and between the moment I wrote the very first word and the last one, mine has made a 360-degree turn…

But today, as I look back, I realize that…

You can lose your health and yet get it back again,
You can actually lose everything and yet succeed in starting everything from scratch,
You can be left heartbroken but then find yourself smiling again and looking into someone else's eyes,
You can have this crazy, farfetched dream and actually see it come true.

But, luckily however, some things, don't change: Indeed, I was very fortunate to have my friends and sons close by: they stuck around even when I didn't call or write back and were all highly supportive of this special project of mine all along the way. My dear friends and amazing boys, may you forgive me for all those times I was busy writing and thus not available. My life, truly, wouldn't be the same without you:

Enzo and Diego, I have raised you both, encouraging you to get up off the couch and get moving to make your dreams come true, and never to expect it all to land on your lap. I am so happy to see you both thrive and slowly fly off on your own. I am blessed. You are both unique and have a beautiful soul. I love you.

Philippe for your incredible support, for your love…for simply being there. The first day I met you, you told me that, true love isn't painful, true love harbors no jealousy and cannot be disrespectful. True love is when both wish the best for the other and help each other become and find that better part of themselves. You have honored your words.

Rachel, you are beautiful inside and out.
Anette, you truly shine.
Sabine, no artifacts, you are beautiful simply being you.
Laetitia, I love that you are so strong and yet have no fear of showing your vulnerability.
Marie, may love come to you in return.
Najet, you are an amazing woman. I have no doubt that you will be an amazing "Mom".
Bianca, so lucky to have seen you blossom from Day 1 into the beautiful woman you are today.

Marie B., you are truly an angel sent from above.

Fiona, my sister, an example in perseverance. Sending you love and hugs.

My parents: C. H. and Georges Ratkoff, thank you for giving me life. I am so grateful and want you to know that I cherish and make the most of every second. Loving thoughts to you and Monique as well.

Michel: in memory of our 17 years together. May you find happiness, love and peace.

My amazing editor: Sabrina, I don't have words enough to thank you. There are no coincidences: your email came to me as a gift. I don't know what I would have done without your help, your ideas, your corrections, your encouragements. (Sabrina Mesko, Founder of Arnica Press)

Linus, you were there holding my hand as I wrote most of these pages. I know that this book wouldn't be here without you. May life bless you.

Marie-Andrée, Dr Gingras, Tante Tony, Oncle Pierre, Colette… you are forever with me, until we meet again.

To that special someone, often called Inspiration, who whispered the idea of this book in my ear one spring day.

ABOUT THE AUTHOR

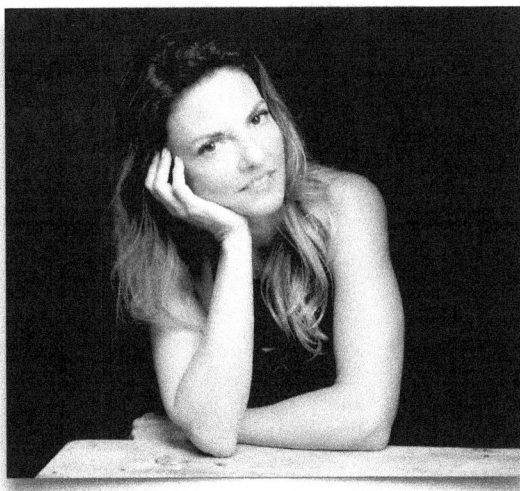

Born in New York in the mid 1960s to a French-American mother, a historian, and a Russian artist father, Barbara had to embrace change from a very early age. She was taken out of the school system, away from the big cities, to live a nomadic life and had to constantly adapt to new environments, moving from one Ojibwe reservation to another. Quite frequently, she was simply droped-off to live with a new family. As a teen, she moved to Paris, France and later Nice. At age 23, she landed, of all places, in Monte-Carlo, where she planned to become a personal trainer. She was certified by the American Council on Exercise (A.C.E.), and the American College of Sports Medicine (A.C.S.M), and became truly passionate about health and fitness.

But life had other plans for her. She got married, gave birth to two beautiful boys, home-schooled them for eight years, and whenever possible, the young family travelled to exotic and unusual places in the world. It may seem that she was living a fairytale, and in many ways she was, but very few people realize the true challenges and demands of such an unusual and unsteady lifestyle.

When she reached the age of 50, she was suddenly faced with a dramatic, all encompassing life-altering change. It seemed that her life as she knew it, started spiraling downward. All at once, she was diagnosed with cancer and faced with a difficult divorce. And it was amidst this life upheaval, that she started to write her book *Change*. Indeed, these devastating challenges never wavered her love of life. Every day, in between job interviews, lawyer meetings and radiotherapy appointments, she would write her book, meditate, eat right and resiliently dive into the ocean for a daily swim. She worked out with tremendous discipline, inner conviction, belief and awareness, that change is a good thing. In fact, change is a necessity. For this reason, she wishes to share with you her inspiring and courageous vision of life, where change is a most positive and powerful tool. Once you learn to embrace it, you will thrive and create the life of your dreams.

Visit Author website at www.BarbaraRatkoff.com

www.ingramcontent.com/pod-product-compliance
Lightning Source LLC
Chambersburg PA
CBHW080602270326
41928CB00016B/2902